Paradigms Lost, Paradigms Found

PARADIGMS LOST, PARADIGMS FOUND

Lessons Learned in the Fight Against the Stigma of Mental Illness

SECOND EDITION

Heather Stuart, PhD, FRSC, CM

and

Norman Sartorius, MD, MA, PhD, FRCPych

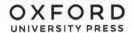

OXFORD
UNIVERSITY PRESS

OXFORD
UNIVERSITY PRESS

Oxford University Press is a department of the University of Oxford. It furthers the University's objective of excellence in research, scholarship, and education by publishing worldwide. Oxford is a registered trade mark of Oxford University Press in the UK and certain other countries.

Published in the United States of America by Oxford University Press
198 Madison Avenue, New York, NY 10016, United States of America.

Library of Congress Cataloging-in-Publication Data
Names: Stuart, Heather L. author. | Sartorius, N., author.
Title: Paradigms lost, paradigms found : lessons learned in the fight against the stigma of mental illness / Heather Stuart, Norman Sartorius.
Other titles: Paradigms lost
Description: 2. | New York, NY : Oxford University Press, [2022] |
Preceded by Paradigms lost : fighting stigma and the lessons learned /
Heather Stuart, Julio Arboleda-Flórez, Norman Sartorius. c2012. |
Includes bibliographical references and index.
Identifiers: LCCN 2022003404 (print) | LCCN 2022003405 (ebook) |
ISBN 9780197555804 (hardback) | ISBN 9780197555828 (epub) | ISBN 9780197555835
Subjects: MESH: Mental Disorders—psychology | Attitude of Health Personnel |
Mentally Ill Persons—psychology | Social Stigma | Prejudice | Social Change
Classification: LCC RC454 (print) | LCC RC454 (ebook) |
NLM WM 140 | DDC 616.89—dc23/eng/20220204
LC record available at https://lccn.loc.gov/2022003404
LC ebook record available at https://lccn.loc.gov/2022003405

DOI: 10.1093/med/9780197555804.001.0001

9 8 7 6 5 4 3 2 1

Printed by Integrated Books International, United States of America

In memory of Julio Arboleda-Flórez, colleague, friend, and partner.

CONTENTS

PREFACE

This book draws on 25 years of experience working with anti-stigma programs internationally, nationally, and regionally. The journey began with the "Open the Doors" Global Program to Fight Stigma Because of Schizophrenia—a program that was delivered in over 25 countries under the auspices of the World Psychiatric Association. Our experiences with Open the Doors and subsequent development of a Scientific Section focusing on stigma in the World Psychiatric Association and regular "Together Against Stigma" international conferences have brought us into contact with an international network of interested researchers and advocates. We have learned much about what can be accomplished with focused anti-stigma efforts and how best to conduct anti-stigma programs even on shoestring budgets. Despite a growing number of large, well-funded national anti-stigma efforts, our experiences have taught us that everyone can contribute something, whether in high-, middle-, or low-income countries.

In the first edition of this book in 2012, we identified paradigms that we thought needed to be replaced. Our emphasis was on recognizing and challenging outmoded approaches, those that had outlived their usefulness or had never really been useful in the first place. At that time, the anti-stigma field was still in its infancy, without a strong evidence base. Programs varied widely in their approaches. As time has progressed, many national anti-stigma programs have adopted some or all of the approaches we initially described in the book *Paradigms Lost*. [1]

In this edition, we continue to emphasize the importance of evidence-based approaches and evidence creation and begin to examine some of the new paradigms that have been developed in recent times—thus, the title *Paradigms Lost, Paradigms Found*. We continue to argue that stigma reduction must be rooted in principles of social equity and result in behavioral change at the individual and organizational levels. The goals must be to eliminate the social inequities that people with a mental illness and their family members face, and to promote full and effective social participation. Awareness raising and mental health literacy are important, but they do little to empower people with a mental illness or their family members to enjoy their civil and legal rights or change the accumulated practices of social groups and social structures that systematically disadvantage those with mental health problems.

This book is written with one eye to the past and one to the future. It will summarize some of the elements and principles articulated in the first edition but will also go into depth in targeted areas (such as healthcare settings, workplaces, schools, and the media) when there was little known about stigma and stigma interventions when we produced the *Paradigms Lost* volume. We expect that this edition will be a useful sequel to *Paradigms Lost*, chronicling what we have learned as a global community regarding mental illness–related stigma and targeted stigma-reduction approaches.

CHAPTER 1
Mental Illness–Related Stigma

INTRODUCTION

In the history of medicine, few conditions other than mental illnesses have cast such a pall on an individual, their family, health providers, health systems, and health research. In addition to having serious consequences for one's social identity, having a mental illness or substance use disorder* results in structural inequities that impinge on one's health, longevity, quality of life, social welfare, civic participation, and access to resources. Stigma also casts a long shadow, affecting all of the supports and structures that people with mental illnesses need in order to recover and embrace socially meaningful roles and relationships. [2] This chapter provides an overview of the nature and nurture of stigma from the era of the asylum to our current recovery paradigm.

A TOUR OF TERMS

The term *stigma* has been variously used to refer to a negative and pejorative attitude that members of the public hold toward people with a mental illness, a mark of shame that someone with a mental illness bears, to a complex sociostructural process that involves a number of interconnected parts, and even to a mark of grace that resembles the wounds of Christ. [2] Some advocates have suggested that the pejorative use of the term *stigma* has outlived its usefulness and we should focus instead on discrimination (e.g., [3]). However, this may be an unnecessarily narrow and polarizing view. Link and Phelan

---

*Throughout this book, we consider *mental illnesses* in the broadest sense to include all neuropsychiatric conditions and substance use disorders.

provide a useful and broad definition of the stigmatization process that incorporates a variety of interrelated elements. [4] The first element involves the identification and labeling of socially salient differences. Next, the label becomes linked, in the public psyche, to a negative stereotype. People who are labeled are placed in a distinct category and viewed as separate from the norm (e.g., us vs. them). They are no longer thought of as unique individuals, but as members of a homogeneous group. Once categorized in this way, labeled people experience status loss and discrimination leading to social inequities in all walks of life. The ability of a social group to stigmatize is entirely dependent on the ability of its members to access social, religious, economic, and political power, as only powerful groups can stigmatize. The various types of stigmas (e.g., structural, public, and self-stigma) are discussed in more detail elsewhere in this chapter.

Stereotypes and prejudicial attitudes are key components of stigma. *Cultural stereotypes* are broadly held beliefs about the defining characteristics of a group. They can be inaccurate, negative, over-generalized, and exaggerated depictions that are applied to all members of the group. Stereotypes are frequently expressed even though an individual may never have met someone from the stereotyped group. *Prejudices* go much farther than stereotypes involving negative feelings and attitudes. Whereas stereotypes form the cognitive scaffolding about a group, prejudices reflect deep feelings of hatred and distrust that may give rise to discrimination. Once developed, stereotypes and prejudices are difficult to change as people will attend to new information selectively and accept only information that is in harmony with their beliefs. This has implications for anti-stigma programming as one way of changing stereotypes and prejudice is to present a more positive perception of the group as a whole, or to promote an understanding that groups contain significant variability and that all group members are not the same. [5] *Misconceptions* are based on wrong information or a lack of knowledge and are changeable with new information. Prejudices do not change when exposed to new information and may even become more entrenched and unyielding. [6]

Mental health literacy is a term that was coined to refer to knowledge and beliefs that aid in the recognition of mental disorders, their management, and prevention. Since then, the term has expanded to include cognitive and social skills related to individual and collective empowerment needed for mental health promotion. Good mental health literacy would include such things as being able to recognize mental disorders in oneself or others, knowledge about the effectiveness of interventions, and knowledge about how to seek help. [7] Members of the lay public often have poor mental health literacy, with the result that they may not seek treatment when appropriate to do so or may not adhere to advice given by clinicians. Seeing mental health professionals as the only persons who can provide help when experiencing a mental disorder is also an indication of poor mental health literacy. Poor mental health literacy may be a consequence of stigma. While mental health literacy is important in its own right, an increasing number of studies show that members of the public can be quite knowledgeable about mental illnesses and about their treatments and still hold negative and socially intolerant views. [8,9] Greater gains in prevention, early intervention, peer support, and self-help could result if members of the public had more mental health literacy. [10]

THE STIGMATIZATION OF MENTAL ILLNESSES

Both in ancient and modern times, labeling someone as "mentally ill" immediately brands them as someone of lesser social value. Lay notions of what constitutes a "mental illness" differ over time, and from culture to culture. Once a behavior is deemed to be indicative of a mental illness, it is open to prejudice and discrimination and this designation varies. [11] In one culture a trance-like state may demonstrate special healing powers, such as that of a shaman; in another, it will be viewed as evidence of a mental illness and considered to be deviant and may be demonized. This could explain why those experiencing psychological or psychiatric phenomena in different cultures may be differentially stigmatized. [12]

The term *stigma* comes from the Greek *stizein*, meaning to brand someone with a sharp stick, or *stig*. Hence the Latin derivative, stigma, conveys the meaning of a mark of infamy or ignominy. The pejorative use of the term most likely appeared in early Christian cultures when mental illnesses became linked with sin. By the 19th century, mental illnesses were irrevocably linked to heredity brought about by a degenerative taint in the family. Degeneracy theory, which was popular until World War II, underpinned the eugenics movement and discouraged physicians from seeking cures. It also made it acceptable to house people with mental illnesses in overcrowded and inadequate asylums. [2] From the 1930s through to the 1980s, countries such as the United States, Japan, Canada, Sweden, Australia, Norway, Finland, Estonia, Slovakia, Switzerland, and Iceland all enacted laws that allowed for the coerced or forced sterilization of marginalized or disabled women, including women with mental or other disabilities. More recently, forced and coerced sterilization of marginalized women has been documented in countries in North and South America, Europe, Asia, and Africa. [13]

Contemporary notions of stigma are rooted in the work of early sociologists, particularly the seminal work of Erving Goffman. [14] In *Stigma: Notes on the Management of Spoiled Identity*, Goffman explored various forms of stigma but concluded that the stigma associated with mental illnesses was the most discrediting. People who had a mental illness were "marked" for social devaluation, status loss, and marginalization. The label had the effect of reducing someone from a whole person to one who was irredeemably tainted. He further described stigma as a contagion that could be conferred on those who were in close proximity to the stigmatized. He termed this *courtesy stigma*, also known as stigma-by-association, which was conferred on family, friends, mental health providers, psychotropic medications, other psychiatric treatments, mental health research, and systems of care.

It is possible to trace three eras of stigma discourse beginning in the mid-1950s to the present day. In the first era, stigma was viewed as a consequence of institutional psychiatry. In the second, it was considered to be the result of a hasty and ill-managed deinstitutionalization process. In the third, stigma was viewed as a consequence of therapeutic nihilism perpetuated by the over-medicalization of psychiatric illnesses.

Stigma as a Consequence of Institutional Psychiatry

Goffman and his contemporaries were particularly critical of institutional psychiatry. He viewed mental hospitals as anti-therapeutic and considered that many of the negative and socially debilitating consequences of mental illnesses were more a result of the way in which mental patients were treated rather than a result of the illnesses themselves. [15] Together with contemporaries such as Thomas Szasz, R.D. Laing, and David Cooper, these thinkers ushered in an era of anti-psychiatry sentiment. As well as challenging the very basis of psychiatric illnesses, they were deeply distrustful of organized psychiatry because they saw it as being the driving force for the creation of the coercive and stigmatizing nature of psychiatric hospitals. [16] Indeed, Goffman grouped psychiatric hospitals together with other "total institutions" such as prisons and concentration camps in terms of their effects on the human spirit. [15] While Goffman has been criticized for an exaggerated and negative characterization of mental hospitals in the same vein as concentration camps [17], the general tenor of anti-psychiatry sentiments was to place the blame for the isolating and stigmatizing qualities of mental health facilities on the psychiatrists who were running them.

The growth in the number of large psychiatric institutions occurred at a time when there were massive social changes in family and community structures brought about the industrial revolution. Prior to the 19th century, support for people with a mental illness had been a family and community affair. Industrialization made it increasingly difficult to manage mentally disordered behaviors using these traditional structures. Families had been disaggregated into smaller nuclear units, and small supportive communities had given way to industrial villages and larger densely populated urban centers. As a result, there was a decreasing tolerance for and ability to manage mentally disordered behavior. The rise in asylums was an efficient method of removing the problem from view. [18,19] From this perspective, institutionalized care grew out of a desire to segregate unwanted groups from society so that they could be effectively forgotten.

Stigma as a Consequence of Deinstitutionalization

The community mental health movement started with the intention to reintegrate people with mental illnesses into society, which then would remove asylums as a source of stigma. However, deinstitutionalization carried out without proper preparation of the community and the necessary reorganization of services placed heavy demands on selected communities that suddenly had to host a group of individuals who were traditionally shunned. As former patients became more visible in unprepared community settings, they became targets for social fear and disapproval. Rather than being welcoming and supportive, many local communities marshaled efforts to exclude the placement of needed mental health services and clients in their midst.

In most countries that have deinstitutionalized, community care has been slow to develop and remains patchy. Still, many people with serious mental illnesses do not receive the supports and services they need. In many settings, community care has become a term indicating neglect, lack of resources, homelessness, the transfer of care to untrained staff, and trans-institutionalization. In many locales there has been a backlash fueled by sensationalized accounts in the media and public inquiries into homicides committed by people with mental illnesses. Perceptions of dangerousness have been at the core of public stigma in the community care era. [20]

The NIMBY Syndrome

As the community mental health strategy has unfolded, it has become common for local municipalities to use zoning bylaws and other restrictive covenants to socially distance themselves from people with mental illnesses, services, and supports; this is dubbed the NIMBY (not in my backyard) syndrome. [21] Dear [22] mapped the evolution of NIMBY sentiments as follows. Initially, news of a proposal to locate a service in a local neighborhood breaks and conflict erupts in the small groups who live near the proposed service. Then, more formal battle lines are drawn, and the issue becomes polarized. Complaints that may have been aired in private now become public. Rhetoric that was initially raw and abusive ("get these bums out of here!") takes on a more rational and objective tone where concerns become centered on property values and public safety. Residents worry that their neighborhood enjoyment will be compromised, and that children and youth will be negatively influenced. As the opposition matures, victory is usually reserved for the group that can stay in the game the longest—often the neighborhood.

Sayce [23] has described the moral panic that has ensued as a result of de-institutionalization and the increase in NIMBY campaigns, noting that some have been quite harsh. In one instance, for example, a "schizophrenics go home" sign was posted on a van near a proposed social housing project, and in another, local people attacked users of a supported housing program, with the result that the project closed immediately to protect its users. NIMBY campaigns exist to ensure that people with mental illnesses remain community outcasts.

A U.S. study involving telephone interviews with 169 mental health agencies in seven states estimated that opposition to mental health services and supports existed in one-third to one-half of all proposed neighborhood sites, with housing in low-income, transient, heterogeneous neighborhoods generating the least resistance. Opposition is typically the strongest when mental health administrators notify neighbors that special services are being planned. In the United States, mental health administrators have the legal right to forgo neighborhood notification; however, many still do because they believe that community outreach facilitates integration. In this study, organizations that notified neighbors were significantly more likely to experience opposition (59% in areas that were notified vs. 35% in areas that were not). Concerns focused on safety, antisocial behavior of residents, and risk to property values. [24] This is despite the fact that research has shown that the establishment of residential facilities and group homes has no effect on the value of properties in the surrounding neighborhoods and that NIMBY sentiments expressed at the outset may change to acceptance over time. [25]

Despite the fact that negative community responses have been widely documented, they are not inevitable. If communities are appropriately prepared in advance, they can be welcoming and supportive to mental health services and their clients. For example, in 1993, after the closure of a large Victorian mental hospital in London, group homes were opened in two urban areas. [26] One area was randomly chosen to receive an educational campaign consisting of a video packet and information sheets about the new facilities, a social component consisting of social events and overtures to residents from staff, and a mixed component including a formal reception and informative discussion sessions. This series of interventions was associated with improved attitudes and behaviors toward the mentally ill residents, with a decrease in fear and exclusion and an increase in levels of social contact. The key driver of change appeared to be the social contact between community residents and the former patients. While educational campaigns have received mixed results, this is one example where community preparedness had a positive effect.

In another example, residents of Long Island had been particularly vociferous with respect to the placement of community residence programs, including sending petitions to public officials, mounting legal battles challenging the site selection process, incidents of suspected arson and physical threats, and holding protest vigils. Between 1987 and 1990, fully 60% of proposals for locating community residence programs were rejected by Long Island municipalities, compared to less than half of that in other parts of the state. Arens [25] interviewed community residents 2 to 3 years after placement and found a striking turnaround in attitudes. Whereas almost a third of residents sampled initially reported negative or strongly negative attitudes, less than 2% expressed current negative attitudes, and 68% reported positive attitudes. Community members cited the negative and damaging role played by the selection process, specifically meetings that raised false expectations about their ability to veto the service placements. When they realized they couldn't prohibit placement, they felt tricked and betrayed. The shift to a more positive attitude shows that strong opposition to community residences for people with mental illnesses is not a predictor of subsequent lack of acceptance. The overwhelming majority of respondents reported that the group home residents were good neighbors, they had no problems, and the homes did not have a negative impact on their property values. These results suggest that a better community preparedness plan may go a long way to alleviate residents' fears.

Criminalization and Trans-institutionalization of the Mentally Ill

The widespread trans-institutionalization of the mentally ill was another unforeseen consequence of deinstitutionalization and amounted to a large-scale resegregation of former patients from psychiatric hospitals to other forms of institutional care, such as prisons and jails. Fazel and Danesh [27] conducted a systematic review including 62 surveys of mental disorders among 22,790 prisoners. They found that the burden of treatable mental illnesses among inmates was substantial. For example, compared with the general U.S. or British population of a similar age, prisoners had a two- to four-fold excess in psychotic illnesses and major depression and a 10-fold excess of antisocial personality disorder. This means that about one in seven inmates in Western countries has a psychotic illness or major depression. One in two males and one in five females has antisocial personality disorder. It is worth pointing out that most of what we know about the prevalence of mental illnesses in jail and prison populations comes from studies conducted in the Western world. [28]

In 1939, Lionel Penrose documented an inverse relationship between the populations of psychiatric hospitals and prisons. "Penrose's Law," as it came to be known, postulated that, in any social group, a certain number of individuals require institutionalization. If one form of confinement (such as mental hospitals) contracts, the other (prisons) expands. [29,30] Penrose's Law has since been examined in several countries using both cross-sectional and longitudinal data, with fairly robust results. Most studies find that a fall in the number of available psychiatric beds coincides with a rise in prison populations, though it is not clear to what extent the relationship is directly causal. Reduced tolerance of criminal activities (including mentally disturbed behavior), community pressures for stricter law enforcement, a rise in the response to substance misuse, and the politicization of law-and-order agendas may all play a role. [31] Kaliski [32] identifies a "quiet unnoticed retreat into institutional care" through the growth of forensic psychiatric beds designed to provide secure treatment for individuals with mental illnesses who have been incarcerated or are in conflict with the law. Forensic beds have been on the rise, with growth in some countries approximating 150% in a span of less than 15 years.

Stigma as a Consequence of Therapeutic Nihilism

The recognition of the damaging effects of stigma that has resulted in poor quality of care, increased mortality, and diminished quality of life for people with a mental illness has given rise to a new treatment paradigm that emphasizes recovery. In this context, the notion of "recovery" has moved beyond its previously narrow clinical focus (emphasizing a cure) to embody a broader understanding that views recovery as the development of new purpose and meaning in one's life following the experience of a mental illness. Recovery reflects a personal journey toward empowerment, self-management, self-determination, and meaning. It involves the right mix of treatments and supports (including supportive relationships from family, friends, and peers) and hope. [33] Recovery-oriented systems are consumer- and family-driven [34], promote person-centered care, and eschew therapeutic nihilism. [35]

On a population level, the process of recovery can work only if the external environment (including healthcare environments) promotes personal empowerment, self-management, and inclusion. Unfortunately, the culture of healthcare settings is often identified as disempowering, where people with mental disorders feel patronized, humiliated, and excluded from treatment decisions or are assumed to lack the capacity to be responsible for their own lives and treatment decisions. Other problems include not being given sufficient information about their illness and treatment options, prognostic negativism, and the threat of coercive treatment. [35] In their examination of recovery competencies for inpatient care, Chen and colleagues underlined the importance of the physical environment for the success of recovery-oriented care, showing that it will not be successful in settings where routines and interactions are experienced as dehumanizing, discouraging, and disempowering. [36] Most would agree that adopting a recovery perspective requires a complete transformation of mental health services, supports, cultures, and relationships.

It is worth noting that the term *recovery* has a different origin and evolution in the substance use field. Early debates pitched abstinence as the hallmark of recovery, whereas more recent dialogue understands a range of outcomes, including harm reduction, improved social supports, and improved social integration. In 2008, a UK Recovery Consensus Panel defined the process of recovery from problematic substance use as sustained control over the use of substances that maximizes health and social integration. [37] Like recovery in mental health care, recovery in the substance use field is person-focused and addresses wider social factors such as housing, employment, and well-being. For some, abstinence may be an important recovery goal, but for others, smaller incremental steps such as feelings of acceptance, taking responsibility, gaining control, or improving mental health are as important. For still others, simply recognizing the need to change may be the focus. [38] In all instances, however, the social environment and the physical environment play an important role.

Peer support is a key component of recovery-oriented care because it focuses on strengths, the positive aspects of people, and their ability to function effectively in social roles that are meaningful to them. The literature supports the idea that peer support workers can be more successful than professionally trained mental health workers in promoting hope, a belief in recovery, empowerment, a positive self-concept, and social inclusion. Employment for peer support workers offers the added advantage of promoting their own recovery (through valued social roles) as well as financial benefits. [39] In addition, however, there is evidence that peer support workers teach non-peer staff about recovery and recovery-oriented care [40] and so can be a key driver of changes in treatment and care culture.

Peer support roles have been introduced into a variety of mental health organizations across the world, and peer workers have participated in a broad range of functions within these organizations. What is considered to be distinctive about peer support is a set of values that stands in juxtaposition to typical mainstream clinical practices that emphasize medical disability. [41] The rise in peer support has coincided with the reduction of extended family size and the difficulty experienced by women who are often employed outside of the home to take on full-time caring and supportive roles for mentally ill family members.

Diagnostic Overshadowing

One important barrier to recovery-oriented care that is attracting growing attention in the literature is the problem of diagnostic overshadowing.

Diagnostic overshadowing is the process by which a person with a mental disorder receives inadequate or delayed treatment for a physical condition because it is misattributed to the underlying mental health challenge. People with mental disorders experience higher rates of physical illness and are more likely to die prematurely compared to members of the general population. At least 60% of premature deaths of people with mental disorders are a result of potentially preventable natural causes, most often cardiovascular disease or cancer. [42] Despite the importance for reducing premature mortality, little research has examined the contributing factors and how they may interact with diagnostic or treatment bias to reduce quality of care. [43] In a qualitative study of 25 emergency department clinicians (15 nurses, two nurse practitioners, and eight doctors), diagnostic overshadowing was commonly acknowledged and complications were often serious, ranging from irreversible side effects to death. [44]

The reasons for diagnostic overshadowing are undoubtedly complex, including healthcare staff who perpetuate a culture of stigma, lack of knowledge and skills in identifying physical signs and symptoms when presented with complex cases involving mental disorders, physical disorders that can mimic mental illnesses, or the questioning of the veracity of physical complaints. [45] Despite the potential complexity, Zun and Rozel [46] have described diagnostic overshadowing as one of the "cardinal dangers" of stigma. People cope with this problem in a variety of ways, including avoiding treatment altogether, bringing someone with them to a healthcare setting to advocate on their behalf, or going to settings, such as emergency departments, where their former psychiatric history is unknown. [47]

It is important to note that diagnostic overshadowing works both ways. An individual with a physical disorder will be treated for that disorder but not examined or treated for any underlying mental health condition. For example, in the case of diabetes, current research suggests that at least one-third of patients will also experience a subthreshold or major depressive disorder. While depression is associated with poor self-care, impaired glycemic control, poor microvascular and macrovascular outcomes, higher healthcare costs, and poorer quality of life, the depression will often go unnoticed. In one study, the majority of nurse specialists failed to document high levels of anxiety or depression in patients who screened above the clinical threshold. [48]

THREE STIGMA MECHANISMS: COMBINED AND INTERTWINED

Stigma is often conceptualized as involving three interrelated mechanisms that work together to create and maintain stigma: structural stigma, public stigma, and self-stigma. Figure 1.1 shows the trickle-down effect of these

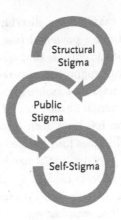

Figure 1.1 Trickle-down effect of stigma processes

stigma processes from the broadest social structural level to members of the general public, to individuals who have a mental illness.

Structural Stigma

Structural stigma refers to broad social and legal frameworks and organizational practices that deliberately or unintentionally create social disparities and inequities for people with a mental illness. Individuals are born into social groups with preexisting structures that help to socialize members with respect to cultural norms. From an early age, members of the public are taught how to think, feel, and behave toward people with a mental illness (as well as other disabling conditions). They entrench stereotypical thinking that perpetuates misconceptions and negative attributions (such as that people with a mental illness are dangerous), which fuels social intolerance and social distance. People who have a mental illness are socialized in the same way, so when they become ill, they may internalize public perceptions and apply them to themselves through a process of self-stigmatization. [4] Structural stigma is the broad social driver that creates and maintains stigma at the level of the social group, through members of the public, and ultimately through individuals who experience a mental illness.

Corrigan and colleagues [49] note that structural stigma can be intentional or unintentional. Intentional structural stigma manifests itself in explicit and discriminatory rules, policies, and procedures that purposefully restrict individual rights and opportunities. Laws that would restrict people with a mental illness from voting, holding elective office, serving on a jury, or parenting illustrate this type of structural stigma. There are also policies and practices that restrict the opportunities of people with a mental illness in unintended or covert ways. These are cases where discrimination occurs without the conscious prejudicial efforts of a powerful few. Examples of unintentional discrimination include economic policies that allocate less funding for psychiatric research and treatment programs compared to other equally disabling conditions, or insurance policies that assign higher risk and therefore higher premiums to people with a mental illness.

Discriminatory legislation has long been recognized as a driver of structural stigma. Bhugra and colleagues [50] focused on property rights as an important enabler of full and effective social participation. Also, as they point out, the right to property is recognized as a human right by the Universal Declaration of Human Rights (Article 17). They reviewed property-related legislation from all United Nations member states (193 countries) to determine if people with a mental illness were disadvantaged in their ability to own or manage property (e.g., had the right to enter contracts, inherit property, or make a will). Over a third of the member states (38%) do not recognize the right of persons with a mental illness to enter into a contract; 20% do not allow people with a mental illness to enter into a contract; and only 16% recognized the right of persons with a mental illness to contract without any restrictions. Member states in low-income countries were more likely to deny property rights.

Structural stigma has been described as a "fundamental cause" of health inequalities. [51] Fundamental causes are social factors that persistently influence health inequalities despite any surface changes in the prevalence of illness, health interventions, or individual risk factors. They are robust over time and place, and they result in inequitable access to resources such as money, power, prestige, or beneficial social circumstances that can be used to reduce or avoid risk or promote recovery.

Globally, mental disorders have received less policy interest than disorders that convey a commensurate burden of illness, resulting in serious structural inequalities. For example, most of the world's psychiatric beds remain in large mental hospitals, many of which have been shown to provide anti-therapeutic environments or violate the human rights of the patients and their families. Per capita spending on mental illnesses is significantly lower than other illnesses with commensurate public health burdens, and large proportions of people who have a serious mental illness fail to receive appropriate treatment. In developing countries, unmet need can be as high as 85%. [52] In Canada (as perhaps elsewhere), psychiatrists are the lowest-paid medical specialty, earning 20% less than the average specialist and 65% less than the top earner. [53] Funding for mental health programming and research is also subpar. [1] These structural inequities impinge on the health, welfare, civic participation, and quality of life of people with mental illness and their families.

Research also shows that people with serious mental illnesses have a much lower life expectancy at birth compared to the general population. For example, in a UK study [54], males with schizophrenia, schizoaffective disorder, bipolar disorder, substance use, or depressive disorder lived an average of 8 to 15 years and females 10 to 18 years less than their general population counterparts. Other studies have reported an almost three-fold increase in premature mortality for people with a mental illness compared to the general population. [55] The causal pathways linking serious mental illnesses to premature mortality are complex but include lack of attention to prevention, side effects of medications, poor lifestyle choices, and death from violent causes. [54] A Canadian study reported that cardiovascular disease and cancer were the most common causes of premature death of people with mental illnesses. [56] These findings suggest that greater access to primary care, risk assessments, and assertive interventions by primary and secondary medical services are needed. [57]

The media have been identified as one of the key structural drivers promoting a culture of stigma. Denigrating fictional images of people with a mental illness are frequent and potent. They do little to convey to the viewing public that people with a mental illness can recover or become productive members of society. Stigmatizing portrayals of mental illnesses are found in a range of fictional and nonfictional media, including children's television. [58] Even children's fairy tales clearly construct villains and heroes based on who is physically or mentally disabled (and therefore evil) and who is not (and therefore good). Fairy-tale transformations typically occur at the individual level, when someone is magically transformed from a disfigured and pitiable character to a beautiful prince or princess. Social structures are never the object of transformation or improvement; thus, fairy tales protect the status quo. Typically happy endings occur when characters who are disfigured become whole again and live happily ever after. [59] Such negative images in the news or entertainment industries are profoundly upsetting for those experiencing an illness and their families. Negative media images leave people feeling angry, hurt, sad, and discouraged, particularly when acts of extreme violence are emphasized, or when derogatory and disrespectful language is used. [58]

Public Stigma

Attribution theory describes the process of public stigma as beginning with a label. The label triggers stereotyped attributions, which then may evoke a negative and prejudicial emotional response and discriminatory behavior. Corrigan and colleagues [60] found that public stigma was worse for people with substance-related disorders compared to those with a mental illness or a physical disability requiring a wheelchair. They recruited a sample of 815 Americans using random-digit dialing from a national sampling frame of all telephone numbers available in an online panel. The sample was stratified to be representative of the American, English-speaking adult population and represented a 71.4% response rate. Respondents were randomly assigned to read one of three vignettes depicting a person with a mental illness, with a drug addiction, or requiring a wheelchair. Respondents were then asked a series of questions to measure two stereotypes often associated with mental disabilities: (1) attributions of dangerousness and (2) responsibility for the health condition. People with a drug addiction were viewed as significantly more responsible for their disorder, less likely to overcome the problems associated with their condition, less often considered worthy of help, and less often deserving of assistance in finding a job. Cultural values concerning the use of drugs, particularly alcohol, may alter public perceptions of these attributions. For example, in a culture where alcohol use is highly prevalent, people with alcohol problems may be less likely to be seen as blameworthy. A more detailed description of cultural variation in stigma is provided in the next chapter.

Using data from a representative sample collected in the 1996 U.S. General Social Survey (n = 1444, 76.1% response rate), Martin and colleagues [61] examined the role of six factors thought to influence the public's willingness to interact with people who have a mental disorder: the extent to which they would move next door, make friends, spend an evening socializing, work closely on the job, have a group home in the neighborhood, or have them marry into the family. Five vignettes describing major depression, alcohol dependency, drug dependency, schizophrenia, and a person with no signs of a mental illness, but described as having "normal troubles," were used to elicit responses. The highest level of social distance was toward people with drug (77.8%) and alcohol (55.7%) dependencies. By comparison, 48.4% would socially distance themselves from someone with schizophrenia, compared to 37.4% for depression and 20.8% for someone with normal troubles. In addition, few Americans defined substance disorders as formal mental illnesses (10.9% for alcohol dependency and 13.3% for drug dependency).

In 2010, the *Opening Minds* anti-stigma initiative of the Mental Health Commission Canada funded a representative survey conducted by Statistics Canada involving 10,389 Canadians 12 years and older (response rate of 72.3%). Six items were used to assess the extent to which the sample thought that people with depression (defined as a prolonged period of sadness or loss of interest in usual activities that interferes with daily life) would be devalued or discriminated against. More than half of Canadians (58.2%) endorsed one or more of the items indicating that they thought someone with depression would be stigmatized. The most commonly endorsed item was that most employers would not consider an application from someone who had depression (38.2%), followed by people being reluctant to date someone with depression (33.7%). One-third of the people who reported being treated for a mental illness in the past year indicated that they had been treated unfairly because of their current or past mental health problem, most frequently with respect to personal relationships such as with family (32%) or romantic partners (30%). Stigma was also experienced in relation to school or work (28%), finances (25%), and housing (18%). [62]

In a large international study of discrimination experienced by people receiving mental health services for depression in 35 countries, discrimination in social situations was also among the most frequently reported. For example, 40% of the 1082 respondents identified discrimination from family members, approximately a third reported they were avoided or shunned by other people or had problems making or keeping friends, and approximately a quarter indicated they had experienced discrimination with respect to marriage or divorce. Other areas of discrimination that were experienced included keeping a job (21%), personal safety and security (21%), dating or intimate relationships (21%), mental health staff (19%), or social life (18%). [63]

Angermeyer and Dietrich [64] reviewed 33 national and 29 regional/local population-based studies of public attitudes toward mental illnesses published between 1990 and 2004. The most prevalent negative attitudes were that people with mental illnesses were unpredictable and violent, which appeared more frequently over time. Stereotypes varied by diagnostic group, with the highest prevalence among those with "alcoholism." People with schizophrenia were considered to be more dangerous than people with depression or anxiety. Perceptions of unpredictability and dangerousness were significantly associated with desire for social distance. Also, those who considered that people with mental illnesses were blameworthy were more accepting of structural discrimination, such as reduced allocation of health resources.

Self-Stigma

Stigma was, for me, the most agonizing aspect of my disorder. It cost friendships, career opportunities, and—most importantly—my self-esteem. It wasn't long before I began internalizing the attitudes of others, viewing myself as a lesser person. In fact, this process began the moment I received a diagnosis. [65, p. 308]

As this quote illustrates, people with a mental illness can internalize the negative attitudes of others and come to feel that they are of little worth. Self-stigma can lead to loss of hope, lowered self-esteem, lowered self-efficacy, disempowerment, poor morale, and lowered quality of life. Self-stigma also has been associated with treatment avoidance, increased symptom severity, diminished social functioning, poorer insight, and lack of recovery. The altered sense of self that embodies the notion of self-stigma has been associated with the "why try?" effect, where people avoid pursuing opportunities such as work, housing, treatment, or other personal goals. [66]

People who self-stigmatize also anticipate negative views and actions in their social interactions with others [67] and may recede from public life in order to avoid these. In the Statistics Canada survey cited above, people who were personally stigmatized were more likely to expect others to be stigmatizing. [62]

Brohan and colleagues [68] described levels of self-stigma experienced by mental health service users with a diagnosis of schizophrenia or other psychotic disorder in 14 European countries. Members of a mental health charity organization recruited participants using a random sample of 500 people at each site (n = 1229, 72% response rate). Almost half (42%) reported levels of self-stigma that met predefined cutoffs for moderate or high, though there was significant country-to-country variation. The majority (69.4%) reported moderate to high levels of perceived discrimination, and this was significantly associated with higher self-stigma. Empowerment and a higher number of social contacts were associated with lower levels of self-stigma, suggesting that interventions that enhance these factors may be effective in reducing self-stigma. Factors associated with lower levels of self-stigma included empowerment and self-esteem. The significant variation across countries suggests that interventions should be tailored to local circumstances and to the specific aspects of self-stigma that are most highly endorsed.

This cycle of stigmatization has an impact on the family, who may experience stress (by feeling shame, guilt, and worry), which can reduce their reserves and undermine their ability to provide the social supports necessary to promote recovery. At the level of the mental health system, the stigmatization of mental health professionals and services means that they are underfunded, making it difficult to provide high-quality, recovery-oriented care. Medications needed for the treatment of serious mental illnesses are often not available because they are deemed to be too expensive, which is just another way of saying that people with mental illnesses are unworthy of this (or perhaps any) expense. These cycles (individual, family, and system) perpetuate disability and, in so doing, promote further stigmatization. Figure 1.2 shows how the cycle of stigmatization can affect the quality of care provided by mental health services. Similar models have been developed for the individual and the family.

An important advantage of these cyclical models is that they imply that an intervention made at any point might disrupt the entire process. So, for example, it may be difficult to change public stigma, but it may be possible to remove discrimination by legal or other means. Similarly, it may be possible to improve treatment and rehabilitation to a level where they can offer the supports needed by people with a mental illness to live full and productive lives in the community. Sometimes it is possible to remove a marker, such as in the case of extrapyramidal symptoms that can appear as side effects of certain medications but do not appear with other treatments.

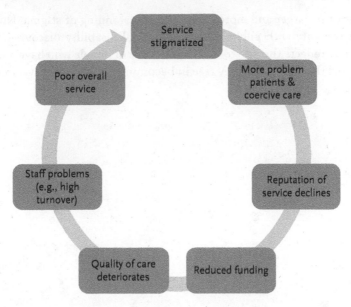

Figure 1.2 Cycle of stigmatization as it affects mental health services
Adapted from Sartorius N, Schulze H. *Reducing the Stigma of Mental Illness*. Cambridge: Cambridge University Press, 2005.

A more detailed analysis of anti-stigma interventions is described in subsequent chapters. Suffice it to say that there are multiple points of entry, making it possible for everyone to contribute to stigma reduction in some small or large way.

SUMMARY

In our modern age, people with mental illnesses are not visibly tattooed, but they still bear the indelible marks of social inequity, poverty, homelessness, and disenfranchisement. They continue to be socially banished through methods such as criminalization, unemployment, and social distancing. Modern stereotypes portray people with mental illnesses as blameworthy, sometimes sinful, incompetent, unpredictable, and violent—all of which echo the historical notions that people with a mental illness are morally tainted and unfit for social company.

As discussed in this chapter, stigma has been defined narrowly, to reflect imperfections in an individual resulting in social labeling, prejudice, and discrimination, and more broadly as a complex social process that involves numerous interconnected and mutually reinforcing parts, all of which work in concert to marginalize and disenfranchise people with a mental illness, their family members, and mental health systems. Throughout this book, we adopt this larger and more complex understanding of stigma. Not only does it resonate with public health and social disability discourse, but it also better reflects the day-to-day experiences of people who have a mental illness and the challenges they face in becoming full and effective members of society.

CHAPTER 2

Cultures Count

They Stigmatize and Destigmatize Mental Illnesses

At its essence, mental illness–related stigma is a cultural phenomenon, created by such factors as shared beliefs, values, and expectations about what constitutes normal, abnormal, and mentally disordered behavior. Stigma has been generally described as being universal. Yet, more recent research shows that it can vary considerably by time and place. Mental illnesses take on a particular significance in relation to local beliefs and norms, and associated stigma may be substantially modified or even eliminated as a result. This chapter reviews historical and cultural perspectives of mental illness and its related stigma. While stigma has been highly prevalent, and often severe, there have been times and places where stigmatization has not been the dominant reaction to people exhibiting mentally disordered behaviors. Cultures can act as both a stigmatizing and destigmatizing force.

HISTORICAL PERSPECTIVES ON STIGMA

At times, societies have responded to people with mental illnesses with violence and barbarism, but at other times with reason and humanism. In early antiquity, up until the time of the early Greeks, people with mental illnesses were not necessarily looked on with scorn, fear, or derision—not because the ancients were necessarily humanistically inclined, but because they did not make an important distinction between mental and physical illnesses. People could be shunned for all manner of reasons (including violent and disorded behaviors), but not because they were perceived to be "mentally ill." [70] From the early Hippocratic treatises to later Byzantine medical texts, there was no established word for "mental illness." From the point of view of the ancients, all medical disorders were affiliations of the body. [71] Rather than being indicative of mental illnesses per se, psychiatric symptoms were often understood as signs of spiritual forces working through the individual, such as possession by gods or demons.

Ancient Greece (5th to 2nd Century B.C.E.)

The term "stigma" is a Greek noun signifying a tattoo used to denote ownership of a slave, criminality, or a religious decoration. In ancient Greek culture, however, decorative religious tattooing was associated with barbarians and not widely practiced. Thus, tattooing usually signified a mark of degradation or punishment—such as tattooing the foreheads of criminals with the name of their crime. Without hygiene, tattooing would have been a dangerous procedure, which likely contributed to its value as a form of punishment. Tattoo removal became an important business, and there were many medical and technical writers of the day who gave prescriptions for the removal of these "stigmata." [72]

Although tattooing and the term "stigma" were not used in ancient Greece in reference to mental illnesses, considerable stigma was attached to being mentally ill, causing a sense of deep shame, loss of face, humiliation, and fear of pollution. If mental illnesses were chronic or severe, or involved unpredictable behaviors, the afflicted individual might be locked up, shunned, or on rare occasions put to death. This was less a function of being mentally ill and more a function of being socially disruptive. There were no dedicated hospital-like institutions to care for people with mental illnesses, so this responsibility typically fell to the family. Contagion was a concern as the "madman" was considered to be polluted and also could pollute others. Interestingly, many Greek doctors were careful to avoid incurable or chronic cases because they made their reputations look worse. [73]

An array of practices was available to address physical and mental illnesses, including interventions that were scientific, religious, and magical. Some temples (such as the cults of Asklepius) specialized in treating mental illnesses and others in treating possession. Included among the temples' treatment approaches to psychogenic disturbances were a balanced diet, daily massage, quiet sleep, and warm baths—all intended to soothe patients. The main therapeutic procedure was the interpretation of dreams by the priests, which revealed both the cause and the cure for the disorder. [74] Patients would sleep in the temple hoping for a miraculous cure or a divine dream that could then be interpreted by the priests. Others reported being cured after being licked by the sacred snakes or holy dogs that were kept in the temple. [75]

Hippocrates is credited for his forthright rejection of the magic and sorcery of the priest-healers of the Asklepian cults. He emphasized a rational scientific approach to diagnosis, with treatments relying on the healing powers of nature. It is interesting to note that many of his ideas about physical and mental illnesses were consistent with the teachings of an ancient Chinese physician known as the Yellow Emperor, born some 2000 years before. [75]

Middle Ages (5th to 15th Century)

In the Middle Ages, mentally ill people were accepted with considerable tolerance. Mental illness was understood to be an expression of God's will. The mentally ill were viewed as living witnesses to the frailty of man and so were largely accepted as part of the fabric of humanity. Rather than being hidden away, they were exposed as a testimony to human frailty, constantly at the mercy of the battle between evil and grace. [76]

While many of the mentally ill were tolerated in their communities, individuals with clear psychotic symptoms were often chased away from home or kept hidden under the supervision of family members, who may have been cruel and abusive. Some of those whom mental illness made completely unmanageable or dangerous were turned over to local authorities and thrown into dungeons, sometimes for life. A few were also cared for by religious orders in institutions that were part hospital, part shelter, part workshop, and part penitentiary (meaning a place to do penance for sins). In feudal society, individual freedom for all but the lords was virtually unknown, and severe punishments for all manner of infractions were daily occurrences and considered as part of the overall divine plan. [76] There are many accounts of large numbers of mentally ill individuals being boarded onto ships, termed "ships of fools," and cast adrift, being turned away at every port. The original metaphor was popularized in Europe by Sebastian Brant's poem "The Ship of Fools," which satirized all manner of sin, such as greed, gluttony, avarice, or carelessness, and folly (e.g., not taking good advice, adultery, the impertinent patient, and the foolish doctor). At the turn of the 16th century, many visual and literary works exploited the "ship of fools" metaphor. [77] These ships were imagined having crisscrossed the waterways; however, scholars have been unable to identify corroborating evidence from historical accounts that these ships ever existed. Thus, the ship of fools may be a literary fiction that expresses the tenor of the times toward people with mental illnesses rather than a reality. [78]

Maristans (meaning "place for the sick") spread widely in the 9th and 10th centuries across North Africa, where they were typically founded by sultans and supervised by physicians. Many were teaching hospitals and focused on specific diseases. The maristan of Cairo (872), was the earliest identified as primarily focusing on treatment of the mentally ill, though others were known to exist in Baghdad, Marrakech, and Fez. In the late Middle Ages, two institutions specifically dedicated to the treatment of the mentally ill appeared in southern Spain, one arising from the Christian tradition (founded in Valencia in 1409) and the other arising from the centuries-long Moorish tradition of medically oriented hospitals and centers of medical learning (founded in Granada in 1365). Both may have been patterned after the Cairo maristan and the Fez maristan (1286). [79,80]

The maristan of Granada and the asylum at Valencia (named the Hospital of Our Lady Mary of the Innocents) were developed out of strong convictions from political or religious leaders who saw a need for better treatment for the insane. While their motivations included hope for spiritual rewards, social benefits, and charitable donations, they also likely included recognition of the need to isolate and remove the mentally ill from urban streets, where they were a social nuisance. [81]

The Renaissance (14th to 17th Centuries)

As the Renaissance emerged, mental illnesses became less associated with God's divine plan and more associated with an array of occult sciences that could affect human behavior. The Inquisition, which emerged sometime during the 12th century, focused on sorcery and meted out the cruelest forms of punishment. [76] The *Malleus Maleficarum*, published in the mid-1400s, embodied a negative and condemning attitude toward witches, but numerous symptoms consistent with mental illnesses, such as schizophrenia or depression, were described among the victims as signs of their communion with the devil*. [2] This period of demonology lasted more than a thousand years and resulted in hundreds of thousands of mentally disordered individuals being abused, tortured, burned, hanged, or drowned. [70]

The Rational Era (17th and 18th Centuries)

Prior to the 17th century, there were two opposing explanations for mental disorders. The medical explanation understood an imbalance of humors as the root cause, whereas the religious (and popularist) understanding emphasized evil spirits taking possession of the sufferer's mind. With the growth in the belief of witchcraft, possession was added to the etiological list. In the 17th century these explanations began to be overturned. Science had been progressing

---

*Clearer descriptions of mental illnesses, such as schizophrenia, did not occur until the 18th century. [19]

and medical knowledge was growing. Older explanations involving the spleen and uterus as the seat of nervous disorders, for example, were becoming increasingly untenable. [82] The belief in witchcraft took much longer to overturn, and accusations of witchcraft were common in 17th-century England and New England. Witches were thought to cause victims to have fits that signified possession by the devil. While any disease could be attributed to the devil, mental illnesses were particularly singled out. [83]

In the 17th century, in parallel to the urbanization in many parts of Europe, there was a marked change in social attitudes toward "lunatics," who had been allowed to wander freely as long as they were not dangerous or socially disturbing. Madhouses began to spring up to restrain them. Early madhouses were largely private, entirely custodial, and harsh, though public opinion later questioned the brutal practices and wrongful detention. In the early 18th century, lunatics began to be admitted to institutions for care, protection, and treatment rather than simple confinement, and insanity began to be viewed as treatable. By the close of the 18th century, workhouses, houses of corrections, and prisons contained a number of "lunatics" and "idiots." However, over time, asylums began to function as long-term repositories for the segregation of the insane from community life. Therapeutic nihilism, owing to deterministic organic and hereditary views of mental illnesses, began to prevail. By the late 18th century, less than 8% of those in asylums were thought to be curable. It is important to note that the afflicted members of the upper classes did not experience the harsh brutalities characteristic of these institutions as they were housed in private asylums with higher standards of accommodation, limited overcrowding, and an atmosphere that was evocative of a substantial country house. [84]

The Era of Moral Treatment (19th Century)

With its advance in treatments for the mentally ill and the decline in the belief that demons caused mental illnesses, the 19th century ushered in a period of humanism, asylum, and moral treatment. Early conceptions of the "asylum" during this time conjure humanitarian images of protection, refuge, shelter, and retreat. The functions of these were to provide a calm shelter against the disquieting effects of a frenetic social environment. The asylum was a benevolent institution where moral treatment was practiced—a dramatic change from the beastly conditions of the almshouses, previous homes for the insane, and prisons that housed an ever-increasing number of mentally ill persons. [85]

With the notable exceptions of the maristans in Spain and elsewhere, early institutions for the insane in Europe were atrocious. There were no provisions for cleanliness, comfort, or treatment. They were custodial institutions where barbarity and ignorance were the rule. Following the French Revolution, a growing body of post-Enlightenment thinkers expressed their disgust for these conditions and the failure to recognize the value of kindness and sympathy. The regular use of chains was considered to be an outstanding fault of the older practices. "Moral treatment," which accorded the mentally ill humane treatment, including unshackling their chains, was a new approach that spread throughout Europe and America. Philippe Pinel is the name most often associated with moral therapy, but he was not the only one experimenting with humane treatment approaches, which were becoming widely adopted. [86]

Rothman provides a detailed historical account of the rise of institutions for the placement of the mentally ill across the United States. [87] No such institutions existed during the Colonial times. Prior to this time, as in Europe, the mentally ill lived with their families, in communities, or, if impossible to control, in jails. Following the Civil War, institutionalization became the preferred way of treating people with a mental illness. At that time, however, institutionalization was not viewed as a last resort by a frightened community. In post–Civil War society, community life was considered to be characterized by unbridled economic and social expansion brought about by the overzealousness with which the Americans of the day sought wealth, power, and education. Psychiatrists, reformers, and their lay supporters claimed that insanity was curable if the individual was removed from the social turmoil of community life. Communities of the day did not feel threatened by the establishment of an asylum in their midst. Rather, they competed for the right to have one as it brought considerable employment, income, and revenue.[†] Also, most institutions were built some distance away from local communities where there would be a better chance of creating a calm, natural environment, and where any disruption to community life would be minimal—a win–win situation.

During the latter part of the 19th century, standards of care in the asylums again began to decline. Admission rates were mounting, finances were dwindling, and staff were too few and ill prepared to care for their patients properly using moral treatment methods. Because mental hospitals were typically isolated from their communities and from mainstream medicine, they were not able to stir public interest. The "cult of curability" that was a centerpiece for the 19th-century asylums had collapsed, and statistics that boasted 80% to 100% cure rates were quickly debunked. Under increasing economic restrictions, custodial care soon replaced active treatment, creating a static environment that promoted passivity and dependency. [88]

[†] When it came time to deinstitutionalize and close large institutions, may small communities in Canada (and perhaps elsewhere) resisted planned closures, citing a loss of income and employment opportunities for their citizenry.

As new medications emerged to treat the most disturbing symptoms of mental illnesses, as human rights models questioned the need to involuntarily remove people with a mental illness from their communities without due process, and as exposés uncovered the brutal conditions in many mental hospitals, attitudes toward the need for institutions changed dramatically, and the community care movement was born. The fall of the asylum era and its aftermath are outlined in more detail in Chapter 1.

Gheel, Belgium: A Special Case (600 A.D. to Present)

The Gheel colony in Belgium has long been renowned for its special relationship with people experiencing a mental illness. According to Tuntiya, the special attitude of the people of Gheel toward those with a mental illness began in 600 A.D. with the legend of an Irish princess. [89] Dymphna was preparing to commit herself to the church and fled to Gheel away from her father who, following her mother's death, wanted to wed her. Dymphna was followed by her evil father (who was considered to be incited by the devil) and, when she wouldn't submit to marriage, was beheaded. [90] In her death she was able to overcome what came to be considered the insane desires of her father.

The martyred princess became a saint and patroness of all people with a mental illness. Rumors of the healing powers of her shrine touched off a pilgrimage from far and wide. Initially pilgrims were kept in the church, but space soon ran out. An additional cottage was built, but even this was not sufficient to accommodate all of the pilgrims. The Church asked the residents of Gheel to provide temporary housing for those waiting for treatment. This began a tradition of families boarding mentally ill pilgrims, which has remained active to this day. The colony existed under religious auspices until 1852 and then was taken over by the state to become the first community-based system for alternative treatment for the mentally ill. This system was built on an unconditional acceptance of people with mental illnesses. [89,91]

As reported by Kilgour, who traveled to Gheel in 1935, the patient population was just over 3000, the bulk of them living in private homes in the community. [92] It was a mark of standing in the community to foster a patient. There were always more homes available than patients who needed them. Families who had never had a patient were held in considerable disrespect. Though families received a small stipend for supporting patients' necessities, the main motivation was to share in the great humanitarian work that had been part of community life for centuries.

According to Siabbald who visited Gheel on several occasions in the late 1800s, no family was allowed to have more than two boarders. [91] This restriction was imposed to prevent the patients from being excluded from family life. It was thought that a household could incorporate two boarders easily into family life, but more than two would be problematic. Observations by Ellis indicated that the patients were generally treated as members of the family. They took their meals at the same table, went to church together, and shared in work and leisure time. Patients who were violent or aggressive or intractably dangerous to themselves or others were not admitted to the Gheel colony.

Though Gheel is often considered to be the single exception to the widespread abuse of the liberty and rights of the mentally ill, the practice of boarding out psychiatric patients in the homes of private individuals was widespread across Europe, beginning in the late 1700s, exceptions being the Iberian Peninsula and England. By the close of the 1800s, in Scotland, for example, about a fifth of all of the "insane" lived in boarding-out arrangements in private homes. [93]

The Village of Aro, Nigeria

To modernize psychiatric treatment in Nigeria, Dr. T.A. Lambo recruited and gained the confidence of local witch doctors. Mental illness was understood as one of many evils that could be bestowed on people by the gods or other supernatural forces. The supernatural was blamed for all manner of evil, and witch doctors acted as intermediaries to help appease the offended spirits, ghosts, or witches. Lambo thought that traditional Nigerians needed to be treated in a village environment with the active participation of local witch doctors. Inhabitants of the village of Aro (and surrounding villages) agreed to receive patients as lodgers. Patients had to be accompanied by a relative whose job it was to see to the patient's needs in terms of food and housework. Each patient was free to socialize with the village inhabitants and to participate fully in village life. The witch doctor helped diagnose and treat the patients, as well as supervised recreation, occupational therapy, and sleeping arrangements, thereby giving him a central role in the village with respect to the care and treatment of the mentally ill. Using this approach, the average patient stayed in the village for approximately 6 months—much less time than patients who were hospitalized in a nearby facility. [94]

PERSPECTIVES FROM NON-WESTERN CULTURES

In addition to the historical forces just described, there are three great non-Western traditions in medicine that are associated with distinct civilizations and religious views that provide different interpretive systems for understanding and managing mental illnesses and mental illness related stigma: Islam, China, and India. [95]

Islamic Culture

In the Koran, the most common word used to refer to those with a mental illness is *majnoon*, which is derived from the Arabic word *jinn*, referring to a supernatural spirit that has the power to assume human and animal forms that can be either good or bad. The traditional Islamic concept of insanity is that one is possessed by a *jinn*. [96] Unlike cultures that are built on individualism, Islamic cultures are more collectivist, where individuals are defined in relation to others in their social group, particularly their family. [97] Historically, Islamic cultures have viewed mental disturbances as illnesses with no particular moral meaning, guilt, or shame attached. The primary responsibility for the care of the mentally ill rested with the family, which appears to have been supportive and tolerant. [98] Individuals would have been placed in hospitals only in extreme cases when the family was no longer able to care for them. These would be cases where individuals were seriously disturbed, probably psychotic. [99]

Early Islamic hospitals included sections for the mentally ill that could be severe but were open to visitors, often family members. The sections had walls that were reinforced with heavy wood and iron, and keepers were equipped with whips, which they used when a patient became agitated or violent. The most seriously disturbed patients were held in restraints. Yet, these mental hospital units were also places where physicians practiced physiologically oriented medicine and where diversions were provided to patients such as dancing, theatrical performances, and recitations. In some hospitals, patients were led to the mosque to pray.

So, while some patients were restrained and sometimes beaten, the systematic abuses that accompanied the rise of European asylums during the "Great Confinement" in the 17th century were not evident, suggesting that mental illnesses did not elicit as much stigma in the early Islamic world as they did in other societies. [98] In fact, less serious psychotic-like behaviors were tolerated in the community and explained as being the acts of holy men. These individuals were treated not as pariahs but with respect and tolerance as individuals who were in direct communication with God. [99]

In modern Islamic cultures it appears that people with mental illnesses (particularly serious mental illnesses) and their families do suffer considerable stigma and are socially marginalized. [100,101] In a study of 100 family members of patients with schizophrenia in Casablanca, Morocco, for example, most family members (87%) reported experiencing stigma because of their relative's illness. This included maltreatment (41%), mockery (29%), and distrust (15%), causing psychological, sleep, and relational disturbances (72%). [102]

Lay understandings of mental illnesses continue to reflect religious or supernatural causes, such as God's punishment, God's will, the evil eye, demons, spirits, paranormal phenomena, supernatural powers, a curse, and magic. However, unlike in the past, mental illnesses are now considered to be shameful, an embarrassment, and incompatible with friendships, marriage, or having children. Social distancing is the norm. People who have greater access to modern mental health services and those with higher education have been found to be less stigmatizing in their views. Stigmatizing attitudes are also held in reference to psychiatric medicines, and families often prefer faith healers as a first approach to treatment. [101]

Chinese Culture

Confucian ethics provides a strong moral framework governing interpersonal relationships in Chinese culture. Confucianism expects social relationships to be harmonious. Mental illnesses are a source of dissonance that disrupts an otherwise ideal state of harmony. In Chinese medicine, the focus is on restoring the balance between *yin* and *yang*. Excessive emotions are considered unhealthy and a threat to social harmony. Views on the causes of mental illnesses include: resulting from moral transgressions toward ancestors; hereditary, ancestral inheritance of misconduct; cosmological forces; wrath of gods and ancestors; possession by spirits, demons, and foxes; hormones; diet; brain dysfunction; and even political ideology. They tarnish the family and ancestral honor, resulting in a strong desire to hide this shame from outsiders. Denial, somatization of symptoms, and avoidance of psychiatric help are common avoidance strategies. Instead of Western medical solutions, herbs, special diets, and traditional medicines are usually sought. People holding traditional beliefs support the idea that those with a mental illness should be segregated in hospitals away from local neighborhoods. [103,104]

Asylums and institutional care were not characteristic of old China. The first psychiatric hospital for the treatment of people with mental illnesses was opened in Guangzhou in 1878 by a Presbyterian missionary. Despite modest growth in available beds over the next 50 to 60 years (estimated to be 1200 in 1931), for most Chinese people, hospital treatment was unavailable or unaffordable, leaving families to cope as best they could at home. By the early 1960s, there were approximately 11,000 psychiatric beds in 46 hospitals and 5000 psychiatric personnel reported to serve an estimated 10 million people with serious mental illnesses—though the number of mentally ill is most certainly an underestimate. By the late 1980s, government policy documents recognized that 80% of mentally ill people received no treatment at all. Psychiatric services, considered to be necessary to preserve social order, were staffed by people who were inadequately trained, poorly paid, and received little respect or support from the general public. By the early 1990s, reforms concerning the management of disability were under way, spearheaded by the

China Disabled Persons' Federation, headed by the older son of the Paramount Leader Deng Xiaoping, who was confined to a wheelchair after being thrown out of a window during the Cultural Revolution. Despite growing policy recognition, psychiatric plans remained unrealistic due to financial difficulties, poor levels of training, and the low motivation of government personnel. As hospital care was inaccessible for most families, they continued doing what they had always done—confining mentally disordered relatives at home with ropes, shackles, and bars if needed. [105] More recently the "686" program focused attention on the treatment of people with severe mental illness, and the adoption of the Mental Health Law (which had been in preparation for nearly two decades) provided a basis for further improvement of care for people with mental illnesses. Traditional Chinese treatments, dating back to the time of *The Yellow Emperor's Classic of Internal Medicine* (ca. 770–476 B.C.E.), such as moxibustion and acupuncture, were also available to treat psychological disorders outside of hospital environments. [106]

Indian Culture

In ancient India, Hindu cultural psychology emphasized the responsibility of the family, caste, and village for supporting people who were ill, including those with a mental illness. Local systems of support sheltered and contained people with mental illnesses, complemented by access to academic physicians, village practitioners of magical and religious medical arts, priests, and monks located in regional temples and religious centers. [107]

There are at least three distinct medical traditions that can be simultaneously invoked in Indian culture to explain mental disorders. In traditional folk medicine, mental illnesses are considered to be the result of supernatural causes, involving punishment by sorcery, gods, or spirits. In Ayurvedic medicine, mental disorders arise from a disturbance of the normal healthy humoral balance. In modern medicine, they stem from a dysfunction of the normal bio-psycho-social processes. These varying interpretations have given rise to a range of alternative treatment approaches, including allopathic psychiatric services, Ayurvedic practitioners, homeopaths, folk healers, and healing temples. [108] In rural areas, where 80% of the population lives, modern psychiatry is absent. People rely on a variety of traditional healers, sometimes following the advice of more than one at a time. Where modern medicine is available, people consult with both traditional healers and doctors without this causing any anxiety for the clients or the therapists. [109]

Bhattacharyya describes a cognitive pluralism that exists with respect to lay understandings of mental illnesses. [110] The first paradigm focuses on possession by ghosts who cannot leave this world. Transformation of an individual's personality (such as expressions of hostility or anger) is considered indicative of ghost possession. Those who are believed to be possessed are brought to a folk healer for an exorcism. In the second paradigm, sorcery is the etiological factor. When individuals act against their own best interests, such as in cases of adultery or jealousy, then sorcery is suspected, and the individual is brought to a folk healer who provides amulets or medicine to counteract the spell. In the third paradigm, physiological explanations (e.g., head disturbance) are invoked. Based on the Ayurvedic tradition, mental illnesses result in an imbalance of three humors (wind, bile, and phlegm). Grief, anger, and frustration are emotions that can disrupt the body's humoral equilibrium. The three paradigms are not considered to conflict. Villagers are pragmatic and use whatever system of medicine is available. It is likely that these different explanatory models for mental disorders influence the way in which stigma is expressed and experienced. For example, in a study of 60 patients with schizophrenia receiving treatment at a psychiatric treatment facility in Bangalore, previous use of allopathic services was associated with less stigma. [111]

Early institutions for the care of people with mental illnesses in India date to the 15th century. Prior to this time, mentally ill people were cared for in various settings, including in their homes, temples, and religious institutions. Modern asylums (dating from the 18th century) were a British conception and were designed to separate seriously mentally ill people from mainstream society. Patients could be treated with opium, hot baths, leeches, and music. At the time of India's independence in 1947, there were approximately 10,000 beds in mental hospitals for a population over 400 million. Since independence, the population has more than doubled (to well over a billion), while the number of beds has increased to only about 21,000, leaving a relatively constant psychiatric bed ratio of 1 bed for every 5,000 people. [112]

CROSS-CULTURAL STUDIES

As we have seen, stigma is deeply connected to social norms, which vary over time and across cultures. Yang and colleagues have proposed that culture affects stigma by threatening someone's ability to participate in the activities that "matter most" to them; what matters most will differ from culture to culture. [113] As an example, they describe how loss of face is a key component of stigma in Asian cultures. Asian families typically require "face" to participate in social exchange networks that enable them to fulfill crucial life opportunities such as finding work or a suitable marriage partner. By comparison, Latino groups in the United States consider that mental illnesses could be willed away through self-reliance and, if not, were indicative of laziness. What mattered most in this cultural setting was that people were hard-working, overcame their problems, and took advantage of the opportunities provided by living in the United States. Taking medications meant one was weak, useless, and small, thus violating fundamental values. In African American groups, privacy regarding one's family business was an important part of the culture, so disclosing a mental illness could have dire social consequences. In a culture that values spirituality, mental illnesses were considered to reflect insufficient faith and spiritual weakness.

Methodologically coordinated attempts to understand variations in stigma across multiple countries are scarce, likely because they are so challenging. [114] In 2008, Pescosolido and colleagues examined stigmatizing beliefs regarding depression and schizophrenia across five European nations (Bulgaria, Hungary, Spain, Germany, and Iceland). [114] Probability samples of adults (18 years of age and older) who were not living in institutions formed the basis of the analysis. The total number of respondents was 3971; national samples ranged from 673 for Iceland to 847 in Spain and Germany. The highest levels of social rejection were reported by respondents in Bulgaria, Hungary, and Spain. More specifically, 73.7% of Bulgarians sampled would be unwilling to have someone with schizophrenia marry into their families, 49% thought they would be unlikely to be accepted into the community, and 32.5% thought that they would not be hired for a job even if they were qualified. Though stigmatizing attitudes were less for depression, a similar "dose-response" pattern occurred, with 56.4% unwilling to have someone marry into the family, 35.2% unlikely to be accepted into the community, and 17.5% unlikely to be hired. The figures for Iceland were significantly lower but with the same pattern, at 50.2% (marry), 23.0% (community), and 10.0% (hired). In this study, residents in countries with lower levels of gross domestic product (GDP) per capita were more rejecting, while those in more economically advanced nations reported less rejection. It is important to note that self-reported stigma beliefs are susceptible to social desirability bias, which occurs when respondents hide their true feelings. Because willingness to speak about true feelings may differ from culture to culture, such variations as reported above are difficult to interpret as reflecting real differences in prejudicial beliefs.

In 2016, Seeman and colleagues used a complex web-based survey technique to assess users' attitudes toward people with a mental illness worldwide. [115] The number of respondents replying to each question varied between 596,712 and 1,099,333. Smaller countries, such as Mauritania or Angola, provided between 300 and 500 respondents. Larger countries, such as Germany or India, provided between 10,000 and 267,005 respondents. The total response rate was 54.3%. The percentage of respondents who considered that they were in daily contact with someone with a mental illness ranged from almost 60% in China to approximately 25% in the United Arab Emirates and Germany. In the higher-income countries such as Canada or the United States, less than 10% thought that people experiencing a mental illness were more violent, compared to approximately 16% in middle- and low-income countries such as Algeria and Mexico, though conceptions of what constituted

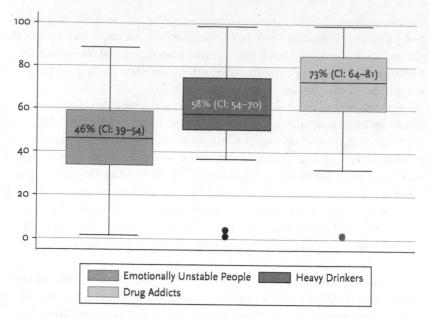

46% (CI: 39–54)

58% (CI: 54–70)

73% (CI: 64–81)

Emotionally Unstable People   Heavy Drinkers

Drug Addicts

Figure 2.1 Boxplot of social distance reported by respondents to the World Values Survey in 36 countries (n = 54,144)

a mental illness may have differed widely. Approximately 50% of respondents from high-income countries such as Australia, the United Kingdom, Canada, and the United States considered mental illnesses to be similar to physical illnesses, compared to 12% to 15% in middle- and low-income countries (Pakistan, Turkey, Algeria, Morocco, Iran, Korea, Egypt, and Indonesia). However, when asked whether people could overcome a mental illness, respondents from high-income countries (United States, Canada, Australia) were more pessimistic: Only about 7% from these countries supported the notion of recovery, compared to almost 20% in middle- and low-income countries such as India, Algeria, or Pakistan.

Figure 2.1 illustrates the variation in desired social distance reported by representative samples of respondents from 36 countries[‡] (n = 54,144) who provided data to the 2004 World Values Survey. [116] In 2004, this survey included social distance questions about people who were "emotionally unstable," "heavy drinkers," and "drug addicts" (the last year for which questions about emotionally unstable people were included). Respondents were provided a card with a number of different groups listed and were asked to

[‡]Countries included in this analysis are Albania, Algeria, Argentina, Bangladesh, Bosnia Herzegovina, Canada, Chile, China, Egypt, India, Indonesia, Iran, Jordan, Kyrgyzstan, Macedonia, Mexico, Moldovia, Montenegro, Morocco, Nigeria, Pakistan, Peru, Philippines, Puerto Rico, Serbia, Singapore, South Africa, South Korea, Spain, Tanzania, Turkey, Uganda, United States, Venezuela, Vietnam, and Zimbabwe.

indicate which groups they would not want to have live in their neighborhoods. The box-and-whisker plots in Figure 2.1 show the weighted percentage§ of respondents who indicated that they would prefer to exclude that individual from their neighborhood. The middle line in the boxes shows the median percentage value across all 36 countries, indicating that half of the countries above this mark reported a higher overall prevalence of social distance and half below reported a lower overall prevalence. The "CI" reflects the 95% confidence interval, indicating that the true value of the prevalence estimate will be within that range in 95 samples out of 100. Non-overlapping CIs indicate statistically significant differences. The box indicates the extent of variation in responses between the 25th and 75th percentiles. The whiskers show the maximum and minimum values, and the circles show extreme values.

Considering the whiskers, the proportion of sample respondents indicating that they would not want to have emotionally unstable people living in their neighborhood ranged from almost none to approximately 90% across the 36 countries polled. The average was 46%, with the bulk of countries falling in the 35% to 60% range—meaning that 35% to 60% of the sample indicated they would not want an emotionally unstable person living in their neighborhood. People who were described as heavy drinkers or drug addicts were more stigmatized, with a clear trend from a median of 58% for heavy drinkers to 73% for drug addicts. The 95% CIs indicate that those with substance use problems (either alcohol or drugs) were significantly more likely to be socially distanced than those with emotional problems. Though not shown, no differences were noted across the 2004 World Bank economic groupings.

These studies show considerable variability across countries in the reported stigmatizing attitudes of people toward those with mental or emotional problems. However, it is not always clear whether self-reported attitudes lead to unfair or discriminatory behaviors. Thus, it may be that attitudes vary cross-culturally but behaviors do not. In 2009, Thornicroft and colleagues examined anticipated and experienced stigma as reported by people with schizophrenia who received treatment in 27 countries (n = 732) as part of the International Study of Discrimination and Stigma Outcomes (INDIGO) research network. [117] Sixty percent of respondents reported anticipating discrimination, but more than half of these (56%) reported they had not experienced discrimination directly. There were statistically significant differences in experienced discrimination by country, but not anticipated discrimination. Positive stigma was infrequent (under 10% for most domains) and occurred largely in relation to obtaining welfare benefits and family supports.

In 2015, Lasalvia and colleagues analyzed differences in discrimination reported by people with a major depressive disorder. [118] Data were collected

§ Each country provided a weight to ensure its samples were representative of the population.

as part of the Anti Stigma Program European Network (ASPEN) study, which was nested within the larger INDIGO-Depression study. Forty sites in 34 countries participated, including both high-income and lower-income countries. Each center investigator was asked to identify a minimum of 25 participants who, in their judgment, were reasonably representative of people with depression who attended specialist mental health services. Countries were then grouped according to the United Nation's Human Development Index, which ranks countries on the basis of (1) a long and healthy life, (2) access to knowledge, and (3) standard of living. Three country groupings resulted: very high, high, and medium/low. Anticipated discrimination varied across countries by Human Development Index, with high-income countries reporting more severe scores. In this context, anticipated discrimination occurred when someone limited their involvement in daily life because of the expectation that they would be discriminated against. Almost twice as many respondents in high-income countries anticipated discrimination in the job domain, compared to those living in lower- and middle-income countries. No differences were reported in the level of discrimination actually experienced.

SUMMARY

This chapter shows how cultures may stigmatize or destigmatize mental illnesses. Mental illness–related stigma emerged historically as cultural understandings separated illnesses of the body from illnesses of the mind. Throughout much of history, people with mentally disordered behavior were accepted as part of community life and, so long as they were benign in their social behaviors, were consigned to their families or were permitted to wander about. When mentally disordered behaviors became understood in the context of Christian notions of sin, they became synonymous with diabolical forces such as the devil and witchcraft. However, as much as religious traditions have been a source of stigma, they have also been a source of healing, as illustrated by the Gheel colony and the practices in early Islamic and Indian cultures. While this chapter highlights the difficulty in drawing firm statements about the universal nature of stigma across time and place, it does reinforce the importance of cultural norms and practices and illustrates how stigma may be substantially modulated by these. It shows us that mental illness–related stigma, while prevalent, is neither universal nor inevitable.

CHAPTER 3

Paradigms Found in Fighting Stigma

In the previous chapter we showed that local environments change and modulate people's reactions to those with mental disorders. This chapter summarizes the key points and guiding principles for anti-stigma programming described in the predecessor of this volume, *Paradigms Lost: Fighting Stigma and the Lessons Learned*. [119] Readers who wish the full scientific justification and research citations for these points will find them there. In this chapter, we provide a high-level summary of the important points to keep in mind when developing anti-stigma programming and outline our model of "enlightened opportunism." Readers who wish more detailed information may also consult the work that we have conducted in the context of the Opening Doors program of the World Psychiatric Association or the Opening Minds program of the Mental Health Commission of Canada. [1,69,120] A more detailed description of national and international programs is contained in Chapter 5.

THE ENLIGHTENED OPPORTUNISM MODEL OF STIGMA REDUCTION

Traditional approaches to public health programming often emphasize the importance of creating long-range plans that can be followed with little deviation. Typically, the measure of success is the extent to which the plan has been implemented as intended, and considerable time is expended in collecting process data to reflect program implementation. We have found this to be overly structured, top-down, and misguided in the sense that too much activity is focused on processes rather than outcomes, and too little on building partnerships and alliances. To be successful, anti-stigma programming must be grounded in grassroots aspirations and nimble enough to use emerging events as springboards to action, even when they weren't predicted or part of the initial plan. An alternative approach is to support individual and collective self-help and mutual aid efforts, thus creating a readiness to use opportunities, where they emerge, to effectively address problems related to stigma. From this perspective, the solution lies in building collaborative relationships among stakeholders based on the shared value of creating problem-solving capacities. The resulting anti-stigma programs will build on people's commitment to their own interests and priorities, provide opportunities for empowerment and engagement, and strengthen relationships. Stakeholders will work together in ways that fit their own needs and address the problems that they deem to be important. We use the term "enlightened opportunism" to refer to the readiness of a group wanting to fight stigma to use windows of opportunity as springboards for targeted action.

In the old paradigm, anti-stigma programming was highly structured and technical, requiring professional input and expert skills. Often groups of professionals would create generic messages about mental illnesses or mental illness stigma and direct these to vast population groups. Messages were developed to fill some perceived gap in knowledge, create awareness of a problem, replace negative stereotypes with positive ones, or promote positive attitudes. Messages were typically fashioned to convey scientific facts, such as the high prevalence of mental illnesses; that anyone could develop a mental illness; that people with a mental illness are not a public risk; that mental illnesses are treatable; or that mental illnesses are illnesses like any other. In some cases, mental health experts would provide lectures to target audiences, such as high school students or community interest groups, about the signs and symptoms of mental illnesses and their causes and consequences.

This approach assumes that development involves a process of "catching up" the public to medical and technological knowledge. It assumes that once people are aware of the burden associated with mental illnesses and recognize how damaging stigma and social marginalization can be, they will overcome their own personal fears and prejudices and reduce the social distance they have created between themselves and people who have a mental disorder, and they will spontaneously change from becoming part of the problem to becoming part of the solution. This "magic bullet" logic overlooks the importance and impact that small-scale focused actions may have on the day-to-day lives of people with a mental illness and the impracticability of making "big bang" changes in the area of social development.

Top-down approaches are cumbersome and inefficient because they often fail to recognize and harness available resources. They are not nimble enough to jump on opportunities when they arise. Because they do not pay attention to stakeholder realities or integrate grassroots knowledge into their workings, they are often perceived by those most directly affected by mental illnesses as being foreign, imposed, or beside the point. People are far more likely to change their behaviors when familiar leaders are helping to spearhead the design and implementation of programs directed to problems that are deemed to be important by the community. In this context, the community may be geographically defined, or it may be a community of like-minded people who are not in geographic proximity. With the advent of social media platforms and rapid urbanization seen in many countries, geographically defined communities are being supplanted as a locus for advocacy and action. We use the term "community" to reflect this broader understanding.

To consider that the stigma attached to mental illnesses can best be reduced through well-structured, long-term programs portrays anti-stigma programming as a highly structured, technical activity that must be reserved for people with expert skills. This approach overlooks the impact that all individuals can make through their actions. A key strength of enlightened opportunists is that they can corral a much wider group of stakeholders. They recognize that anyone and everyone can take advantage of opportunities to improve social inclusion for people with a mental illness, either through direct personal action or by supporting others. Also, outside of large government-funded programs, most anti-stigma efforts will be made up of volunteer labor. Grassroots initiatives have a better chance of surviving because they build on the common interests of a wide range of participants and do not depend on a single individual or source of funding to make things work. Small, quick wins, which are more likely using the more nimble and focused enlightened opportunism model, will keep volunteers interested and enthusiastic.

THE IMPORTANCE OF BUILDING NETWORKS

Networks can be composed of individuals and organizational representatives who share common values and objectives and who work together to achieve these. In the past, networks were predominantly geographically based, located in specific communities. With the expansion of web-based social networking platforms, this is no longer the case. Networks can be composed of individuals from across a country or the globe who share a common purpose and who interact regularly to achieve their goals. Because internet communities can have greater reach, they can take anti-stigma advocacy to a broader constituency, such as lobbying international organizations or national governments and bodies to give higher priorities to mental health and anti-stigma programming.

Networks are highly fluid and depend on the ongoing trust relationships that have been developed between network members to promote collective action. Because networks can straddle a number of organizations and interests, they can bring a wide range of expertise to solve complex public health problems. Unlike bureaucratic organizations, community networks are borderless and flexible, making them particularly well suited to anti-stigma work that uses enlightened opportunism to guide activities. They can change quickly to be responsive to community members' needs and priorities and can quickly invent new structures and activities as needed. New members may be enlisted when required to address emerging opportunities. Networks also provide important training grounds for new members, which fosters sustainability. They build collaboration, consensus, and continuous learning.

Many positive outcomes stem from the sense of community that is generated by a successful network, including strong feelings of empowerment and commitment, satisfaction with group activities, pride in successes, and an easy flow of information between members. Decisions do not rest on hierarchical structures, making networks adaptable and flexible. Sharing experiences creates a strong sense of joint enterprise. Network members learn through critical reflection about the problems they have faced, the roadblocks that may have slowed or thwarted their progress, and any unintended effects of their interventions. Members can draw on each other's knowledge and experiences to become more effective problem solvers. Exposure to a wide range of views can challenge and motivate. Tools and solutions developed in one part of the network can be disseminated among all of the partners, eliminating the need to begin everything from scratch.

It is crucial for anti-stigma programming to take a long view. To maintain sustainable development, networks must remain open to newcomers and provide them with opportunities for training and development so that they can move from an initial peripheral status in their role as newcomer to a more central role, including network leadership. Learning from people who have conducted successful programs is better remembered, is seen as more credible, and can more easily lead to action.

Maintaining a unifying vision is important, particularly when network partners represent autonomous organizations. When considering who will lead the network, it is important to remember that anti-stigma activities can be best served by grassroots leaders who are respected for their contributions to mental health advocacy and who are capable of providing a democratic style of leadership that engages and empowers network partners. Otherwise, networks may degenerate into a process of political and social control. In the mental health arena, this may mean a tug of war between hospital and community agencies, professional and lay communities, and specific professional disciplines, or among advocacy organizations. Network members must be clear that they are not "representing" the interests of their respective organizations but are joining forces to achieve a common aim, whether that be local, regional, national, or international.

THE IMPORTANCE OF TARGETING EFFORTS

Smaller intensive interventions that target specific groups and are tailored to the culture and practices of these groups are our recommended approach to stigma reduction. The experience of someone with schizophrenia in the emergency department is quite different than the experience of someone with depression in high school. It seems axiomatic that anti-stigma programs should be tailored to the specific needs of target groups. Indeed, one of the most important changes that has occurred in the past 10 years of anti-stigma programing and research has been the realization that targeting interventions to specific groups—such as judges, police officers, or teachers—pays off. Not only are interventions tailored to meet specific needs, but evaluation strategies are also easier to mount and effectiveness is more easily assessed than in the case of large population-based campaigns. In many settings it will be most useful to target groups that have frequent contact with people who have mental disorders and who have been experienced as behaving in stigmatizing ways. For example, groups that have been targeted have included youth (through teachers), healthcare providers, the media, the police, first responders, employers, policymakers or legislators, and people with lived experience of a mental illness (e.g., to address self-stigma). Even small improvements in the behaviors of target group members can make an important difference. Locally implemented programs that are shown to be effective can be widely disseminated to create regional or population-level change. In most cases, members of the general public will be too heterogeneous to provide useful primary targets for anti-stigma activities, though they may be considered important secondary targets.

While science may not be helpful in defining local target groups, scientific methods are useful for assessing local needs and exploring the personal perceptions and priorities of people who have been stigmatized by members of a particular target group. For example, a *situational analysis* (Box 3.1) can be used to conduct a systematic investigation of a complex problem that impacts people and systems. It offers a method for selecting target groups that is systematic and evidence-informed and thus is well suited to anti-stigma activities. It is both consultative and collaborative and recognizes and values multiple stakeholder views. It encourages engagement from people who have local knowledge and integrates these views into a strategic decision-making process. Once targets are chosen, reference to the scientific literature and experience from other anti-stigma programs may further inform intervention approaches.

1. **People with Lived Experience**: What is the current situation with respect to stigma? What are stakeholder perceptions and priorities? What is their capacity to act?
2. **Influencing Factors**: What factors are making the situation better? What factors are making the situation worse?
3. **Opportunities**: Which settings offer the best opportunities for successful action? Are there emerging opportunities for action? What are other organizations doing? Are there obvious partners?
4. **Actions**: What actions can we take to address the situation? What is the evidence to support these actions? What is our ability to affect the situation within existing constraints (e.g., time, resources)?
5. **Resources**: What resources are available to support these actions? How can these be accessed? Which approaches are most cost-effective? Which approaches are likely to get broad buy-in from stakeholders?
6. **Data**: What information is available to answer these questions? How will this information be gathered and from whom? Who will organize and synthesize this information?
7. **Communication**: How will the results of the situational analysis be communicated to key stakeholder groups?

HEALTH PROFESSIONALS SHOULD TAKE A BACK SEAT IN COMMUNITY ANTI-STIGMA PROGRAMS

Health and social service professionals often expect to instigate and lead community-based anti-stigma programs because they consider that their advanced education in psychiatry and related disciplines will have equipped them with the requisite knowledge and skills to improve knowledge and change opinions. They may doubt the competency of laypeople and people who have experienced a mental disorder. Their working assumption is often that they exercise power on behalf of their client communities and work in their best interests. They learn about client needs through indirect means such as surveys and other community assessment techniques that are designed to rise above the clamor of vested interests.

Against this backdrop, advocacy groups may be viewed as a problem rather than a resource, asking for things that professionals may consider to be unrealistic or of lower priority. For example, mental health professionals often like to focus on inequities in funding for mental health treatment services or the stigma that they themselves experience.

A second and more intractable issue is that mental health service systems and the professionals who work within them have been viewed by service users as having perpetuated stigma through disempowerment, coerced care, and social exclusion. From the perspective of many service users, health professionals are an integral part of the problem, making it difficult for professionals to inspire confidence and trust. In addition to the trauma associated with forced hospitalization and coercive care, recurrent themes include feeling punished, patronized, humiliated, spoken to as if they were children, being excluded from decisions, and being assumed to lack the capacity to be responsible for their own treatment decisions and lives. Mental health professionals are often unaware of the facets of their own behavior that are pejorative and stigmatizing. Because stigma is seen as something that others do, professional blinders make it difficult to accept responsibility for being part of the problem. Rather than being leaders of anti-stigma programming, many service users would consider that health professionals and health systems are worthy targets for anti-stigma initiatives. In a subsequent chapter we address the contribution of healthcare providers and systems to stigma and stigma-reduction strategies.

An increasing criticism of health systems is that they are not recovery-oriented. Professionals working within them express a sense of therapeutic nihilism that undermines their ability to engender hope and recovery. In this context, recovery means not just the abatement of clinical symptoms but also the ability of the individual to assume roles and responsibilities that are meaningful to them despite ongoing symptoms or relapses. Mental health professionals often base their views on their own personal experiences working with people with a mental illness who are quite unwell. People who do not recover keep coming back for help and treatment while those who recover tend to vanish, not returning to the service. By spending much more time with people who do not recover than with those who do, mental health professionals often become pessimistic about the outcomes of treatment and acquire a distorted impression about the prospects of recovery. People who recover from mental illnesses rarely maintain ties with the service system and, in order to avoid stigma, may not speak about their illness or its successful treatment. Being pessimistic about recovery, mental health professionals are often not at their best as leaders of anti-stigma programming. Instead of assuming a leadership position, mental health professionals are better positioned to adopt a supportive role.

LISTENING TO THE EVIDENCE

Though science cannot be (and should not be) the only driver of anti-stigma programs, it is still important to listen to the evidence where it exists. A decade or so ago, scholarly interest in anti-stigma programming was just beginning to emerge as an important field of study. Since that time, the field has blossomed and there is now considerable knowledge about what works, where, and when. Still, anti-stigma programmers regularly confront the unbridled enthusiasm of volunteers and advocates and the difficulties that sometimes occur when trying to curb the desire to act rather than reflect. Using the enlightened opportunism model of stigma reduction, stakeholders are often strongly committed to intervention approaches that may or may not be supported by evidence or, in the case of new innovations, by any evidence at all. Too many anti-stigma initiatives have been initiated out of good intentions but with little understanding of the evidence, or more often lack of evidence, supporting these approaches.

A key challenge is that evidence, like beauty or art, is in the eye of the beholder. The nature and quality of evidence used by program developers versus researchers can vary widely, so it can be challenging to bring scientific and community partners together. It requires bridging different knowledge cultures. Community agencies and advocacy groups rarely have the opportunity for in-depth monitoring, reflection, and learning. Typically, they cannot invest in formal research. They need knowledge that is contextualized, easily accessible, decision-oriented, and pragmatic, making it possible for them to accept a much broader range of evidence than researchers, and share it much more informally. In assessing effectiveness, researchers pursue formal, objective knowledge that has been decontextualized and carefully cross-examined following a lengthy peer-review process and shared through the academic literature, which may be inaccessible to community groups. A third knowledge community involves people with lived experience of a mental disorder. Their personal stories, testimonials, and qualitative reports also must factor heavily. Failing to incorporate experiential evidence has been the norm. The way forward is to take steps to understand each other's knowledge cultures and work toward pragmatic compromises.

BUILDING BETTER THEORIES OF CHANGE

In the next generation of anti-stigma programming, advocates will be required to clearly understand and be able to articulate the principles and procedures underlying their program activities in ways that will allow them to be meaningfully tested using a variety of research methods and techniques. Policymakers and funders face unprecedented pressure to justify their decisions with systematically collected data supporting an intervention's effectiveness. Evidence-hungry policymakers and funders will use the lack of evidence to restrict funding opportunities for anti-stigma programming.

Understanding why a program works or does not work and demonstrating that it produces the right kind of change will become more important than showing that it does work. It will be increasingly important to show *why* a program works, as understanding the active ingredients is key to scaling up programs within regions or across entire countries—something that funders are wont to do. This will mean clearly articulating program theories (the principles and procedures underlying program activities) in ways that will make them amenable to testing using a variety of methods and techniques. Only by understanding why an intervention is likely to work and by articulating and testing its various assumptions will it be possible to build generalizable theories of change.

Careful ongoing evaluation of anti-stigma initiatives will be necessary to build better practices that are policy-relevant and of interest to potential funders. Systematically collected data will become an important advocacy tool. In addition to traditional forms of data, it is also important to record stories illustrating ways of working and successful initiatives. Such stories can be invaluable when initiating programs or describing them to potential donors of resources.

Improved Mental Health Knowledge Will Not Eradicate Stigma and May Increase It

As previously mentioned, most conventional practices for developing anti-stigma programs pay little attention to the underlying theory of change. Program planners often operate with repertoires of established approaches. Program design often means using "off-the-shelf" packages without a close analysis of the match between the nature of the problem and the capacity of the intervention to bring about change. A common theory of change underlying many anti-stigma interventions (indeed, many public health programs) is that improving knowledge will change attitudes, which in turn will change behaviors. Nuggets of knowledge, such as "One in five will experience mental illness in their lifetime" or "Depression is treatable," are considered to be sufficient to demystify mental illnesses, explode myths, and normalize their occurrence, and, in so doing, unseat prejudicial beliefs and discriminatory behaviors.

To date there is no supporting evidence from social psychology that knowledge can change deep-seated prejudices, particularly when they are rooted in fear. Indeed, the opposite seems to be the case. People will selectively attend to information that supports their entrenched beliefs and actively ignore or discount information that contradicts them. People can maintain their prejudices even in the face of considerable contradictory evidence. There is also a growing body of evidence showing that high levels of mental health knowledge and literacy coexist with high levels of social intolerance—think of mental health workers, who have been identified as among the most stigmatizing of all groups.

There is no compelling reason to believe that literacy designed to increase knowledge about the etiology, classification, and treatments for mental illnesses could alter the burden of social disability experienced by people with mental disorders or improve their quality of life and social inclusion. Indeed, there is every reason to believe that increased understanding of the neurobiological bases of mental illnesses will sharpen divisions between "normal" and "abnormal" and increase stigma and social rejection. Although still widely used, the knowledge—attitude—behavior theory of change model is unlikely to produce fruitful results and should be retired in favor of change models that more directly target behaviors.

Mental Illnesses Are *Not* Like Other Illnesses

Many anti-stigma programs are built on the theory of change that it is important to convey the message that mental illnesses are like any other illnesses, in that they are brain diseases. This assumes that once the public comes to realize that mental illnesses and physical illnesses are similar, they will naturally adopt a more benevolent view. This perspective overlooks the historical and social facts (presented in the first two chapters) that set mental illnesses apart from other illnesses and deeply misunderstands the nature and effects of mental illness–related stigma. Mental illnesses are *not* like other illnesses because they regularly cause people to lose their rights and freedoms in ways that are unimaginable in other health conditions. In addition, most mental illnesses are not accompanied by physical weakness or incapacity, as in the case of many physical illnesses. They may result in behaviors that estrange family and friends and may lead to social or moral errors. These factors have to be kept in mind to understand why mental illnesses are not like physical illnesses.

Consumer-survivor groups, which emerged at the turn of the last century, have played an important role in drawing attention to the human rights issues raised by the practice of psychiatry, in particular involuntary and coercive treatments. Former patients provided some of the earliest and most radical critiques of psychiatric authority. The mental health field has some of the most vociferous and angry service user movements. Consumer-survivor groups have expressed considerable hurt and anger and have denied that the care and treatment provided within mental health systems were effective or appropriate. Moreover, they have forcefully proclaimed that they are the best qualified to judge whether and how they should be treated. Unlike other illness constituencies that have developed their own support groups, people with mental and substance use disorders have established their own self-help and treatment groups as alternatives to hospitals and community-based programs. These alternatives to mental health systems embrace core principles that overturn medical authority, promote self-determination, and resist stereotypes.

Though many branches of medicine have been criticized, psychiatry is the only specialty where members of its own ranks—eminent psychiatrists of the day—have questioned the very existence of mental illnesses. Various social and historical currents have coalesced to place psychiatry on the defensive in a way that is unlike any other medical group. For example, it would be unthinkable to see protesters and placard-waving antagonists picketing outside of a medical conference, yet this is the norm for psychiatric conventions. Busloads of protesters regularly descend on psychiatric conferences with slogans, noise-making apparatus such as drums and loudspeakers (to drown out the congress proceedings), and leaflets to be thrust into the hands of conference-goers who may be jostled and spat at as they enter the conference facility. It would be difficult to imagine a similar ruckus at a conference on cancer or diabetes. Even the term "psychiatric survivor" is meant to denote someone who has survived a traumatic event at the hands of abusers, rather than someone who has survived an illness.

Neurobiological Explanations Are Stigmatizing

Many anti-stigma advocates believe that stigma could be reduced if we could educate people that mental illnesses are brain disorders—real biological diseases like any other. Stigma-reduction efforts using information about the biological bases and biological treatments for mental disorders have become a mainstay of many anti-stigma efforts. The problem with this approach is that the public is deeply aware that mental illnesses are not like any other. As depicted in the entertainment and news media, people with mental illnesses are considered to be a public risk, responsible for mass shootings the world over, and perpetrators of other unspeakable crimes. The persistence with which the "brain disease" model has been proffered has significantly eroded public confidence in these advocacy efforts. Emphasizing a brain disease model may lead to the belief that people with mental or substance use disorders will have no control over their behavior. This is because the illness has eroded the very brain structure of the individual, with the result that recovery is not possible: Once mentally ill, always mentally ill, unpredictable, and dangerous.

There has been considerable research examining the relationship between biological explanations of mental illnesses and stigma. Biological explanations are more likely to be associated with social intolerance and rejection. When biological theories have been successfully challenged, social distance has been reduced. Thus, anti-stigma programs that promote the "illness like any other" or "mental illness as brain disease" models likely do more harm than good. Such models rarely provide a good vantage point from which to assess the broader determinants of mental health such as poverty, unemployment, and homelessness.

WHAT COUNTS AS SUCCESS?

One of the key challenges in this area is determining how much change could be considered to reflect "success." Program advocates typically proclaim lofty goals (such as eliminating stigma) without critical analysis of the extent to which the program intervention is sufficiently potent to achieve the desired ends. If expectations are grand but effects are small, program participants may become discouraged. The message to funders and policymakers may be that stigma cannot be beaten. Thus, choosing reasonable goals and managing expectations are central to the success of anti-stigma efforts. Cultures do not change overnight. Small, incremental changes over long periods of time are the norm.

A second issue is deciding what should be the yardstick of success—the general public's knowledge and attitudes; health professionals' care practices; or the experiences of people with lived experience of a mental disorder? A central premise of our approach is that anti-stigma programs can only be judged to be successful when (1) people who are stigmatized feel that their lives have been improved, (2) the impact of stigma on various life domains has been diminished, and (3) structures that promote inequity are removed or replaced with structures that protect and promote social entitlements in areas such as education, housing, healthcare, disability supports, training, or employment. Focusing on knowledge or attitude change as a consequence of anti-stigma programming is likely to yield disappointing results, both because these changes tend to be small and sometimes fleeting, and because they are not predictive of changes in discriminatory behaviors. It is unlikely that anti-stigma programs that solely target changes in knowledge or attitudes will bring meaningful improvement in social inclusion or social equity for those with mental or substance use disorders.

PRINCIPLES TO GUIDE NEXT-GENERATION ANTI-STIGMA EFFORTS

A feature of the enlightened opportunism model is that detailed, long-term plans are not needed (and may not be helpful) to guide anti-stigma programming. Rather, it is important to be able to capitalize on opportunities as they arise. Thus, having a shared vision and general principles to guide activities will provide a better basis for interventions than a long-range plan. We have found the following six principles useful for guiding next generation anti-stigma activities.

Put People First

People who have a mental illness and their family members must be central to the process of stigma reduction. They must be the ones to set the targets for change, and they must be involved as equal partners in every level of planning, programming, and evaluation, including helping to decide which are the most meaningful outcomes to address and how best to measure them. Not only will this approach ensure that program targets are meaningful, but it also offers opportunities for social interaction, knowledge exchange, mutual development, and cultural change. Most importantly, it can raise the self-confidence and self-efficacy of people who have experienced a mental illness and their family members.

Plan for Sustainability

The social and cultural processes that create and maintain stigma are complex, pervasive, mutually reinforcing, and resistant to change. This means that "one-off" interventions will do little to unseat stigma. Programs must take a longer view and plan for sustainability at the outset. This means that program developers must refrain from depicting their activities as "campaigns," as these often involve short bursts of activity that may or may not be repeated. Campaigns are typically time-limited, are not in themselves sustainable, and do not create sustained change. Because anti-stigma programs are often working with shoe-string budgets (if they have any real budget at all), they must retain the loyalty of their supporters over the long haul. They must consider and plan for ways in which new generations of activists will be recruited, trained, and move into leadership positions. Having training opportunities, tool kits, and apprenticeships will help newcomers acclimatize to the program and continue promoting anti-stigma initiatives. While it is possible to engage in anti-stigma activities with few resources, it is useful to be able to count on some stable resources to support someone to assist with the coordination of network activities.

Focus on Activities That Change Behaviors

Many programs attempt to improve mental health literacy by increasing knowledge about mental illnesses and their treatments, or correct stereotypical beliefs and attitudes by replacing misinformation with accurate portrayals.

However, the deep-seated prejudices that are the emotional scaffolding for stigma are highly resistant to change and do not respond to new information. Thus, interventions that aim to remove stigma by changing knowledge or attitudes are problematic as these are not predictive of behavioral change. In order to create meaningful changes for people who experience mental disorders and their family members, structural and behavioral changes must occur. Programs that change discriminatory laws, inequitable organizational practices, or unfair and discriminatory behaviors are necessary. Once these are in place, knowledge and attitude change will likely follow—and if they don't, it won't really matter because people with mental disorders will be able to enjoy the social rights and entitlements enshrined in legal and social frameworks and will have accessible avenues of redress if their rights and entitlements have been breached. Once these are implemented, public knowledge and attitudes may be ancillary to these protections.

Target Activities to Well-Defined Groups

How we want a police officer to behave is not how we want a doctor or nurse or teacher to behave. Therefore, one-size-fits-all programming is likely to miss the mark and leave even the most well-intentioned professionals without a roadmap for change. Programs that take the local contexts of players into consideration and ground their activities in the interests and skills of their target groups are more likely to be successful in bringing about behavioral change. Helping teachers devise lesson plans to assist their students in understanding mental illness stigma is quite different from assisting healthcare providers in understanding and practicing person-centered or recovery-oriented care. And, while both of these may contain an element of literacy, the key change-maker will be the creation of useful tools and the skills required to use these tools effectively.

Think Big But Start Small

The long-term goal of every anti-stigma program must be to eliminate discrimination experienced by people with mental disorders so as to promote their full and effective participation in social roles and relationships that are of value to them. Wholesale cultural change is difficult to create, so smaller successes should be the initial goal. These go a long way to reaffirming that stigma can be beaten, and they maintain the enthusiasm of all participants and stakeholder groups. Accumulating and celebrating quick wins will create and maintain program momentum and avoid burnout.

As important as it is to create quick wins, it is equally important to communicate them to the wider community, including local funders, program planners, media, and other key constituents, as these will provide an important source of positive news and may generate much-needed funding. Such communication must be evidentiary so that successes are not just rhetoric but are backed by data.

Build Better Practices

Building better practices is all about making false starts and learning from mistakes, which every program will make and which they often live in fear of. This requires critical reflection, systematic evaluation, and a genuine spirit of inquiry. It is based on the philosophy that we cannot know everything in advance and each new program is, in essence, a natural experiment requiring careful examination and understanding. Because the best practices that catch the eye of policymakers and funders are those that are supported by scientific evidence and culled from the scientific literature, it is important to ensure that program experiences are translated into usable information that can be exchanged with these key stakeholder groups. Unless anti-stigma programs have scientific or evaluative expertise within their ranks, they will need to collaborate with external researchers. Not only are third-party studies considered to be more credible, but external researchers will also have the expertise to ensure that evaluations are methodologically sound and that results make it into scientific publications, where they can become part of policy-relevant systematic reviews and meta-analyses.

SUMMARY

In this chapter we have summarized some of the key components of a new paradigm for fighting the stigma associated with mental disorders. We used the term "enlightened opportunism" to refer to the readiness of grassroots groups to use windows of opportunity as springboards for targeted action. It means that anti-stigma programs are best when they are nimble, able to pivot quickly, rather than constrained by top-down plans that are entrenched in rigid processes. We also argued for the importance of long-term, sustainable activities that make the most of emerging opportunities.

Within this context, we promoted the use of community networks because they can change quickly to be responsive to community members' needs and priorities and can quickly invent new structures and activities as needed. We understand "community" as broadly based networks of individuals working toward a common goal, whether they be geographically located or internet-based. Because many mental health professionals do not know what recovery looks like, or how their own biases influence therapeutic relationships and recovery goals, they are poorly suited to be opinion leaders or role models in anti-stigma interventions. Instead of leading anti-stigma programs, we argued that health professionals should adopt a supportive role. Though science cannot be (and should not be) the only driver of anti-stigma programs, it is still important to listen to the evidence where it exists. Too many anti-stigma initiatives have been initiated out of good intentions but with little understanding of the evidence (or more often lack of evidence) supporting their approach.

The model of enlightened opportunism, though not mired in scientific evidence as a basis for long-term planning, does require ongoing evaluation of anti-stigma initiatives to build better practices that are policy-relevant and of interest to potential funders. This will require program planners to understand why an intervention is likely to work and be able to articulate and test its various assumptions to build generalizable theories of change.

In the new paradigm, it is recognized that mental illnesses are not like other illnesses by their characteristics—they can damage communications and family and social relationships, they do not lead to physical weakness, and they may make people who experience them break moral or social rules. They regularly cause people to lose their rights and freedoms in ways that are unimaginable in other health conditions. Second, emphasizing an illness model is likely to entrench, rather than erode, stigma. Biological explanations are more likely to be associated with social intolerance and rejection. The success of anti-stigma programming should not be measured against improvements in the public's knowledge of medical mechanics of mental illnesses but when (1) people who are stigmatized feel that their lives have been improved, (2) the impact of stigma on various life domains has been diminished, and (3) structures that promote inequity are removed or replaced with structures that protect and promote social entitlements in areas such as education, housing, healthcare, disability supports, training, or employment.

Finally, the six principles that should be used to guide anti-stigma programming in the next generation are (1) putting people first, (2) planning for sustainability and readiness to use opportunities as they arise, (3) focusing on activities that change behavior (such as revising legislation), (4) targeting activities at well-defined groups, (5), thinking big but starting small, and (6) building better practices as you go.

CHAPTER 4

Eleven Steps to Build an Anti-stigma Program

Growing numbers of community groups and coalitions are interested in undertaking anti-stigma activities, often with limited resources and volunteer labor. In this chapter we provide a non-technical summary of a more detailed training resource provided in *Paradigms Lost*. [1] It is intended to help local groups through the process of setting up an anti-stigma program. It draws on our experiences working with international, national, and local anti-stigma groups and is intended to broadly serve as a "how-to" resource. The advice is meant to be pragmatic and expresses our view that everyone can take part in anti-stigma programming, at some level—modest efforts are possible for anyone to achieve. What is important to remember is that anti-stigma programs can be implemented even if there is not specific funding that has been made available, using volunteer resources. The following text offers suggestions for how this can be done. It is offered as a narrative overview, but it could be converted into a manual for action.

STEP 1: DEVELOP A PROGRAM COMMITTEE

Anti-stigma programs often begin with a small group of interested people who will provide the leadership needed to launch a program. These initial organizers will need a larger group of people to help with development and carry out the program's activities. One of the first tasks, therefore, is to develop a "program committee" or "action group" that is willing to serve as a motor for this work. It is important that the group has a chairperson with tested leadership skills and, if possible, community prominence. Members of the committee must have direct access to expertise needed to plan and deliver the program; often this will be achieved by including among the members someone who has participated in (or studied) programs elsewhere. Other members will include people who have experienced stigma, representatives of the groups that will be targeted for anti-stigma activities (e.g., judges, police officers, teachers), people in community agencies and advocacy groups that may be working in the area, media or communications experts, a financial expert, and a researcher skilled in program evaluation. The group must be task-oriented, and its size cannot be so big as to be unwieldy. Program committee members must be willing to follow through with program assignments and report on their activities to the group. Regular meeting attendance is essential. The members of the group must see their membership as a long-term commitment rather than a short-lasting campaign.

STEP 2: CREATE AN ADVISORY COMMITTEE

The second step is to develop a broader advisory committee to support the program committee. Members of the advisory committee should give input into program activities (but not direct them) and help provide visibility and political support for the program. The advisory committee should act as a political sounding board for program activities, develop good will in the community, and provide additional technical advice if needed. In setting up advisory committees, program developers should look for individuals who (a) have lived experience of a mental disorder or cared for a person with a mental disorder, (b) are in positions of power in the community or in the organization in which the program will take place, (c) are opinion leaders who can command respect, provide broader political support, and give credibility to the project, and (d) have some technical expertise that may be required in order to conduct activities, such as financial or accounting skills, media or communication skills, research expertise, or public relations skills. When recruiting for advisory committee roles, it is important to be specific about time requirements (they shouldn't be too burdensome), the nature of the involvement, and the expectations surrounding contributions. Advisory committee members must see that they can make a meaningful contribution—that they are not simply a window dressing.

STEP 3: UNDERSTAND THE NATURE OF STIGMA

The term "stigma" has been used in a variety of ways to refer to (a) the attitudes and behaviors of members of the general public, either toward people with a mental or substance use disorder (termed public stigma) or their family members (termed stigma by association); (b) the way in which individuals with mental or substance use disorders face insurmountable social obstacles once it becomes known that they have a mental illness, which eventually erodes their self-confidence and faith in their own capacities, causing them to share the opinion of others about their own value (termed self-stigma); and (c) the way that social structures (for example, laws) and organizations (for example, healthcare authorities) behave to entrench inequities (termed structural stigma). Because each of these types of stigmas will entail different types of activities, it is important to be specific, at the outset, as to which type of stigma will be addressed. Indeed, it is better to avoid the generic use of the term "stigma" altogether in favor of one of the more specific designations. In previous chapters, we have argued that goals should be behaviorally oriented such that the ultimate aim is to reduce social rejection and social inequities experienced by people with mental disorders or improve their quality of life and sense of social or personal empowerment. Changes in these situations will be the ultimate yardstick against which the program will be evaluated, so careful consideration must go into their choice to ensure that the program activities are sufficiently potent to bring about measurable change. For example, the declared goal of the group might be to change a discriminatory law; this goal would be replaced by another, also well-defined goal after the change in law has happened.

STEP 4: CANVASS LOCAL NEEDS AND PRIORITIES

Before setting specific goals and objectives, it is important to understand the perspectives and experiences of local service users and others who may be experiencing stigma because of a mental or substance use problem. As identified in previous chapters, effective anti-stigma programming must be relevant to the needs of people who are stigmatized. Thus, the group should plan to conduct face-to-face discussions with people who have been stigmatized, either by one-on-one interviews or in group discussions, to determine which consequences of stigma are most distressing and how they are manifested. Qualitative accounts such as these will produce a rich body of information that is expressed in participants' own words. People can explain their reasoning and qualify their responses in ways that structured surveys can never do. In addition, they can (1) empower people who have experienced a mental disorder and their family members by acknowledging their expert role and by soliciting their advice concerning important program targets; (2) identify and recruit interested and qualified individuals to participate in committees and undertake program activities; (3) balance the interests of program planners with the perceived needs of intended beneficiaries of the program; and (4) create community buy-in from agencies that are also mandated to meet the needs of people with mental disorders.

STEP 5: PICK TARGET GROUPS

Having canvassed local needs, it will be possible to identify the key target groups that may be contributing to stigma. This is an important step because program activities must be matched to target group members' particular needs and activities. It is also a strategic decision because not all target groups may be equally accessible to the stigma action group. Using the enlightened opportunism model, target groups should be those that can be easily accessed, have a reasonable chance of accepting the proposed intervention, have frequent contact with people who are stigmatized, and have representation on the program and advisory committees. Groups that have been targeted in past anti-stigma efforts have included the following:

- *Journalists*—It may be important to connect with local journalists who cover health stories to provide them with background information about mental illnesses that they can use in the case of an incident involving someone with a mental illness to provide relevant context (e.g., people with mental illnesses are more likely to be victims than perpetrators of violence). Journalists may also promote the program and its activities if they have clear action-oriented messages. Finally, journalists may benefit from a list of local resources along with a list of individuals who are willing to be interviewed or act as advisors.
- *Youth*—Youth are an important and frequently targeted group for anti-stigma activities. Not only are they at high risk of experiencing mental ill health, but they are also accessible through educational settings. Youth are also highly receptive to meeting someone with a mental disorder and hearing about their recovery journeys. They can be eager and enthusiastic learners. Working in educational settings also offers the opportunity to change the teaching curriculum, correct misinformation, and provide teacher resources to enhance lesson planning about mental health topics. For example, working with medical students will result not only in their help in conducting programs but also in making doctors aware of stigma and its consequences and of ways to reduce it.
- *Health and mental health professionals*—People with mental illnesses and their family members often identify health and mental health professionals as among the most stigmatizing of all groups. Health professionals represent one of the most strategically located but challenging groups for anti-stigma efforts because they are in contact with service users who are at their most vulnerable. Stigmatizing attitudes or behaviors presented by health professionals during these difficult times (such as talking down to someone or letting them know they are not a priority) can be highly devastating for service users and their families. Also, most health systems are committed

to quality improvement activities, and this may represent an entrance for anti-stigma programming.

- *Employers and workplaces*—It has become clear that workplaces that have policies and practices to promote the mental health of their workers are more competitive and financially robust. Studies have demonstrated an important return on investment for employment-related mental health supports and programs. In some countries, such as Canada, workplace guidelines exist to help employers create the structures needed to promote psychological safety in the workplace. There are also a growing number of anti-stigma programs that can be accessed to promote mental health of workers. In addition, large numbers of workers can be accessed by targeting a small number of large companies. A more detailed description of workplace programs is contained in Chapter 9.

- *Police*—The police are among the important first responders when someone is in a mental health crisis. They usually have little training and may be misinformed about the nature of mental illnesses and about the public risk that people in crisis may pose, leading to the use of undue force. Given the high frequency with which police come into contact with people in mental health crises, and given the negative news associated with an incident gone bad, police departments are often highly receptive to training opportunities.

- *Policymakers and legislators*—In many parts of the world, mental health policy and legislation is inequitable, has stagnated, or is absent altogether. Anti-stigma programmers can target policymakers and legislators to raise awareness about existing inequities with an eye to encouraging more progressive policies and laws. Policymakers and legislators are highly influenced by what receives attention in the news, so working with local reporters and researchers to document and report inequities can be an important anti-stigma strategy. In addition, judges and other policymakers are often highly receptive to well-prepared information about mental illnesses and can use this to make decisions that will be of lasting significance.

- *Community neighborhoods*—Targeted interventions designed to influence the behaviors of small neighborhood groups can be highly effective in reducing community hostility surrounding the implementation of community-based mental health supports and services. Establishing a community mental health program without taking the time to forewarn and educate community members is likely to raise considerable hostility and provoke NIMBY responses (see Chapter 1). Carefully thought-out and implemented community engagement plans can reduce fear and hostility and provide a receptive and supportive environment for people with mental disorders in need of these support systems.

STEP 6: SET GOALS AND OBJECTIVES

Once local priorities are clear and target groups have been specified, it is possible to identify the program's specific goals and objectives. Goals are broad statements about the desired result you want to achieve (e.g., a reduction in self-stigma among service users), whereas objectives are specific and measurable actions (e.g., a reduction of 10% on a self-stigma scale over a period of 1 year, or change of a law). Some objectives may be difficult to specify if there is no previous research to draw upon. If this is the case, the program may consider first operating as a pilot project to explore what magnitude of reduction is possible given the intervention. However, there are many objectives that can be clearly specified and whose achievement will be a major boost to the program.

Program outcomes (objectives) are strategically important. They must be measurable, achievable, and locally relevant. It is important that they reflect a consensus of committee members and stakeholders, because if these individuals are not working to achieve the same ends, program success will be jeopardized. Important questions to ask are (1) "In what ways will program participants (i.e., targets) be different following the program?" and (2) "What will change in the environment so that stigma and its consequences are reduced?" Box 4.1 provides examples of changes that may be identified by anti-stigma programs as a measure of success. The specific outcome will depend on the nature of the program and its target group.

STEP 7: IDENTIFY A PROGRAM APPROACH

Once program objectives and target groups are clear, it is important to conduct a scan of existing program approaches for their effectiveness. This will require a thoughtful review of published scientific literature, technical reports, and other documents. Accessing scientific and other literature and exploring evidence-informed options will be greatly facilitated by including researchers on the program and advisory committees. Ideally, the program approach selected will:

- Have evidence demonstrating the effectiveness of the intervention taken to achieve the program's objectives.
- Have been applied to members of the target audience and demonstrated to fit the needs of that group.
- Have been shown to be acceptable to them and its effectiveness based on a sound theory of change.

If there is insufficient evidence to inform program development, then a pilot program to develop a credible theory of change linking the various program activities to the outcomes and to explore potential effectiveness is required. Because it is possible that an ill-conceived program could entrench stigma, it is important that new programs be sufficiently tested before they are scaled up within a community or region. Adopting an evidence-based or an evidence-generating stance will be important in attracting funding and other resources to the program.

Again, it is important to include people with lived experience of a mental disorder in the program delivery. Stories told by service users and family members about the recovery process are powerful and compelling. Many anti-stigma programs use speakers to tell their stories as these can evoke empathy and understanding, reduce fear, and reduce the desire for social distance among audience members. Stories can also help health professionals understand how their behaviors may unintentionally stigmatize their clients, and what to do differently. It is important to remember that public speakers require significant training to undertake this task and may find repeated storytelling stressful and triggering. Therefore, it is important that speakers be protected from burnout and unnecessary stress. Burnout may be minimized by (1) training numerous speakers so the demand on any one person is not too great; (2) introducing speakers to the experience gradually; (3) debriefing speakers after events to explore whether they have found the experience stressful and, if so, plan activities accordingly; and (4) creating a supportive culture among speakers to ensure that everyone feels free to turn down a speaking engagement if they feel unable to manage it. A successful speakers' bureau is likely to develop a strong sense of shared mission and mutual respect. This sense of community is valuable for the recovery process and should be nurtured through regular meetings, rehearsals, social events, and celebratory occasions to mark important milestones and reinforce camaraderie.

STEP 8: CREATE AN EVALUATION PLAN

Program evaluation is helpful to ensure that the program interventions make sense, in light of available evidence; that they have been implemented as intended; and that they are achieving the specified goals. Pilot program evaluations, which are exploratory, are helpful when little is known about the intervention or how it works. Program evaluations are intended to identify strengths and weaknesses, so considerable effort should be expended to use the results to improve program processes. Evaluation plans should be developed at the same time as the program approach—not left as an afterthought, as is often the case. A common mistake is to wait until program activities have been implemented before developing evaluation activities. This can result in lost information and jeopardize the program's ability to demonstrate change. Results and subsequent quality improvement can be an important advocacy tool for funders who are looking for evidence-based interventions.

Including program and advisory committee members with research and evaluation experience will facilitate this process. Evaluators who are external to the program also may be required, often by funders. They are perceived as more objective, so their results hold greater sway. In cash-strapped programs, however, evaluation may need to remain an internal activity designed to promote a culture of critical self-reflection and quality improvement.

Evaluation is an iterative process, and different questions may be posed depending on the program's stage of development (new, middle-aged, or mature). These include the following:

• Did the program successfully reach all members of the target group? If not, what proportion was not reached? Why?
• What activities did the program undertake? When?
• How much was invested in terms of time, money, and other resources to mount and operate the program? Was the lion's share of resources directed toward the program's key activities?

- Did the program make an important difference in the desired outcome(s)? How do program effects compare with similar effects outlined in the literature?
- Were there any negative or unanticipated consequences?
- Was the program cost-effective? How do costs compare to other anti-stigma programs in the literature?
- Could the program be replicated elsewhere? If so, what key processes should be followed? What can be adapted to local needs and what should not be changed?

STEP 9: SITUATE THE PROGRAM ALONGSIDE OTHER ANTI-STIGMA EFFORTS

Enthusiasm for a local program can be enhanced if the program situates itself alongside larger national or international efforts. As there are many of these ongoing (described in the next chapter), program committee members should identify prominent anti-stigma efforts and develop associations with them.

Many prominent people are comfortable disclosing family experiences with mental illnesses and will lend their support to local initiatives. Press conferences, features on local community television channels, and social media profiles are additional ways of reaching audiences. Programs will not survive if they do not generate enthusiasm or meet the common interests of their members and partners. The program must be seen as bringing tangible benefits to the community. This is why it is so important to canvass potential stakeholder interests thoroughly before finalizing program structures and goals. Broad communication of program activities and results is an important way of garnering political support and the attention of policymakers and potential funders.

STEP 10: DEVELOP A RESOURCE PLAN

The single greatest challenge for anti-stigma programs is to acquire sufficient funding to maintain activities over a long period of time. Programs that have sustainable program structures and steady funding are the most likely to create permanent change. This often means working within existing agencies through in-kind resources such as staff time or institutional supports (administrative support, physical space for meetings, etc.). Many socially responsible agencies do not want to lead anti-stigma programs but are happy to be involved in existing initiatives as a way of meeting corporate responsibilities. Most healthcare organizations have stigma reduction as part of their mandate, and most include promoting recovery and quality of care among their goals. Thus, it may be possible to develop partnerships with local programs and organizations to support coordinated initiatives. Indeed, such in-kind resources may be the most important source of sustainable funding. In these situations, anti-stigma activities may be included as part of the normal routines of health services, even though they may not be specifically designated as "anti-stigma" activities. They may fall under the umbrella of quality of care. For example, adding a staff member who will pay particular attention to client complaints, particularly those suggesting unfair treatment or inequity, does not need to be labeled as an anti-stigma activity. This may be easier for some organizations to implement as formal anti-stigma work may not be in their mandate.

Many different funding entities populate the mental health space, so it may be possible to identify an agency or foundation that would look favorably on a well-organized, clearly articulated anti-stigma initiative, particularly one involving community partnerships. Typically, a formal request will be required following a format outlined by the potential funder. This is where it is helpful to draw on expertise from across the program and advisory committees. An agency with recognized financial systems will be an important partner if external funding is obtained. This will ensure program accountability and financial transparency. However, something can be done about stigma even if additional resources are not immediately available, as has been shown by many grassroots programs. In fact, a key message of this book is that anti-stigma activities can be undertaken even when there is minimal funding. Action is necessary now.

STEP 11: IMPLEMENT THE PROGRAM

Implementing the program means implementing the various activities that are designed to reduce stigma and the activities that are intended to evaluate program implementation and outcomes. It also includes any training or orientation that may need to be done in advance to ensure a smooth delivery. Regular meetings of key program staff will be required to identify program processes that are cumbersome or ineffective and identify means of improving these. In the initial stages of implementation, many course corrections may be required. As the program matures, fewer course corrections will be needed, processes will become more stable, and participant capacity should be reached. Any outcome data collected during this time, when program activities may still be in flux, is informative in terms of identifying problematic processes but should not be used to assess program success. Only when the program has stabilized should data be used to formally examine outcomes.

Few programs are perfectly good or perfectly bad. Thus, identifying and learning from one's mistakes in the early implementation phase is one of the most important activities to be undertaken. Areas where performance is lack-luster and unexpected occurrences (either good or bad) should be examined closely. Only in this way can the active ingredients of the program be identi-fied and the connections underlying the theory of change be fleshed out.

Creating a culture of self-reflection can be difficult when there are com-peting pressures to demonstrate that a particular program has "worked," such as when overly enthusiastic committee members harbor larger-than-life ex-pectations—not an uncommon problem. Piloting programs—even mature programs that have been imported from elsewhere—can offer a safe haven where mistakes can be made, readily acknowledged, and examined without fear of retribution. Thus, it is recommended to consider the first year of op-erations a pilot year with the expressed goal of monitoring, evaluating, and correcting.

There are a number of situations that may impede a program's ability to adopt a quality improvement stance. Trained researchers know to look out for these and identify methods for mitigating them:

- Funders have mandated an evaluation be conducted in order to make de-cisions about future funding. Not only will this reduce the willingness of program personnel to be frank about problems they are having, but also the opportunity to make program improvements on the basis of evaluation re-sults may not exist.
- Opposing factions exist within the program that are strongly polarized. In this context, evaluation findings are unlikely to support critical reflection or planned program changes and, instead, may be fodder for finger-pointing and blaming.
- The evaluation did not incorporate sufficient qualitative data to pinpoint the program processes that should be improved.
- Political pressures may be such that evaluation findings will be over-shadowed by other concerns.

NOTES ON RESEARCH APPROACHES

This section provides an overview of research approaches for conducting needs assessments using qualitative and quantitative means. It is not intended to replace a qualified researcher but will provide an orientation to program and advisory group members who have not had previous experience with these methods. The goal is to help them become more fully engaged in the needs assessment process and become more savvy consumers of needs assessment reports.

As we have mentioned, effective anti-stigma programs need to be relevant to the needs and priorities of those who are stigmatized. Both qualitative methods (such as in-depth interviews and focus groups) and quantitative methods (such as surveys) can be used to understand local contexts. It is important to note that these should be conducted by individuals with specific training in these approaches.

Focus Groups

Focus groups involve facilitator-guided discussions, ideally with no more than six to eight participants. The purpose is to examine a limited number of issues in depth using broad, open-ended question formats. The goal is not to achieve or provoke consensus among group members (though this is sometimes a natural occurrence) but to elicit a range of opinions and ideas. The group format helps to stimulate thinking and promote a wider range of contributions than might be the case in an individual interview or in a more structured survey. In addition to using the information accumulated in focus groups to target local problems and priorities, focus groups can be used throughout the life span of the program to:

- Generate new ideas and concepts to be used to solve problems and troubleshoot when things do not go as planned.
- Create anti-stigma themes and messages concerning what information the program will provide about its own activities, the process of stigmatization, or how the program will position itself with respect to key topics addressed.
- Identify and create support for program activities by inviting people with expertise and leadership to become part of the program development.
- Monitor program activities among program recipients and broader community stakeholders.
- Develop and refine evaluation instruments and scales by reviewing survey instruments for relevance, meaning, clarity, and logic.
- Taking stock of how the program and the groups are doing.

Focus groups require careful planning and execution to ensure that clearly defined questions and concepts are addressed within the conversation, an appropriate range of group participants are canvassed, trained facilitators and co-facilitators are enlisted, focus group questions are relevant and likely to provoke discussion, and appropriate space and amenities are provided. It is important to make sure that the topics that are addressed are not too abstract or they may not resonate well with participants' experiences. This often happens when participants are asked to go beyond relaying personal experiences of stigma. It is important to avoid questions that ask participants to solve problems or otherwise move beyond their realm of experiential knowledge.

What is key is to understand the activities that would make a difference to their quality of life or social participation. In our experience, focus group participants will often identify a range of issues, some of which will make appropriate targets for anti-stigma program activities and some of which will not. It then becomes the job of the program committee to sift through these to identify those that may be addressed.

Much information about how to conduct a focus group (and individual interviews) is available on the web and in the scientific literature. Manuals also exist that can be used to structure focus group activities. In addition, the involvement of local talent on a voluntary basis to assist with focus group training and implementation may be sought.

Individual Interviews

When it is difficult to get the number of people needed for a focus group together at one time, or when you want to protect the confidentiality of people, a semi-structured interview is a good alternative. Like focus groups, these typically follow a set of broad, open-ended questions. It is important to note that focus groups and individual interviews can be conducted by phone or other meeting platform. Meeting platforms offer an option of recording the meeting, which is convenient for transcribing comments.

Surveys

Once problem areas have been identified using individual or group discussions, it can be helpful to follow with a survey to determine the scope and magnitude of the problems identified. Ideally, programs will want to target problems that are important and that occur frequently. In addition, surveys can provide important baseline information that can be used to assess the program's success. Survey results are also an important way of raising community consciousness about a problem, and results may be important in justifying funding requests. Journalists are often interested in reporting survey results.

Most programs do not have the skills or time to conduct their own surveys. An easy alternative is to contract a survey (or marketing) firm that specializes in population-based surveys. Typically, these firms have access to large panels of people that they have recruited to conduct survey research. Most external firms will help you refine and test the survey questions to be used, conduct the analysis, and generate a report. In order to ensure that the survey meets the program's needs, members of the program or advisory committees with research expertise must work closely with the survey firm professionals to appropriately guide their activities. This may include specifying the target populations(s) to be sampled, the size of the sample, the nature of the questions to be asked, and the type of analyses to be conducted.

Population surveys can be expensive and may be beyond the budget of many program committees. The cost of conducting a survey is driven by the number of respondents who need to be sampled to achieve a reasonable margin of error (such as plus or minus 3%). Large numbers will be necessary if programs want to demonstrate change at the population level, as program effects are likely to be small and difficult to detect in smaller samples. Program committees should not undertake a survey without appropriate internal expertise. Several national anti-stigma programs have been able to work with national statistical reporting agencies to add relevant questions on their regular surveys. This can be a cost-effective method of acquiring population-based survey data that ensures regular collection and minimal costs.

Ethical Considerations

People who provide critical information to evaluations may be hurt if their comments are identified or if they can be connected back to them. This is particularly true when asking people who have used health or mental health services to comment on stigma experiences. They may worry that their care may be affected. It is also true of program staff, who may worry about how their supervisors or members of the program or advisory committees may react if they make negative comments. It is especially important to ensure that qualitative interview comments cannot be traced back to the source and that all participants remain anonymous. This may necessitate having some of the comments altered (e.g., to remove organizational names or locations) and names changed.

Sometimes, formal evaluations will need clearance from an ethics committee, such as when the results are expected to be published, or when experimental manipulations, such as withholding service from a control group, are part of the research design. In addition, many organizations, such as schools or health facilities, will require a formal ethics review and clearance before allowing researchers to collect data. It is important to be aware of these processes and seek out knowledgeable people from the organizations targeted for program activities to be included on program and advisory committees. Creating partnerships with these individuals can greatly facilitate the process. Researchers on the advisory and program committees will be an invaluable source of information about ethical requirements and may have access to university-based ethics committees.

Communicating Evaluation Results

There are many different ways to communicate evaluation results from anti-stigma programming. If the goal is to create best practices in stigma reduction, then two considerations are paramount.

The first is that evidence-based policy and practice typically begin with a systematic review of the scientific literature. The strongest evidence comes from high-quality studies that show comparable results across different locations and circumstances. Unpublished technical reports that summarize the results of an evaluation are common but rarely persuasive, particularly if the evaluation was conducted by program staff, who will be seen as having a vested interest in finding positive results.

A second way of communicating results is to make sure they are also packaged so as to be understandable and interpretable by policy audiences. Whereas scientific presentations may be highly technical, policy briefs will be more approachable for audiences who do not have specialized scientific expertise and who are less interested in the methodologic details. These reports should contain a brief executive summary outlining key findings and recommendations. Often, policymakers will prefer a verbal presentation with time for questions. The strongest position to be in is to summarize the results of a report that has been published in the peer-reviewed scientific literature, as this will give greater credibility to the findings. Strong evidence in favor of a particular approach will make it increasingly difficult for funders to overlook funding requests.

SUMMARY

This chapter has outlined the key steps necessary to develop, implement, and evaluate an anti-stigma program. Careful planning is needed in order to ensure that programs maximize their chances for success. As in previous chapters, we argue for a targeted approach and provide an overview of some commonly used techniques to learn about local contexts and priorities. Throughout, we have recommended that program and advisory committees include people who can build bridges to local organizations or groups who may be targeted for anti-stigma interventions as well as individuals who have particular skillsets that will be needed by the program to provide, monitor, and evaluate service use and impact. A key message is that anti-stigma programs may be mounted with limited funding and resources. Everyone can contribute something.

CHAPTER 5

Fighting the Good Fight

This chapter examines initiatives to reduce stigma and promote social equity for people with mental and substance use disorders. It begins with a broad view of human rights legislation, examines selected activities of various international organizations to implement programs and toolkits, and closes with a review of national, regional, and targeted anti-stigma efforts. Initiatives illustrate stigma-reduction activities at the three levels of structural stigma, public stigma, and self-stigma.

INTERNATIONAL COVENANTS AND LEGISLATION

It is widely recognized that legislation alone is insufficient to eliminate stigma. However, legislation does have significant symbolic and authoritative power and, if enforced, can change discriminatory policies and behaviors. International conventions, charters, and treaties are "hard law," which means they are binding for countries that ratify them. Declarations, standards, resolutions, and recommendations issued by international bodies, such as the United Nations (UN), are "soft law" and, while they carry no legal obligations, they do confer moral obligations on signatories. Along with pronouncements and guidelines issued by international professional bodies such as the World Health Organization (WHO) or the World Psychiatric Association (WPA), these can exert a significant influence on national and regional legislation and regulations, as well as on judges and policymakers. [121] There have been a number of international covenants and agreements put forward by international organizations to promote the rights of people with disabilities (including mental disabilities) and, more specifically, those with mental illnesses, as follows.

In the wake of World War II, 50 countries drafted and signed a charter that created a new international organization, the UN, that was dedicated to maintaining international peace, giving humanitarian assistance to those in need, protecting human rights, and upholding international law.* Under the auspices of the UN, an international system of human rights was developed, centered on the International Bill of Human Rights.

Although the International Bill of Human Rights forms the basis of international human rights law, it does not explicitly address the rights of people with mental illnesses. However, the UN has adopted additional declarations, resolutions, and guidance documents to more specifically articulate the human rights of people with mental illnesses. [122]

Universal Declaration of Human Rights—1948

Prior to the Universal Declaration of Human Rights, an array of laws and declarations existed throughout Europe and the individual sovereign states of America that identified the inalienable rights of man. "Inalienable rights" are those that belong to the individual by the unchangeable laws of nature, not rights that are provided at the pleasure of the state. These were intended to limit the power of the state, which in more ancient times determined what rights, if any, a citizen would have. [123] By 1798, both America and France had formal declarations of individual rights—the American Declaration of Independence (1791) and the Bill of Rights of Man and Citizen (1793). While there has been considerable discussion in the literature and throughout history about how each may have influenced the other, both countries heralded declarations that gave primacy to individual freedoms and equality. [124]

Building on these, the Universal Declaration of Human Rights was adopted by the UN General Assembly in 1948. [121] The Declaration set out principles of dignity, liberty, equality, and brotherhood and recognized civil and political rights (such as those relating to liberty and freedom from torture) as well as economic, social, and cultural rights (such as the right to a standard of living, health, medical care, and other supports). The Universal Declaration of Human Rights is not legally binding, but it is authoritative and usually considered to be part of international law that is binding and enforceable. Though it does not specify mental illnesses directly, three articles are particularly relevant to people with mental illnesses [121]:

---

* https://www.un.org/en/about-us/history-of-the-un

- Article 1: All human beings are born free and equal in dignity and rights.
- Article 5: No one shall be subjected to torture or to cruel, inhuman, or degrading treatment or punishment.
- Article 25: Everyone has the right to a standard of living adequate for the health and well-being of himself and his family, including food, clothing, housing, medical care, necessary social services, and the right to security in the event of unemployment, sickness, disability, widowhood, old age or other lack of livelihood in circumstances beyond control.

Shamoo has argued that it would have been a more compelling document supporting the rights of people with mental illnesses if Article 2 had specifically articulated these rights by including "illness" and "disability": "Everyone is entitled to all rights and freedoms set forth in this Declaration, without distinction of any kind, such as race, color, sex, *illness, disability*, language, religion, political or other opinion, national or social origin, property, birth or status." [125, p. 208] Despite this lack of specificity, it is impossible to overestimate the importance of the Declaration in having brought about two major developments. [126] The first was the notion of universality itself—that human rights are not tied to country or citizenship. Second, the Declaration included economic, social, and cultural rights in the notion of universality, thus laying the groundwork for the landmark International Covenant on Economic, Social and Cultural Rights.

International Covenant on Economic, Social and Cultural Rights—1976

This was adopted and opened for signature by the UN General Assembly in 1966 and entered into force in 1976. Article 12 of the Covenant requires governments to recognize the highest attainable standard of physical and mental health for all citizens. The right to health is understood as a right to facilities, goods, services, and conditions that are conducive to the realization of the highest standard of health. In this way, the Covenant sets a foundation for positive rights such as family protection, an adequate standard of living, and the right to education. [121] Article 12 of Resolution 22000A (XXI) requires states to take the necessary steps for everyone to attain the highest standard of physical and mental health, including the creation of conditions to ensure that all medical services and medical attention are available in the event of sickness.[†]

[†] https://www.ohchr.org/en/professionalinterest/pages/cescr.aspx. Accessed June 9, 2021.

The Covenant touched off considerable debate, and many in the international community contested the legitimacy of economic, social, and cultural rights as legal rights. For example, the U.S. government maintained that economic, social, and cultural rights belonged to a "qualitatively different category" from other rights—that they should be seen not as rights but as goals of social policy. At this time economic, social, and cultural rights were perceived by many as deeply ideological, an encroachment on domestic affairs of states, incompatible with a free market economy, and something that required a major and costly commitment of resources on the part of governments to realize. Critics argued that the changing economic circumstances characteristic of the 1980s rendered the Covenant provisions unrealistic, obsolete, and utopian. [127] As a consequence of the 2008 economic and financial crisis and subsequent austerity measures, many countries cut back public spending on healthcare, education, and social benefits; labor protections were diminished; and restrictive pension reforms took place. These cutbacks threatened the right to work; the right to have an adequate standard of living; the right to social security and social protection; the right to shelter, food, and water; and the right to education. [126] It is interesting to note that in some countries (such as Eastern European countries), the "right to work" meant that a job must be available for everyone. In others (such as Canada or the United States), it meant that no one must be stopped from having a job for which they are qualified if a job is available.

Harris describes the importance of the Covenant as a tool that can be used to bring pressure to bear on governments to act to protect positive rights by mobilizing shame through publicity. [128] Signatories to the Covenant were to provide national reports, which were viewed as a way of shining a light on government compliance with the Covenant's principles. However, in the first 10 years of its operation, national reports lacked so much information or were submitted so late that little useful information could be harnessed toward this effort. Given these difficulties, the Covenant has remained largely aspirational, and in many parts of the world, problems persist in accessing even the most basic resources. Despite these problems, the Covenant has been described as "universally authoritative" with respect to the protection of economic, social, and cultural rights. [126]

Principles for the Protection of Persons with Mental Illness and the Improvement of Mental Health Care—1991

Adopted by the UN General Assembly in 1991, these 25 non-enforceable principles (commonly referred to as the MI Principles) apply to those with a mental illness and anyone in a mental health facility. They outline minimal human rights standards for mental healthcare and, in particular, protection against abusive and coercive care. In addition to procedural safeguards for involuntary admission to hospital (such as independent reviews with representation), the principles specify treatment in the least restrictive environment and the right to the best available healthcare. The Principles also outline a number of civil and political rights, such as privacy, confidentiality, freedom of communication, access to information, the right to health and social services appropriate to health needs, an individualized treatment plan, recreational and educational services, and resources for mental health facilities comparable to other health facilities. As they are nonbinding, they are intended as an interpretative guide to other UN conventions and declarations. They expressed the most direct description of human rights in the context of mental illness issued by the UN up until that time. [122]

United Nations Convention on the Rights of Persons with Disabilities—2008

Adopted in 2006 and entering into force in 2008, this was the first comprehensive human rights legislation in the 21st century to protect people with disabilities from inequitable and discriminatory treatment. Created with extensive input from people with lived experience of a mental illness and nongovernmental organizations, it obliges signatories to enact laws and other measures to improve the rights of people with disabilities and in particular to abolish discriminatory legislation, customs, and practices. The UN Department of Economics and Social Affairs reports that currently 182 countries and regional integration organizations (such as the European Union) that have ratified the convention.† Critics of the Convention note that it does not define the term "disability," thereby leaving open the question of whether all people with mental illnesses—such as those with intermittent impairments—qualify as having a disability under the Convention. It is unlikely that all people with a diagnosed mental illness would classify themselves as disabled. [129] In this way, the Convention may homogenize people with mental illnesses and reinforce stereotypical thinking about their untreatability.

The Convention explicitly adopts a social model of disability that uses a human rights perspective to promote full social inclusion for people with disabilities, including mental disabilities. Unlike previous frameworks, disability is viewed as a failure of the social environment to meet an individual's needs. From this perspective, disabilities flow not from physical or mental impairments but from structural factors that promote social inequity. In so doing, it rejects the view that people with disabilities are objects of charity, medical

† https://www.un.org/development/desa/disabilities/convention-on-the-rights-of-persons-with-disabilities.html

treatment, and social protection. It affirms the view that people with disabilities have the right to be full and effective members of society, making the Convention a major departure from previous international instruments. The substantive provisions are sweeping, covering both negative rights (such as freedom from torture and abuse, informed consent, and protection of persons) to positive rights (such as the right to education, employment or political participation). [130]

United Nations Sustainable Development Goals—2015

The Sustainable Development Goals look forward to 2030. Seventeen goals cover key global challenges such as poverty, hunger, clean energy, and good health and well-being. For the first time, the prevention and treatment of noncommunicable diseases, including behavioral, developmental, and neurological disorders, have been included under the health goal (Goal 3). Countries are asked to reduce premature mortality from noncommunicable diseases by promoting mental health and well-being, and to strengthen the prevention and treatment of substance abuse, including narcotic drug use and harmful alcohol use. Mental and substance use services are poorly resourced, so it is hoped that the sustainable development goals will increase the policy relevance of these areas so that they will become part of countries' development plans.§

INTERNATIONAL ORGANIZATIONS

A number of international initiatives have developed over time in an effort to promote the dignity and human rights of people with mental disorders.

The World Federation of Mental Health—1948

One of the first international organizations to promote the human rights of people with mental illnesses was the International Committee for Mental Hygiene, first organized in 1919 by Clifford Beers, a former mental hospital patient. Beers planned an international network of national mental health associations devoted to the protection of "the insane." The first International Congress on Mental Hygiene, held in 1930 in Washington DC, attracted an estimated 4000 people: psychiatrists, psychologists, health planners, and

§ https://www.un.org/sustainabledevelopment/sustainable-development-goals/ and https://www.who.int

others. In 1948, at the third International Congress on Mental Hygiene in London, the organization became officially known as the World Federation of Mental Health. In the ensuing years, the Federation provided an important platform promoting the human rights of psychiatric patients, the promotion and prevention of mental illnesses, the destigmatization of people diagnosed with a mental illness, and the elimination of totalitarian abuses of psychiatry. [131]

World Mental Health Day, established as an annual activity by the Federation, was first observed on October 10, 1992.** The goal was to promote mental health advocacy and to educate the public about relevant mental health issues by sparking a range of activities across the world. It wasn't until 1994 that specific themes were identified for each day. Themes that have specifically highlighted human rights and social equity issues have included Mental Health and Human Rights (1998), Making Mental Health a Global Priority: Scaling Up Services Through Citizen Advocacy and Action (2008), The Great Push: Investing in Mental Health (2011), and Dignity in Mental Health (2015). Other topics have focused on mental health in workplaces, depression, schizophrenia, aging, children, and women. As other mental health organizations, such as the World Psychiatric Association (described below), have taken a major role in fighting stigma and promoting mental health policy and practice, the Federation has lost some of its international centrality.

The World Health Organization—1948

In 1945, during the conference to create the UN, an international health organization was proposed. A development committee drew up proposals for the constitution of this new agency and presented them to the International Health Conference in New York City in 1946. On the basis of these proposals, the conference participants drafted and adopted the Constitution of the WHO as a specialized agency of the UN responsible for international public health. The Constitution came into force on April 7, 1948, a day that is now celebrated as World Health Day.††

From its beginning, the WHO has had an administrative section devoted to mental health. Indeed, its first Director General, Dr. Brock Chisholm, was a Canadian psychiatrist who stated that there was no health without mental health. Chisholm was instrumental in creating the broad definition of health that we now know, framing it as more than the absence of disease but as complete physical, mental, and social well-being. [132] The 1973 Expert Committee report highlighted the importance of primary care systems as a

** https://wfmh.global
†† https://www.who.in

means of improving population health and mental health. Using a series of case examples from developing countries that had implemented primary care systems in local communities, it argued against a strict sectoral segmentation of health services, an exclusive focus on curative medicine, and an overreliance on highly trained medical personnel such as doctors or nurses when minimally trained community workers could be more cost-effective. [133] This was followed a review of available information on mental health services in developing countries. The study group concluded that mental healthcare could be extended to primary healthcare using health workers who had received limited psychiatric training. [134]

In 2001, the WHO dedicated its annual report to mental health; in that same year, the theme of World Health Day focused on social inclusion for people with a mental illness with the slogan "Stop Exclusion, Dare to Care." [135] The report, *Stop Exclusion: Dare to Care*, contained wide-ranging messages designed to improve knowledge of mental illnesses and their symptoms and treatments and to raise awareness about the human rights violations and inhumane care occurring in psychiatric institutions in many parts of the world. [136] A key message was to deinstitutionalize the mentally ill from harmful hospital settings and to provide community-based alternatives to support their recovery and reintegration into society. This recommendation was based on the many decades of work by the WHO (e.g., through expert committees on mental health) and the primary care movement, which culminated in the landmark Declaration of Alma Ata in 1978.[‡‡]

To support World Health Day activities, toolkits were widely circulated in various languages to assist with activity planning. These included press kit materials that had been produced by the WHO and its regional offices, as well as audiovisual materials. Posters, stickers, pins, T-shirts, calendars, cafeteria placemats for trays, and website addresses were among the materials circulated. Various events were also held across the world, including:

- Public and scientific seminars
- Awareness-raising activities (such as walks, festivals, and rallies)
- Cultural events (such as art exhibitions or theater performances)
- Mental health service events (such as open houses in psychiatric hospitals)
- Religious meetings (notably, the pope made a statement on mental health and human dignity in his April 8 sermon)
- Political and legislative activities (including adopting new legislation and new mental health units within governments)
- Live webcasts

‡‡ https://www.who.int/teams/social-determinants-of-health/declaration-of-alma-ata. Accessed June 10, 2021.

- A global school contest on mental health, which included submissions from 86 countries representing some 500,000 children.

Proclamations and public statements were also made by important dignitaries such as prime ministers and elected officials. Finally, media coverage was carried out in almost all countries in the form of radio, TV, and/or print media campaigns. [137] In more recent years, the materials provided for World Mental Health Day have lost some of their comprehensiveness and, therefore, usefulness.

From the beginning, the WHO has viewed legislation as a critical factor that could impede or facilitate the development of mental health services. As early as 1955, the WHO conducted its first international survey to compare legislation on hospitalization and, in response to inquiries by member states, provided references to legislative recommendations contained in various Expert Committee reports. [138] This work has continued and, in the past decades, has resulted in a series of documents and materials relevant to the protection of the human rights of people with mental illnesses. One important document in this series is the QualityRights toolkit to support countries in assessing and improving the quality and human rights of their mental health and social care facilities. [139] The toolkit draws on five rights included in the UN's Convention on the Rights of People with Disabilities:

- The right to an adequate standard of living and social protection
- The right to enjoy the highest attainable standard of physical and mental health
- The right to exercise legal capacity and the right to personal liberty and the security of person
- The right to be free from torture or cruel, inhumane, or degrading treatment or punishment, and from exploitation, violence, and abuse
- The right to live independently and be included in the community.

Each of these rights is expressed in terms of a series of standards, then further articulated into a series of criteria that form the basis for an assessment. The toolkit includes assessment tools and reporting forms that can be used to undertake facility or country-wide assessments. It also includes information such as how to establish a project management team; objectives; the scope of the assessment framework; developing assessment committees and their working methods; training for committee members; establishing the committees' authority; obtaining ethics approval; conducting the assessment; observation of facilities; documentation review; interviews of service users, family members, and staff; reporting results; and using the results to improve quality of care.

Systematically collected data can be an important tool for mental health advocacy, and the WHO has been collecting data and supporting international studies since its inception. The Global Burden of Disease study catapulted mental health promotion and prevention onto the world stage by showing the extent of disability associated with mental illnesses (five of the top 10 leading causes of disability worldwide were from mental illnesses). Data from the WHO's Mental Health Consortium Surveys show that 35% to 50% of people with serious mental illnesses living in the community in high-income countries have not received treatment in the year prior to the survey; in low-income countries, the figure is as high as 85%. [52] Most notably, the Mental Health Atlas project[§§] collected, compiled, and disseminated information on mental health resources across the 194 WHO member states. A 2017 iteration of the atlas compared 2014 with 2017 data to assess the extent to which social equity targets, such as those outlined in the WHO's Action Plan, had been met. [140] For example, the first objective in the Action Plan was to strengthen leadership and governance with a target of 80% of countries having developed or updated their policies or plans for mental health in line with international and regional human rights instruments. In the 2014 Atlas, 45% of 88 responding countries had met this goal. By 2017, this had increased to 48% of 94 countries. Similarly, 34% of countries in 2014 had developed or updated their law for mental health in line with international and regional human rights instruments, increasing to 39% in 2017. Though none of the action targets have been fully met as yet, the data provided by the 2017 Atlas project show important movement toward these goals. [141]

The World Psychiatric Association—1950

The WPA came into existence in Paris in 1950 at an international congress and was legally established in 1961. The purpose was to advance mental health and psychiatry worldwide.[***] Aside from congresses, the WPA has initiated educational programs for psychiatrists and other mental health workers, created scientific sections to address themed areas in depth, developed collaborative programs, and published books, chapters, and the journal *World Psychiatry*. *World Psychiatry*, which was initiated in 2002, is now published in 10 languages and has the highest impact factor of any social science journal. [132]

Members are national psychiatric associations worldwide (currently 145 national member societies and 36 affiliate member associations representing some 250,000 psychiatrists). Since its inception, WPA General Assemblies have formulated and approved ethical guidelines for the practice of psychiatry

[§§] https://www.who.int
[***] https://www.wpanet.org/history

and psychiatric research, including the Declaration of Hawaii (1977); its amendment in Vienna (1983); and the Madrid Declaration (1996), expanded in 1999 and amended in 2011. In 2021 the General Assembly of the WPA adopted the WPA Code of Ethics concerning the activities of psychiatrists worldwide. The organization has collaborated with the UN and the WHO to protect the human rights of people with mental illnesses and maintains a standing ethics committee.

In 1996, under the leadership of Professor Norman Sartorius, then the WPA president, a global program to fight stigma related to schizophrenia was initiated (see [69,142] for a more complete description). The program was subsequently implemented in over 20 countries with over 200 interventions. The lessons learned from the Open the Doors program formed the basis for *Paradigms Lost* [1] and are described in earlier chapters of this book. More important than any specific intervention were the demonstrations that (a) anti-stigma activities could be undertaken in any country, including those that had only minimal resources, and (b) small, devoted groups of people, often grass-roots community volunteers, were central to advancing stigma reduction. Table 5.1 summarizes the target groups addressed by the first 18 countries to join the Open the Doors global program.

In 2005, in Cairo, the WPA General Assembly ratified the development of a scientific section focusing on stigma of mental disorders. (Sections form the backbone of the scientific activities of the WPA and regularly contribute to the scientific programs of international and regional congresses.) The Stigma Section (1) disseminates information about stigma and stigma reduction through scientific publications, presentations, and workshops, (2) advances scientific knowledge about stigma by fostering collaborative research and

Table 5.1 TARGET GROUPS ADDRESSED BY THE FIRST 18 COUNTRIES IN THE WPA'S OPEN THE DOORS GLOBAL PROGRAM

Target group	Total countries
Healthcare and mental healthcare providers	27
Service users and their supports (people with schizophrenia, family members, and friends)	22
Students (primary, high school, university)	16
Journalists and the media	13
General public	11
Religious communities and clergy	6
Government workers and nongovernment agencies	5
Businesses and employers	5
Judicial and law enforcement officials	2

Adapted from [69] and [142]

evaluation, and (3) provides training opportunities to support the development of effective programs to fight stigma because of mental disorders. (See the Appendix for a bibliography of recent publications of Stigma Section members for 2019–2020.) Section members also work with local hosts to offer a biennial "Together Against Stigma" conference. The location changes depending on the host, and conferences attract stigma researchers and advocates from around the globe. Nine face-to-face conferences have been held to date, most recently in Singapore (2019), and one virtual conference coordinated by colleagues in Prague.

NATIONAL ANTI-STIGMA PROGRAMS

With the growing certainty that mental illness–related stigma represents an important public health program, anti-stigma programs have been created by national governments, nongovernmental organizations, for-profit corporations, regional organizations, and grassroots community groups. Table 5.2 summarizes some of the most visible of these national programs and provides a brief description of their activities; it is not meant to be a comprehensive list.

The Global Anti-stigma Alliance (GASA) was established in 2012 at the "Together Against Stigma" conference in Ottawa, Canada, with the help of the WPA Stigma Section, as a way of bringing together these national and regional programs. Members share learning, methods, best practices, materials, and the latest evidence to achieve improved outcomes for individuals facing prejudice and discrimination because of mental illnesses. As Table 5.2 illustrates, the majority of programs are nongovernmental, meaning they can accept funding from range of sources, philanthropic and government. Only one—the Canadian program Bell Let's Talk—represents a for-profit company, and the remainder are government-funded. One UK program, Time to Change, obtained a considerable amount of funding through government and other sources but was closed in March 2021 when government funding was discontinued.

In addition to the programs described above, there are a number of smaller anti-stigma initiatives under way across the world that have been spearheaded by local advocates, health providers, students, family members, and people with lived experience of a mental illness. Typically, these programs are difficult to identify and monitor because their activities remain unpublished. An exception is a special supplement describing programs fighting stigma in midsize European countries. [144] What is evident from this review is that anti-stigma efforts are defined broadly in many locations, including literacy and health-promotion activities. In other countries, anti-stigma efforts are being undertaken but not conceptualized as such. Eight of the 14 countries surveyed had country-wide anti-stigma programs and all of them had regional

Table 5.2 EXAMPLES OF NATIONAL AND REGIONAL ANTI-STIGMA PROGRAMS

Program name	Origin	Funding source	Goals/activities
Beyond Blue	Australia	Co-funded across 8 government departments	Stigma reduction Improving mental health literacy Getting people support at the right time Public awareness Support services Training programs and resources
SANE Australia	Australia	Nongovernmental	Stigma reduction for complex and serious disorders Policy development and advocacy Public awareness Training materials Online help 24/7
Opening Minds	Canada	Government funding through Health Canada	Change Canadians' attitudes and behaviors toward people with mental illnesses Ensure that people with mental illnesses are treated as full citizens with equal opportunities to contribute to society Contact-based educational and training programs targeting youth, workplaces, healthcare providers, and journalists
Bell Let's Talk	Canada	Bell Canada Corporation (for-profit)	Open a national conversation about mental illness and mental health Raise funds for mental health programming and research through Bell Let's Talk Day Public awareness
One of Us	Denmark	Nongovernmental	Improve life for all Danes by promoting inclusion and combating mental illness–related discrimination Increase knowledge about mental illnesses Reduce stigmatization Promote social inclusion Targets activities to youth, the workforce, service users and relatives, health and social service staff, journalists.

Table 5.2 CONTINUED

Program name	Origin	Funding source	Goals/activities
Samen Sterk (Together Strong Against Stigma)	Netherlands	Nongovernmental	Eliminate prejudice and discrimination Targets mental health professionals, the workplace, media, the community, and youth. Increase awareness Promote workplace discussions Encourage media to report responsibly Works with educational professionals. Contact-based education Training tools
Like Minds, Like Mine	New Zealand	Government funding	Removal of barriers to social inclusion by targeting people who have the potential to exclude, particularly in workplace and community settings Primary targets are the media, workplaces, and the community. Public awareness campaigns, media reporting guidelines, and online resources for stigma reduction
UPA Movement	Portugal	Nongovernmental	Aim is to reach the entire Portuguese population, with specific efforts targeting youth and the workplace. Awareness raising through music, television, radio, and billboards School-based interventions Community-based psychosocial rehabilitation programs
See Me	Scotland	Nongovernmental	Focus on policy and practice within targeted settings of workplaces, schools, and health/social care Awareness campaigns, training, improved knowledge in target areas Lived experience talks

Continued

Table 5.2 CONTINUED

Program name	Origin	Funding source	Goals/activities
Idecada4 (1 in 4)	Spain	Multi-agency government funding	Combat prejudice, discrimination, and violation of rights A population approach with specific targets including healthcare professionals, service users and families, schools and universities, media, and workplaces Media campaigns, documentary films, media reporting, training courses, workshops
Obertament (Open Mind)	Catalonia, Spain	Nongovernmental	Population-based approach to reach all of Catalonia Campaigns reach 9–11% of population. Target groups include media, youth, primary healthcare, and the workplace. Media observatory and media guidelines Educational workshops and toolkits Activism training for the population Awareness raising Mental health literacy
Time to Change	UK	Government and philanthropic funding. On March 31, 2021, Time to Change closed following the government's decision to end funding.	In light of closure, asked government to agree to a three-point plan going forward: (1) put anti-stigma and discrimination work at the heart of mental health planning, (2) work toward equity, (3) Monitor and publish public attitudes data in an annual survey. To date, the government has not released plans to deal with stigma in the future.
SANE UK	UK	Nongovernmental	Reduce the impact of mental illnesses (reduce stigma, distress, increase support) Improve treatment and care by increasing knowledge about mental illnesses Influence policy and public attitudes by increasing understanding of mental illnesses
Bring Change to Mind	USA	Nongovernmental	Encourage dialogue Raise awareness, understanding, empathy Create national advocacy and awareness campaigns; develop national student-led high school club program; and build a storytelling movement that works to end stigma

Program name	Origin	Funding source	Goals/activities
The Carter Center	USA	Nongovernmental	Fellowships for mental health journalism because, indirectly, journalism affects the general public and policymakers

Table 5.2 CONTINUED

In alphabetical order by country.
Information summarized from [143].

projects or campaigns. Targeting programs to a particular group was not the rule and, when done, was often done out of convenience. Patient and family groups were not usually involved in the planning or execution, and evaluation was not given much attention.

Social Contact

Social contact has become an increasingly popular approach used by anti-stigma programs to promote and normalize social relations between people who have experienced a mental illness and those who haven't. The theory that meaningful social contact will improve relationships between groups was first proposed by Allport in 1954. [145] Meaningful social contact was considered to be based on equality, cooperation, personal interactions, and support from authority to establish a norm of acceptance. It has been used widely to reduce prejudice against a range of minority groups, including disability groups, such as in the case of school-based Paralympic programs. [146] The rapid desegregation of the U.S. Army following President Truman's executive order abolishing racial segregation (on July 28, 1948) provides a powerful example of the social contact theory in practice. Surveys conducted with military personnel prior to and following desegregation (1943 and 1951, respectively) showed improved attitudes. Among white armed forces personnel, 84% opposed integration in 1943, but this number had dropped to 44% in 1951. Among African American soldiers, opposition dropped from 36% to 4%. In 1943, 14% of white soldiers were either indifferent or favorable, increasing to 56% in 1951. Among African American soldiers, attitudes improved from 64% to 96%, respectively. [147]

Corrigan and colleagues conducted a meta-analysis of 72 studies examining three anti-stigma approaches: education, contact, and protest. [148] Educational approaches challenge misconceptions and negative stereotypes. Contact-based approaches create opportunities for interpersonal contact, and protest approaches involve social activism. Significant effect sizes were found with respect to behavioral intentions (a proxy for behavioral change) for both education and contact, but contact effects were larger. Compared to video contact, in-person contact was greater, though both were statistically significant. A problem for the analysis was the large variation between studies in terms of rigor, methods, approaches, and measures. Based on this analysis, face-to-face contact emerged as the most promising practice for reducing stigma. In-person contact was particularly effective for adolescents, with an average effect size showing a moderate effect (Mean Cohen's d = 0.46). Following these results, the use of contact-based approaches, now largely considered to be a "best" practice, has increased.

It is one thing to know that contact works and another to understand why it works. This could not be determined from the meta-analysis described above, given the heterogeneity across studies and the lack of details in most of them concerning the nature of the intervention provided. To begin to fill this gap, Chen and colleagues conducted a study to develop a grounded (qualitatively derived) model outlining the critical domains for contact-based education. [149] Their focus was on 18 school-based programs where trained speakers with lived experience of a mental illness told their personal stories to students and engaged them in a question-and-answer period. Results demonstrated that contact-based interventions varied in the quality of the contact provided. The most successful interventions were engaging. Speakers acted as role models to embody recovery and interacted and connected with youth on a humanistic level. Successful interventions provided students with accurate information about mental illnesses (especially in response to questions), reduced anxiety about interacting with someone with a mental illness (normalized the interaction), and helped students take the perspective of the person with the mental illness (promoted empathy). To accomplish this, speakers had to be in recovery and ready to share their personal stories, equipped with skills and knowledge to provide the intervention, deliver a recovery message, correct misperceptions, connect students with additional resources, and create a positive interaction. Engaging and connecting with students also meant empowering them to advocate against stigma in their schools and communities.

Despite these promising results and the growing popularity of contact-based anti-stigma interventions as a "best" practice, there are also some important caveats to consider. [150,151] The bulk of evidence to date comes from high-income countries. There has been a lack of rigorously implemented randomized controlled trials needed to support the claim that contact-based education is a "best" practice (rather than a promising practice), and little is yet known about the long-term effects of contact-based approaches in changing discriminatory behaviors. Improved study designs, greater attention to isolating the key ingredients of contact-based approaches, and follow-up investigations are needed. Gronholm and colleagues also warn of the danger that contact-based approaches will reduce attention on changing structural stigma. [150] Effect modifiers, such as nature of past contact with people with a mental illness or gender, are also important for improving the effectiveness of contact-based programming. Finally, as pointed out by Ashton and coworkers, evaluation measures and methods could be significantly enhanced through collaborative relationships between providers of stigma-reduction interventions and experienced stigma researchers. [152]

Good Storytelling Is a Key Ingredient

Good storytelling is a key ingredient in contact-based approaches. Humans are storytelling animals. We tell stories to give order to human experiences and to induce others to establish common ways of living. Through stories, values, goals, and ways of being in the world are negotiated and reinforced. They allow us to empathize and identify with others. They are moral in nature and offer a mode of discourse that helps us confront important social and moral problems. They are more effective than rational arguments as they appeal to emotions, imagination, and values. Stories can invoke and challenge the mental schema the listener brings to the conversation. [153,154] This makes them a particularly valuable tool for stigma interventions.

Contact-based education centers on telling a good personal story. However, stories have been told in different ways—some with excellent results, and others with little impact or even negative effects. Effective stigma stories have been described as having three components [155]:

1. The "on-the-way-down" component summarizes the personal challenges of living with a mental disorder—what it's like to have depressive symptoms or hallucinations, for instance. However, stories err if they focus only on this component as it is the piece that is most frightening to listeners.
2. The "on-the-way-up" component describes how the individual overcame the symptoms and obtained the right mix of supports to achieve personal goals. A good story is aspirational, pointing out that achievements are measured not by external standards but by what is important to the individual. They show that everyone can be successful on their own terms, even in the face of a serious mental illness.
3. Finally, the "moral" of the story reiterates three facts: (1) my story is real and not an exception—people recover from mental illnesses; (2) despite my achievements, I still experience stigma—prejudice and discrimination have robbed me of opportunities and have been a bigger hurdle to overcome than the illness itself; and (3) stigma has to be stopped. Affirming attitudes and behaviors have to be promoted to overcome this cultural injustice.

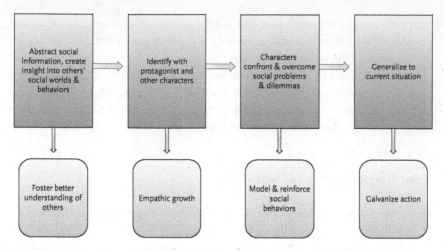

Figure 5.1 How stories can galvanize action

Figure 5.1 offers a theory of change to depict how stories can galvanize action to reduce stigma (see [59,153,154,156–158] for more detailed background information).

The negative side of storytelling is that it can also be used to nefarious ends. Stories can create prejudice and discrimination. They can be used to create and reinforce unconscious biases and negative stereotypes of certain people and groups, promote hatred and division, and reinforce discriminatory social structures and behaviors. One of the best examples are media portrayals of people with mental illnesses that promote negative stereotypes and stigmatized responses. The media's contribution to stigma is discussed in detail in Chapter 6.

PROGRAMS TARGETING SELF-STIGMA

The programs discussed so far have targeted structural stigma (through legislative or policy change) or public stigma (through raising awareness and providing education). There is also a growing interest in developing interventions to address self-stigma among people who have a mental illness. While this field is still new, it seems to hold some promising results. Much work is yet needed to solidify theoretical orientations, key ingredients, efficacy, and sustainability.

Corrigan and Rao offer a staged model of self-stigma that can be used to define the concept and understand how self-stigma occurs. [159] People who live with mental illnesses, particularly those with serious mental illnesses, understand how the broader society has defined negative stereotypes about mental illnesses. If they endorse these stereotypes as applying to themselves, they can experience changes in self-concept such as diminished self-efficacy and self-esteem. Self-discrimination can lead to self-isolation, treatment avoidance, and a host of negative health and quality-of-life outcomes. Self-stigma can interfere with the achievement of life goals, resulting in what these authors call the "why try" effect. Diminished self-esteem results in a sense of being unworthy of opportunities and internalized beliefs that one is incapable of achieving goals. They argue that disclosure is an important first step in overcoming self-stigma and self-shame, though they also recognize that "coming out" can lead to further discrimination. They have outlined a hierarchy of disclosure strategies:

1. Social avoidance (staying away from others who may be stigmatizing)
2. Secrecy (telling no one about the illness)
3. Selective disclosure (telling only people who will understand)
4. Indiscriminate disclosure (telling everyone)
5. Broadcasting (being proud and letting people know).

Using this model, the Coming Out Proud program[†††] was designed to help people with mental illness address disclosure and identity. [160] This 3-week peer-led program examines (1) the costs and benefits of coming out, (2) the range of strategic approaches to disclosure (as described above), and (3) the augmenting effects of peer support. Preliminary evidence from a meta-analysis suggests that this approach effectively supports people with mental illnesses in making disclosure decisions and coping with stigma stress. However, it is not yet clear to what extent the program reduces self-stigma, as findings have been mixed. [161] It is also important to note that cultural context will influence the extent to which individuals can or will "come out." As discussed in Chapter 2, cultural views of mental illness range widely from more accepting to highly punitive.

Russinova and colleagues have noted that peer-led groups may be more powerful in reducing self-stigma, given research demonstrating the effectiveness of general peer-led initiatives in increasing self-confidence, empowerment, and self-efficacy. [162] Peers may serve as counterexamples of social stereotypes and thus may be seen as particularly credible role models. They developed a 10-week peer-led program using Photovoice, a technique designed to facilitate participatory action that has been used to particularly good effect in marginalized groups. Individuals take pictures of objects or events in their daily lives that concern them and generate narratives for these pictures through a group discussion and facilitator-guided questions. The program also

---

[†††] Subsequently renamed *Honest, Open, Proud*. [161]

incorporated psychoeducation about stigma and experiential exercises designed to reduce negative stereotypes about mental illnesses. In a randomized trial of 82 people with a serious mental illness, participation in the photovoice intervention was significantly associated with reduced self-stigma, greater use of proactive coping with stigma, greater increase in a sense of community activism, and perceived recovery and growth.

In 2016, Tsang and colleagues conducted a systematic review and meta-analysis of 14 intervention studies targeting self-stigma, including the Coming Out Proud and Photovoice programs, the only two peer-led programs. [163] Most programs included a psychoeducational approach with additional components such as cognitive–behavioral therapy, social skills training, goal attainment, or narrative therapy. Programs ranged from 10 to 40 sessions and sample sizes were small, ranging from 21 to 205 (totaling 1,131 participants). A reduction in self-stigma was the primary outcome measure in all but one study. Nine studies reported significant reductions in stigma, though only two showed sustainable effects over 1 to 3 months. Many of the studies reviewed had important methodological shortcomings, making it difficult to draw firm conclusions. An earlier systematic review showed similar mixed results. [164] Thus, while programs targeting self-stigma appear promising, particularly those that are peer-led, much more work is needed to articulate the theory of change underlying self-stigma and identify the key ingredients for change.

Because usual treatment regimens typically fail to include instruction about self-stigma, its consequences, or coping strategies, it would be important for health systems to promote peer-led training to help combat the negative effects of self-stigma. Healthcare staff could also include self-stigma as a topic of psychoeducation and discussion within the helping encounter.

SUMMARY

This chapter has shown that interest in protecting the human rights of people with mental disorders has a long and illustrious history and can be traced back to many developments that emerged shortly after World War II. Since that time international legislative frameworks and international organizations have worked to ensure that people with mental disorders are treated humanely and equitably. Yet, data from organizations such as the WHO and other sources show that there is much work to be done. Against this timeline, interest in national and regional anti-stigma programs is a relatively recent and welcome development. While there is still much to learn, evidence is accumulating to highlight promising practices in reducing both public and self-stigma and articulating the program models (or theories of change) that underlie successful interventions. Toward this end, the "Together Against Stigma" conferences have provided an important vehicle for researchers, advocates, people with lived experience of a mental illness, family members, policymakers, and others to come together to share successes and identify barriers. Together, we are moving ever closer to knowing what works, what doesn't, and why.

CHAPTER 6
Media

Mental illness–related stigma can come from many sources, including family members and caregivers, teachers, health professionals, legislators, storytellers, journalists, entertainers, members of the public, and even people who have mental illnesses themselves. The news and entertainment media have produced some of the most sensitive, educational, and award-winning material on mental illnesses and the mentally ill. Investigative journalists have laid bare some of the most serious psychiatric abuses and civil rights infringements (such as during the civil rights movement in the United States or the Cold War in the USSR) and have created award-winning movies that have helped to improve public understanding and empathy for those experiencing mental illnesses. On the other hand, the media also have been responsible for creating a vast store of negative imagery with some of the most malignant depictions of madness and horrifying descriptions and illustrations of psychiatrists and psychiatric treatments. The fact that the latter greatly outweighs the former, and is more memorable, is of immense concern to people with mental health problems, family members, and mental health professionals. This chapter examines the ways in which stigma plays out in the news, entertainment, and social media. It outlines media resources that have been developed to help reduce sensationalized views of mental disorders and promote first-person perspectives of people with lived experience. The role of the media as allies in anti-stigma activities also will be discussed in order to promote a greater awareness of the importance of advocacy in this field.

NEWS MEDIA: TELLING OR SELLING THE NEWS?

News media are among the most frequently cited sources of mental health (and health) information, giving journalists great scope for dispelling inaccurate and stigmatizing stereotypes—or reinforcing and amplifying them. Often, a reporter's job is to *sell* the news, not necessarily to *tell* the news. [58] A good story, particularly a sensationalized one, catches public attention.

One of the ways in which the media can promote negative and stereotypical thinking is to use psychiatric terms metaphorically and pejoratively, as a synonym for something characterized as incoherent, unpredictable, or untrustworthy. For example, a 2010 study of leading Spanish newspapers revealed that 48% of the total texts reviewed (333 of 695) used clinical or psychiatric terms in this way. [165] The bulk of the terms were used to refer to irrational fears (81%), incoherence or contradiction (71%), or eccentricity (64%). In the 362 non-metaphorical articles, more than half (51%) associated psychiatric terms with dangerousness. People with a mental illness were depicted as victims in only 4% of the stories.

In the wake of Serbia's tumultuous socio-political situation, including wars in which Serbia was involved, newspaper stories frequently likened the spread of post-traumatic stress disorder (PTSD) as akin to a virus sweeping across Serbia reaching epidemic proportions. [166] Journalistic accounts of people with PTSD committing violence used phrases such as "bloodstained streets" (to emphasize violence) or "personal and family tragedies" (to emphasize the impact of PTSD on broader family and community networks). Often, perpetrators were portrayed as "quiet and modest people," making their violence seem more unpredictable and scarier. In addition, people with mental illnesses were portrayed as a homogenous group without individual characteristics and lacking in social identity, thus consolidating the separateness of "us" from "them" and giving the impression that they all pose a public risk. Finally, the accounts of service users and people with lived experience of a mental illness were notably absent, with psychiatrists most often heralded as the experts who predominantly attributed mental illnesses to biological causes, giving the impression of inevitability and inalterability and thereby promoting social distancing.

News stories reinforce cultural stereotypes by using them to provide the context for any materials presented. Stories are written such that the reader must draw on negative cultural stereotypes and commonsense understandings of what it means to be mentally ill to co-create the message. Narrative frames promote recognizable stereotypes for audiences who easily identify the frames and fill in the gaps. Deliberately sketchy or generic depictions implicitly link mental illnesses to violence and unpredictability by encouraging audiences to draw on this accumulated storehouse of cultural stereotypes. While not every story is negative, a neutral or balanced story about an unusual incident could be even more vivid, anxiety-provoking, and memorable by providing "factual evidence" that reinforces sensationalized (and fictionalized) depictions contained in the narrative frames. In the case of broadcast news, real-time translation of violent incidents involving people with a mental illness into visual images by news cameras that "don't lie" provides overwhelming authentication for negative cultural stereotypes linking violence and mental illness. Moreover, the global reach of the nightly news ensures that the public will have an endless supply of real-life incidents. Finally, few journalistic accounts of incidents involving someone with a mental illness include the voice of people with lived experience of a mental illness, mental illness advocates, or mental health professionals. This means that messages of hope and recovery are rarely presented. [58]

However, giving voice is not enough. In a content analysis of 1 year of news content about people with schizophrenia in major U.S. newspaper articles, one in five (n = 121) quoted an individual with schizophrenia, whereas the majority (n = 435) did not. [167] Articles quoting someone with a mental illness stood a greater likelihood of being accompanied by stigmatizing statements from readers. Articles that quoted someone with a mental illness were more likely to be stigma-framed (45%) compared to those that used frames to challenge stigma (35%) or provided a neutral frame (21%). These findings are important as they illustrate that reporters must make a deliberate effort to present a positive or neutral frame to dispel stigma when they quote someone with lived experience of an illness.

Media Guidelines

Concerns about the impact of negative news on the public's attitudes and behaviors has led to the development of guidelines for media professionals, though these have largely been confined to the area of suicide, where research shows that incautious reporting can lead to imitative acts. For example, studies have demonstrated that there are imitation effects following broadcasts or movies depicting suicides, particularly among groups whose gender and age are closest to the model. [168]

Guidelines for suicide reporting have been shown to have a positive impact, particularly when developed in collaboration with media professionals or when accompanied by activities such as media awareness initiatives. [169] Several national anti-stigma initiatives have developed or co-developed media guidelines for reporting on mental health and mental illnesses. For example, Everymind in Australia has produced media guidelines specifically to address stories relating to mental illness and crime, including violence. [170] They were developed with input from an expert panel of media professionals, mental health professionals, and consumer advocates. They provide some useful facts about mental illness, its frequency, causes, treatability, and supports and services available. Definitions for a list of key terms, such as "psychosis," "not fit to stand trial," and "psychopath," are provided to help reporters understand terminology that may be used in the context of a story about mental illness and crime. Facts about mental illness in relation to violence are presented to show that violent incidents are rare and that most acts of violence are committed by people without a mental illness. Risk factors for violence, such as history of violent behavior, alcohol use, poverty, and use of drugs, are provided. Reporters are asked to consider the impact of their stories on the people with mental illnesses and how negative and inaccurate reporting can lead to cumulative damage on public attitudes and behaviors. In addition to considering the impact of their stories, reporters are asked to report accurately, provide relevant context, use appropriate language, provide help-seeking information, and avoid stereotypical images and video footage.

The Canadian Journalism Forum on Violence and Trauma, with support from the Mental Health Commission of Canada and the Canadian Broadcasting Corporation, created an extensive journalist-to-journalist guide to highlight the role of reporters in reducing stigma. [171] The guide highlights three fundamental propositions: (1) Most stigma is generated and reinforced by rare, highly shocking, and well-publicized instances of violence by people with serious untreated mental illnesses, (2) attempts to counter the emotional impact of such stories by generating positive news are commendable but unlikely to succeed on their own, and (3) censoring or playing down coverage of major incidents of psychotic behavior leading to serious harm or death is not an option in an open society. Thus, editors and reporters should be aware of the damage that can be done by negative stereotypical images and should strive to minimize this. They have a responsibility to investigate and probe why violent incidents continue to occur. The guide provides extensive checklists, tailored to specific story types (such as suicide) or target groups (such as young or Indigenous people), to promote responsible and non-stigmatizing coverage. This guideline has been circulated widely throughout Canada, and elsewhere, and is now in its third edition.

The Mental Health Foundation of New Zealand and "Like Minds, Like Mine" has noted that respectful and accurate reporting can change public misconceptions, challenge myths and educate people, change discriminatory attitudes and behaviors, promote help-seeking, and provide messages of hope and recovery. [172] They ask reporters to avoid stigmatizing language, check the veracity of their sources, create story balance (including voices of people with lived experience), observe cultural sensitivities and worldviews on mental well-being and mental illness, and avoid using stereotypical images.

The UK's Time to Change anti-stigma initiative included a first-person story of someone who was living with a mental illness to highlight the characteristics of positive and negative media engagement in its media guidelines. [173] The group also provided a brief mental health language guide showing words not to use and offering alternatives and examples of responsible media representations, such as those including sympathetic representations of real-life experiences, an exploration into the causes of mental health problems, inspirational stories of recovery, expert comment from mental health professionals, discussions about the impact of stigma, and information on the frequency of mental illnesses. They identified negative and stigmatizing stories as those that link mental illnesses to violence, portray people with a mental illness as victims, describe people as "strange" or "odd," share details about a suicide method, or use disrespectful language, sensationalist headlines, stereotypical images (such as head-clutching or out-of-date treatments), and triggering images of self-harm or severe distress. Examples of disrespectful language and misuse of terms included using the term "schizophrenic" to mean a split personality or being of two minds, using the term "psychotic" to refer to someone who is angry, or referring to someone who is tidy or clean as "a bit OCD." Table 6.1 highlights some of the specific recommendations contained in these guidelines.

As these guidelines illustrate, there is considerable consistency of messaging with respect to:

- Not automatically linking mental illness to criminality and violence
- Use of "person-first" language—use "a person who has experienced schizophrenia" not "schizophrenic"
- Avoiding derogatory and colloquial terms
- Not speculating about the existence or nature of a diagnosis
- Relying on authoritative sources, such as mental health professionals or criminal justice proceedings, when reporting on incidents involving people with a mental illness
- Avoiding oversimplification of cause-and-effect relationships by providing broader context, such as for frequency of violence or the role of other contributory factors
- Not using negative story frames and stereotypical imagery, including sensationalized headlines
- Appreciating diversity, including cultural diversity, so that people with a mental illness are not homogenized into a single group.

Are Media Guidelines an Effective Anti-stigma Strategy?

It is difficult to know whether media guidelines have the desired effect of improving newspaper coverage of stories about people with a mental illness because most studies have documented broad secular changes that may be due to a number of different factors. Few studies have attempted to time changes in media coverage to a specific anti-stigma intervention. However, countries have differed in the way guidelines have been developed and implemented. Some have supported the media to develop their own guidelines, while others have provided guidelines and resources to the media on the assumption that

Table 6.1 EXAMPLES OF RECOMMENDATIONS OFFERED IN
MEDIA GUIDELINES

Source	Examples of do's and don'ts
Australia, Everymind [170]	To ensure accuracy when reporting, don't assume that the cause of a crime is a mental illness or imply that everyone with a mental illness is violent or a risk to the public. Don't excuse bad behavior of high-profile people on the basis of a mental illness unless this has been established by an authoritative source.
	Don't speculate about or attribute a mental illness to someone purely because their actions are shocking or inexplicable. Don't generalize about people on the basis of their diagnosis.
	When reporting on crime, rely on authoritative sources when reporting a person's mental health status and exercise caution in reusing information about someone's mental health.
	In cases where a diagnosis has been verified by an authoritative source, do not assume that everything the person does is a result of their mental illness, and only report on the mental illness where it is relevant to the criminal proceedings, such as when a mental illness has been verified as playing a role in the criminal act.
	Don't oversimplify the situation where mental illness is presented as the sole cause of a violent incident. Provide relevant context by examining additional factors that may have been contributory. Seek out professionals to provide context.
	Avoid using language that sensationalizes or is derogatory (e.g., schizo, wacko) and use person-first language so that people are not defined by their diagnostic label. Don't use colloquialisms to refer to treatments (such as happy pills or *shrinks*), and don't describe mental health facilities in terms that make them prison-like.
Canada, Mindset [171]	Don't reinforce stereotypes (especially in headlines).
	If violence is involved, put it in context. Violence by people with a mental illness is rare. Don't imply that all people with a mental illness are violent. Avoid referring to people with schizophrenia as "schizophrenic." Don't label someone with the name of their disease. Use person-first language. Strive to include quotes from those experiencing the illness or others affected by it.
	Be careful not to be specific about the diagnosis. Make sure it is confirmed by a professional and avoid vague terminology that homogenizes people with a mental illness and links them to stereotypical images.
	Include comments from professionals and seek professional advice when needed.

Continued

Table 6.1 CONTINUED

Source	Examples of do's and don'ts
	Demonstrate empathy and respect when interviewing people with a mental illness. Don't retraumatize them by pushing too hard.
	Don't romanticize suicides, go into detail about the method used, accept single explanations uncritically, publish suicide notes, or automatically mention suicide in every story about a mental illness.
	Appreciate diversity among Indigenous communities and avoid stereotypical story frames and assumptions. Appreciate the impact of intergenerational trauma and focus on underlying systemic problems. Recognize the importance of traditional culture to self-determination and emotional resilience.
New Zealand, Mental Health Foundation of New Zealand and Like Minds, Like Mine [172]	Regarding language, don't (1) label a person by their mental illness or cultural background (e.g., Māori mental patient); (2) use derogatory descriptions (e.g., deranged, madman, psycho); (3) use names of mental illnesses metaphorically to mean something else; or (4) portray people living with a mental illness as victims or mental illnesses as a life sentence.
	With respect to images, don't use dark, distressing images that reinforce negative stereotypes or images that show people isolated. Don't use generic hospital ward pictures, as most people are treated in the community. Don't use images of pills, as some people choose not to take them.
	Don't speculate about someone's mental health or whether they have a diagnosable mental illness, and don't emphasize violence.
	Include the voices of people who have a mental illness alongside other experts.
UK, Time to Change [173]	Don't undermine the seriousness of depression by referring to "happy pills" instead of antidepressants, medication, or other prescription drugs.
	People are more than an illness label, so don't refer to them by their diagnosis (a schizophrenic or depressive). Instead use people-first terminology such as "has a diagnosis" or "is being treated for."
	Don't use derogatory terms that are linked to popular culture or dangerousness such as "psycho," "schizo," or "maniac." Instead, refer to "a person with a mental health problem."
	Don't use the word "committed" when referring to suicide or attempted suicides as it suggests that a criminal act has occurred. Instead use "died by suicide" or "attempted suicide." Suicide is not a criminal offense.

they would be gratefully accepted and widely used. In some cases, active dissemination strategies have been used, including face-to-face briefings, while in other cases, dissemination has been more passive. It is also difficult to separate out the effects of one intervention from the broader social and cultural forces that may operate to change the type of incidents that garner media attention.

Whitley and Berry followed trends in newspaper coverage in Canada over a 6-year period (2005–2010) when the country was undergoing intensive anti-stigma activities, including the release of media guidelines, online education for actual and aspiring journalists, and educational seminars provided to journalism schools. [174] In perhaps the largest media monitoring study today, a total of 11,263 newspaper stories from major high-circulation Canadian papers were analyzed for content and theme. As commonly described in the literature, danger, violence, and criminality were direct themes in 40% of the articles where mental illnesses were discussed in the context of crime, deviant behaviors, prisons, courts, and the police. Treatability and recovery themes were notably lacking, appearing in slightly less than one in five of the stories. There was an almost complete lack of voice for people with a mental illness— 83% of the articles did not include a quotation or a paraphrased statement and 75% did not include a quote or statement from a mental health professional. Trend analyses showed that media coverage was not improving: Positive stories did not increase, and negative stories stayed about the same. During this time a gruesome incident caused a spike in the number of stories linking mental illnesses to dangerousness and criminality.

By 2017, there were more optimistic results to report. [175] Just under 25,000 articles published between 2005 and 2015 were analyzed. Articles about mental illnesses doubled in the last year of the study compared to the first. There was a significant change over the 11-year period suggesting that coverage had improved. There were increases in articles with a positive tone that discussed a shortage of resources, quoted people with a mental illness, included comments from a mental health expert, and discussed mental health interventions. There was a significant decreasing trend in articles that were stigmatizing in tone or content or that linked danger and negativity to mental illness. As found in other research, articles in tabloid newspapers had the most negatively oriented coverage. Significant differences were noted in the nature of the coverage before and after the implementation of the Mental Health Commission of Canada, which, as described above, identified journalists as one of their key target groups. Articles with an overall positive tone significantly increased from 17% to 22%; those with a stigmatizing tone decreased from 34% to 27%. The largest increase occurred with respect to discussions of shortages in mental health resources, from 16% to 32%. The study supported the notion that newspaper coverage was improving and also suggested that the concerted efforts made by the Mental Health Commission of Canada to educate journalists had a positive effect. However, it is important to note that many organizations in Canada were launching anti-stigma activities at the same time, including large-scale interventions such as the Bell Let's Talk campaign, and many grassroots initiatives. Thus, it may be that the combined efforts of all of these groups contributed toward these changes. Results also highlighted that there is still room for improvement and need for continued work with journalists and newsrooms.

In 2016, Rhydderch and colleagues examined changes in newspaper coverage during the Time to Change anti-stigma campaign in the United Kingdom between 2008 and 2014 (n = 9792). [176] Time to Change could have influenced reporting by including newspaper journalists and editors as a target group for advice, training, and lobbying, and through its social marketing campaign including journalists as members of the general public. Results were mixed. For example, over the 7-year period, the absolute number of stories about mental illnesses increased, with a slight increase in the proportion of non-stigmatizing stories and no statistical difference in the proportion of non-stigmatizing articles. In addition, there was a statistically significant decrease in the depiction of people with a mental illness as dangerous to others and a decrease in the articles providing a sympathetic portrayal of people with a mental illness. These inconsistencies and the lack of any discernable pattern over time undermined researchers' optimism about continued positive change.

A number of studies have examined trends in media coverage without attempting to link changes to any particular set of interventions, with mixed results. As one example, Goulden and colleagues analyzed newspaper coverage across a range of broadsheet newspapers in the United Kingdom in 1992, 2000, and 2008 (representing 30% of the newspaper market) (n = 1361). [177] Bad news stories declined from 59% in 1992, to 44% in 2000, to 37% in 2008, and this was statistically significant. Stories designed to increase understanding of mental illnesses significantly increased from 26% to 45% to 50%, respectively, and stories about services and advocacy remained unchanged (ranging from 11% to 15%). There was also a small but statistically significant increase in the number of articles featuring a quote from an individual with a mental illness. However, there was considerable variation by diagnosis. Reporting of depression, anxiety, bipolar disorder, and eating disorders either improved over time or remained largely favorable. Articles about schizophrenia, personality disorders, and general references to mental illnesses appeared mainly in the "bad news" category, where there was little or no change over time. Thus, the strength of the association between mental illnesses and violence in newspapers may be partly a function of the diagnoses included. Selective searching among news databases that focus on a single highly stigmatized disorder, such as schizophrenia or personality disorder, may be skewing results. [178,179] If a broader net were cast, including conditions such as mood or anxiety disorders, the strength of the association may be diluted. [180]

These studies suggest a slow progression toward improved news coverage that is consistent with the recommendations of guidelines and that has occurred during a time of vigorous anti-stigma activities. While it is difficult to link changes in coverage to any particular activities, it does suggest that cumulative anti-stigma activities are beginning to bear fruit.

Language Change: Semantic Sleight of Hand or Effective Anti-stigma Strategy?

Because so many of the media guidelines called for careful use of language, we thought it would be important to understand whether language changes could be an effective anti-stigma strategy. However, the jury is still out on whether good connotations can drive out bad. Indeed, the Allan-Burridge Law of Semantic Change holds that bad connotations drive out good. Innocent words become just as objectionable as the words they oust, which can then be rejected in their turn. Steven Pinker has termed this the *euphemistic treadmill* and notes that the lifespan of a euphemism can be short or it can be long. In many cases, the euphemistic value of a term can be quickly diluted and negative connotations reattach. [181] This line of argument calls into question whether euphemistic terms for mental illnesses will have the long-term desired effect or whether, in time, they themselves will need to be replaced.

In the mental health field, there has been an ongoing debate as to whether those who receive mental health care should be referred to as *patients, consumers, clients, self-advocates, survivors, consumer/survivors, service users, people with lived experience*, and so forth. Cheung suggests that current discussions can be differentiated from historical attempts to change labels in that they give greater prominence to calling people what they want to be called. [182] Having an opportunity to self-identify is a first step toward redressing power imbalances that have been the result of centuries of social, cultural, and political marginalization. However, this can lead to a confusing array of terms. While many people advocate person-first language, there are increasing numbers of those who prefer identify-first language, and they are reclaiming words like *mad* or *crazy*. Thus, words that are empowering to one group can be disempowering to another, making it difficult to know how to use language change as a generic anti-stigma strategy.

One good example of language change as a deliberate anti-stigma strategy comes from Japan. In an effort to eliminate negative connotations, the diagnostic term for schizophrenia has been changed, accompanied by a complete reformulation of the illness. [183] The Japanese National Federation of Families with Mentally Ill requested the Japanese Society of Psychiatry and Neurology to change the name of schizophrenia. They thought the name, which meant *mind-split disease*, evoked negative stereotypes that reinforced images of dangerousness, unpredictability, and untreatability. In 2002, the name of schizophrenia was changed to reflect an *integration disorder*, which was considered to give a better impression that the condition was reversible and controllable. The name change was accompanied with a significant reformulation in the concept of the disorder that was newly defined by a cluster of symptoms that were amenable to treatment. Previously the condition was described as hereditary and untreatable, without chance of recovery, and a Eugenic Protection Act (1940–1996) that contributed to their inhumane treatment. With the reformulation, patients and family members could expect a full and lasting recovery if treated with modern pharmacological and psychosocial care. Countries such as South Korea and Taiwan have followed suit. [184]

In Japan, Aoki and colleagues conducted a retrospective review of nationwide newspaper articles about schizophrenia and danger in the 10 years before the name change (n = 1241 articles) and the 10 years after (n = 3436). [183] While the absolute number of stories highlighting dangerousness increased, the proportion of articles with themes of dangerousness decreased from 43.2% to 37.4%, and positive news stories increased from 44.0% to 48.0%.

Only time will tell if the Law of Semantic Change will hold. However, in the interim, the name change has been accompanied by important improvements in clinical practice, including 78% uptake in the use of the term in psychiatric practices in the first 7 months following the change, and an increase in the percentage of people who were informed about their diagnosis (from 37% in 2002 to 70% in 2004). The new term made it easier for psychiatrists to inform patients, which facilitated education about the illness and use of psychosocial interventions. [184,185] These results suggest that the full reformulation, rather than the name change alone, was the active ingredient in bringing about change. It is not clear whether changing diagnostic labels alone, without an accompanying reformulation, would have a similar effect.

MOVIES AND MADNESS

The green skinned, leather-clad warrior woman and her blue skinned robot sister battle on the precipice of a rocky cliff as spaceships swirl in the brightly colored sky behind them. "Sister!" yells the green skinned woman, "fight Ronan with me—you know he's crazy." The popcorn pauses on its way to my mouth. My mind disentangles itself from the film. In the darkened theatre I am painfully aware that I am alone, even though the theatre is crowded and I'm with a date. I'm pretty sure that I'm the only person watching The Guardians of The Galaxy who's really pissed off right now.

As we left the theatre, my date and I argued over the merits of the film. It was a funny movie and there were some interesting progressive elements, inter-racial alien families, for example. But why, I wondered couldn't the green skinned girl just have said, "you know Ronin's evil" instead of, "You know Ronin's crazy"? My date said I was making a big deal out of the use of the word crazy because, "Crazy means a lot of different things," but it doesn't. Not according to the dictionary.

Denigrating images of people with a mental illness are not restricted to the news media; they are also a staple of moviemaking. The message that mental illness causes violence has been consistent throughout the entertainment media. [58]

Movies reflect a "cultural reservoir" of norms, attitudes, stereotypes, expectations, and beliefs that influence what we take for granted in society both directly and indirectly. Movies have the ability to maintain worldviews by setting boundaries of normality and confirming typologies. Movies also have the ability to construct worlds, meaning they can shine a light on activities that are not normally publicly available for viewing, such as sexual activity, drug use, or drug treatment. [186,187]

In an effort to simplify the concepts surrounding mental illnesses, filmmakers often confuse symptoms, lump various psychiatric conditions together, or depict exotic and esoteric conditions such as multiple personalities or trances, giving us the impression that these occur frequently. [188] They also overemphasize grossly disorganized and bizarre behaviors, particularly of characters with schizophrenia, who are often shown experiencing florid visual or command hallucinations. Owen examined English-language commercial movies released between 1990 and 2010 featuring at least one character with schizophrenia. [189] Forty-two characters from 41 movies were included in the analysis. The majority displayed bizarre delusions (67%), auditory hallucinations (62%), and visual hallucinations (52%). Most (83%) displayed dangerous or violent behaviors toward others, and nearly a third of those who engaged in violent behavior (31%) were homicidal. Seventy-one percent were portrayed as unpredictable and 69% showed some form of self-harm. Ten characters (24%) died by suicide. These findings illustrate how contemporary movies misinform, support negative stereotypes, and promote stigmatized views of people with serious mental illnesses.

Of particular concern are films targeting young children, who may learn prejudicial attitudes and distancing behaviors that can carry into adulthood. Lawson and Fouts examined the 40 full-length animated feature films created by the Disney Network between 1937 and 2001. [190] Eighty-five percent contained references to characters with a mental illness, and 21% of all principal characters were referred to as mentally ill. The most common words used to refer to mental illness were *crazy*, *mad* or *madness*, and *nut* or *nutty*. These words were used to denigrate, segregate, and denote inferior status. In

*Personal communication, Julie, August 15, 2014.

Beauty and the Beast, for example, the townspeople frequently refer to Belle and her father as mentally ill. As the film progresses, the frequency of mental-illness words increases, climaxing in a scene where the father is chained and hauled off in a *lunacy wagon*. In *The Lion King*, the three hyenas are depicted as mentally ill through their rolling eyes, high-pitched hysterical laughter, and the antics of Ed, the *craziest* of them all, who mistakenly gnaws on his own leg. The hyenas are portrayed as the lowest group in the animal hierarchy and are to be feared and avoided. The generic nature of mental illnesses portrayed in children's television—lacking in symptoms or diagnoses—invites negative generalizations to all mentally ill people. [58]

Movies rarely portray psychiatrists or psychiatric treatment in a positive light. Psychiatrists are either wildly malevolent or benignly friendly but incompetent. Psychiatric treatments, particularly electroconvulsive therapy, are depicted as brutal, harmful, and of no therapeutic benefit. Psychiatric medication is akin to mind control. Gharaibeh examined 106 American movies depicting psychiatrists and psychiatric treatments and found that almost half the psychiatrists or therapists committed a boundary violation, with almost one in four committing a sexual boundary violation. [191]

A widely used taxonomy has been developed to describe on-screen portrayals of mental health professionals. For example, Dr. Dippy is a comic character, often with an Australian accent, who is bumbling, idiotic, incompetent, and sometimes sanctimonious. Dr. Evil is a sinister scientist who is often outwardly charming but inwardly malevolent, manipulative, and untrustworthy. Dr. Wonderful is an attractive, selfless, dedicated, extraordinarily skillful therapist who often transgresses boundaries. Dr. Sexy is a seductive female therapist whose sexuality is portrayed as integral to the patient–therapist relationship and whose therapeutic outcomes are more a result of her sexual relationships than her competency as a mental health professional. Finally, the rationalist foil is a therapist that typically comes up with logical, scientific arguments and formulations that explain supernatural phenomena, only to be proved wrong as the plot develops. [192] Given the negative portrayal of therapists and therapeutic interventions, it is not difficult to understand why individuals who are experiencing mental health symptoms might avoid seeking treatment.

ENGAGING THE MEDIA FOR POSITIVE CHANGE

It is widely accepted that the largely negative media portrayals of mental illnesses, mental health professionals, and treatments promote public stigma and act as a barrier to help-seeking for people who have a mental illness. Given that the news and entertainment media are among the most important structural elements that create and maintain stigma, it is important to consider how the mental health community can work more closely with news and entertainment people to raise awareness about the damaging effects of stigma and provide support for more positive and realistic portrayals of people with mental illnesses and their family members. Indeed, interventions directed to news and entertainment media are often high on the list of "to do's" for anti-stigma programming and mental health advocates. It is important to engage media because journalists may be unaware of their contribution to stigma or minimize the important public health role they play.

News Media

Few studies have attempted to educate journalists on mental health–related issues. In a systematic review with an initial screening of 6291 papers published between 1960 and 2017, only two studies were subsequently identified for detailed review. [193]

The first, by Stuart, was conducted as part of the World Psychiatric Association's Open the Doors global anti-stigma initiative. [194] Local mental health advocates worked with local news reporters to help them gain access to more accurate information to develop more positive storylines. Positive mental health stories increased by 33% in the post-intervention period and their word count increased by 25%. Stories about schizophrenia increased by 33% but their word count declined by 10%. Negative stories about mental illnesses also increased, by 25%, and their word count increased by 100%. The greatest increase was in negative news about people with schizophrenia, which increased by 46%, and their word length increased from 300 to 1000 words per month. Thus, the immediate effects of the intervention seemed to be positive, resulting in more positive news stories. However, from a broader perspective, locally focused efforts yielded meager results in light of the larger increases in negative news, particularly involving people with schizophrenia—the target group for the anti-stigma program. Results of this evaluation were deemed to be both positive and negative. Despite the increase in positive news, the steady flow of global news—dubbed the *CNN effect*—was no match for the local efforts. These results highlighted the importance of having counterstrategies in place when media incidents occur, such as having background briefs available so reporters can quickly obtain accurate factual information, maintaining a list of local experts available for interviews, and keeping in close contact with local reporters. Results also highlight the importance of implementing industry-wide standards such as media guidelines.

The second study was a small qualitative description of the events that unfolded in the press following a knife attack by a man with schizophrenia involving a minister at a Remembrance Day event in a small village in northern

Scotland. [195] In an effort to aid reporters in presenting a balanced story, local mental health providers gave a lecture on schizophrenia at a press conference prior to the release of the results of a formal inquiry into the event. Eight out of the 10 journalists were contacted subsequent to the conference. While the lecture was well received, few of the journalists considered that it had altered their storyline. The attempt to provide background information seems to have come too late in the process to affect the news coverage. It may have been more impactful when the incident occurred (when most of the stories were aired) rather than later (after the inquiry was completed). On a positive note, several of the reporters had remembered points from the backgrounder weeks later. These results suggest a missed opportunity on the part of the National Health Service to operate proactively—a lack of enlightened opportunism!

There are also several promising examples of interventions that have targeted journalism students. In 2011, for example, the Opening Minds initiative of the Mental Health Commission of Canada provided a half-day contact-based educational intervention to journalism students. Three individuals who had experienced a mental illness and two media experts talked about the media's pivotal role in creating and maintaining stigma, particularly in adopting storylines that portray people with a mental illness as violent and unpredictable, or using negative and disrespectful language to sensationalize the story content. Pretest data (n = 89) showed that students reported positive and non-stigmatizing attitudes and agreed that people with a mental illness are often treated unfairly. However, only about half (55%) disagreed with the stereotype that people with a mental illness are dangerous, unpredictable, and untreatable. There were significant positive shifts in the extent to which students failed to endorse negative stereotypes as well as social distance items. An unanticipated consequence was that 14% fewer students indicated on the posttest that they would go to see a doctor if they were experiencing a mental illness, perhaps because they had become more aware of the stigmatizing attitudes and behaviors people with mental illnesses face in the healthcare system.

Campbell and colleagues developed a collaborative curriculum for journalism students (n = 5) and psychiatric residents (n = 14). [196] Over a weekend, students received seminars from prominent journalists and psychiatrists focusing on mental illnesses and mental illness–related stigma. At the end of the workshop, two integrated student teams were formed and were required to compete to develop a print or radio anti-stigma campaign over the next 3 months. Teams met biweekly with journalism faculty. The winning team had its campaign run in the local media during the next semester. Pre- and post-surveys revealed that knowledge and attitudes improved. For example, prior to the workshop three (60%) of the journalism students agreed that stigma was a problem for people with a mental illness, but in the post-survey all five agreed. All of the psychiatric residents agreed with this statement in both pre- and post-surveys. In the pre-survey 11 (64%) of the psychiatric residents agreed that they had the ability to affect society's ideas about people with a mental illness; this figure rose to 13 (92%) on the post-survey. While this is a small project involving a selected group of students, it does suggest that attitudinal change can occur as a result of collaborations between the media and mental health fields.

Entertainment Media

The sheer scope of the entertainment media makes anti-stigma interventions seem a daunting if not impossible task. However, Pirkis and colleagues argue that the mental health sector (i.e., policymakers, mental health professionals, people with mental illnesses, and their families) should collaborate more with the film and television industries (i.e., producers, directors, scriptwriters, and actors) to minimize negative portrayals and maximize positive ones. [192] A previous section of this chapter outlined the impact of media guidelines. In this section, we focus on interventions that target media personnel directly.

There are precedents for enlisting members of the entertainment media in anti-stigma activities. In Australia, for example, producers and scriptwriters of a popular teenage soap opera (*Home and Away*), with a viewing audience of 1.5 million, created a storyline in which one of the main characters, Joey, experienced schizophrenia—a story that developed over 3 months. Working with members of the local advocacy group, Sane Australia, non-stigmatizing behaviors and recovery messages were reinforced. Local clinicians consulted with producers and scriptwriters to ensure that the story was both realistic and positive. A helpline number was given, a chat site was created, and the actor who played Joey became involved in the publicity for the campaign. In the 3 months following, there was extensive national media coverage, resulting in a 100% increase in helpline and online contacts. By working with local anti-stigma programs, the show was able to illustrate how someone could recover from schizophrenia. In addition to transmitting the important message that schizophrenia was treatable, it also showed how people with schizophrenia could be stigmatized and highlighted the effects of stigma on the person and family. More importantly, the actors and actresses modeled non-stigmatizing behaviors. [1]

In 2021, a groundbreaking coalition of media companies and mental health experts was announced in the United States that included media partners such as the MTV entertainment group, Viacom CBS, The Walt Disney Company, Amazon Studies, NBCUniversal, Sony Pictures Entertainment, Endeavor Content, and others. The coalition will create a guide to support storytellers in any phase of the production process, across topics, and across genres. It will officially be kicked off at a Mental Health Storytelling Summit in May 2021.[†]

SOCIAL MEDIA

Social media platforms (such as Facebook, Twitter, YouTube, etc.) have become important sources of health information but are also a frequent source of health misinformation (fake news), including stereotypical and stigmatizing content, which cannot be easily corrected or deleted, only commented upon. For example, Li and colleagues used linguistic analysis to detect depression-related stigma in over 15,000 Chinese social media posts referencing depression. [197] Six percent of the 15,879 web posts indicated depression stigma, the most frequent being that people with depression are unpredictable (39.3%) or depression is a sign of personal weakness (15.8%). It is important to keep in mind that social media users are not representative of all Chinese people, and the content of the stigmatizing statements is culturally intertwined with beliefs about mental illnesses and their causes, so the findings would not be broadly generalizable. Nevertheless, this study illustrates how analysis of language patterns could be used to screen for stigma and monitor it over time.

Robinson and coworkers quantified the frequency of stigmatizing and trivializing attitudes across physical and mental health conditions in random-sample tweets. [198] For the five health conditions studied (AIDS, asthma, cancer, diabetes, epilepsy), the average prevalence of stigmatizing statements was 8.1% compared to 12.9% in the five mental health conditions (autism, depression, eating disorders, obsessive compulsive disorder, schizophrenia). Trivializing comments minimized the seriousness or severity of the condition. These occurred in 6.8% of the health conditions compared to 14.3% of the mental health conditions. Mental health conditions were 1.5 times more likely to be stigmatized and 2.1 times more likely to be trivialized. Schizophrenia had the highest frequency of stigmatizing content and OCD was the most frequently trivialized.

Social media channels are increasingly used by anti-stigma programs to share their work and influence public perceptions. For example, New Zealand's Like Minds, Like Mine Facebook page has a Stigma Watch component that allows members to post and discuss media articles of concern because of their stigmatizing content. Other programs, such as Beyond Blue in Australia,

[†] https://www.businesswire.com/news/home/20210406005936/en/Groundbreaking-Coalition-of-Media-Companies-and-Mental-Health-Experts-Unite-to-Tackle-Growing-Mental-Health-Crisis. Accessed June 7, 2021.

provide space for people to post their stories of recovery. However, what is most interesting about social media is that an individual can post a comment about a stigmatizing experience that can go viral and be picked up by conventional media and then backed by anti-stigma organizations. In this way, individual experiences can be amplified and exploit traditional media channels. Spontaneous bursts of protest can bring about significant change in organizational behaviors. [199]

While the bulk of suicide and mental health guidelines are targeted to news reporters, social media platforms are of increasing interest. In Australia, for example, the Entertainment Industries Council has produced media guidelines for mental health promotion and suicide prevention for organizations and individuals using social media. [200] While many of the recommendations echo those presented in other guidelines (e.g., use of language, stereotypes, story balance, portrayal of violence), some are specific to social media platforms, such as:

- Use reliable sources and links.
- Check the entire content of a message before passing it along to be sure there is no stigmatizing content.
- Be transparent if you are working for an organization with a commercial interest in the topic.
- Talk matter-of-factly about personal experiences with mental illness.
- When you see someone else posting a stigmatizing or disparaging message, explain why the post may be harmful.
- Add the phrase "trigger warning" when linking to graphic stories or images.

SUMMARY

Long before a person ever meets someone with a mental illness or encounters a mental health professional, they will have formed mostly negative opinions and attitudes. The media perpetuate mental illness–related stigma through repeated use of negative and inaccurate images. Regardless of the genre studied, the media have provided overwhelmingly dramatic and distorted images of mental illnesses and the mentally ill, emphasizing dangerousness, criminality, and unpredictability. The media also model reactions to people with a mental illness, including fear, rejection, derision, and ridicule. News, entertainment, and social media communicate and employ dominant cultural stereotypes, giving vivid examples of the language and behaviors that are expected. Programs aimed at children act as a powerful socializing agent. Factual and fictional images are mutually reinforcing. News coverage—even balanced news coverage—of adverse events involving someone with a mental illness anchors cultural stereotypes in day-to-day events and provides real-life, close-to-home examples of how mental illness *is* linked to violence or criminality.

It is also important to recognize that the media may be enlisted as a for-midable ally in helping to challenge public prejudices, initiate public debate, and project positive human-interest stories. Media professionals may be eager and responsive targets for anti-stigma programming, particularly if this improves communication between media professionals and psychiatric experts. If appropriately enlisted, media professionals may challenge stigma and promulgate mental health messages. This chapter has reviewed some of the approaches that have been used to improve media portrayals of the mentally ill. Though vastly underused, they provide examples of activities that may be taken to work together with media professionals to reduce mental illness–related stigma.

CHAPTER 7

Health Systems

Healthcare systems, including healthcare providers, have been consistently identified as major contributors to mental illness–related stigma at both interpersonal and system levels. Stigma occurring within health systems is particularly impactful to people who have a mental illness and their family members because it occurs at a time when they are at their most vulnerable. It not only undermines access to and quality of care, but it can also create and reinforce self-stigma and result in negative health outcomes, including increased morbidity and premature mortality. This chapter examines key ways in which health system stigma occurs and reviews examples of novel interventions that could be used to create a non-stigmatizing, person-centered care experience.

STRUCTURAL STIGMA IN MENTAL HEALTH SYSTEMS

The healthcare system has been consistently identified as a contributor to structural stigma that occurs two levels: the organization of the health system and the functioning of healthcare services. At the level of system organization there are decisions about how much funding to provide to healthcare systems of which mental health programs are a part. Then, there are decisions about how much of the budget will go to mental health infrastructure and care. Individuals within the mental health system then make decisions about how to spend their respective budgets. Finally, mental healthcare personnel make decisions about how they will deal with their clients. These decisions lead to various inequities, including insufficient funding for mental health programs and research; fragmentation and underservice; overuse of coercive care practices; poor knowledge of health providers about mental illnesses and possibilities for recovery; and diagnostic overshadowing, where physical and psychiatric needs are not adequately met. Structural stigma in the healthcare system contributes to poor quality of care, disability, and premature death. [201] Surprisingly, given the magnitude of the outcomes, structural stigma in healthcare settings has not received much scientific interest—nor has it been an important focus of anti-stigma programs, which typically target stigma at interpersonal or individual levels.

A recent focus group study involving 20 individuals with mental or substance use disorders in Canada identified a number of dimensions of structural stigma. [202] Participants did not have any difficulty identifying examples of structural stigma they had experienced within healthcare settings. Many experiences centered on the poor quality of care and a culture of care that could be described as "broken." Physical and social spaces were experienced as disempowering, as were a range of behaviors exhibited by clinical staff that diminished self-esteem, personhood, and recovery. Participants blamed stigma on the narrow clinical focus on diagnostic labels and symptom reduction instead of a broader social focus including recovery principles such as empowerment, self-management, and meaning-making. Participants were acutely aware of the power differential between staff and clients and the overly controlling and at times punitive approaches to the treatment encounter. In addition to a lack of transparency regarding treatments and medication side effects, there was a lack of attention to clients' physical health. Diagnostic overshadowing was frequently identified as a cause of inadequate or delayed treatment for a comorbid medical condition (though the reverse could also be true when medical patients' mental health needs are not addressed). People with substance use disorders felt particularly stigmatized. Lack of consistency in care across geographic regions (e.g., when someone moved and needed a methadone prescription), inadequate access to family physicians, and stigma surrounding methadone treatments were identified as significant problems.

The "Architecture of Madness"

Physical structures can send powerful messages that reinforce negative social stereotypes and promote social exclusion. Historically, psychiatric hospitals were large, usually Victorian-styled edifices that were located outside of city centers, many of which are still visible today. The original hospitals were not intended as places to segregate the mentally ill, but as places of asylum to protect them from stigma and abuse from the community and from the terrible conditions in the workhouses and jails. For example, in 1410, Father Gilbert Jofré established the first asylum in Valencia, Spain, after witnessing a gang of young people taunting and hitting a mentally ill man (depicted in Figure 7.1). He demanded they stop and was so outraged that in his next sermon he

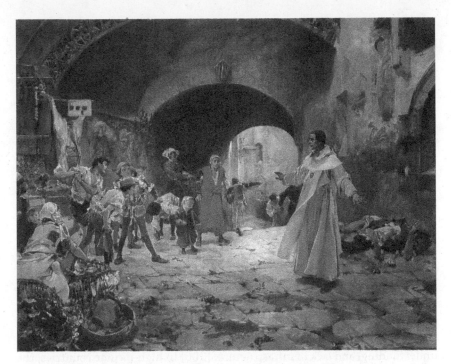

Figure 7.1 *Father Jofré Protecting a Madman* by Joaquín Sorolla (1863–1923)
Public Domain: Sorolla J. Father Jofré Protecting a Madman. 1887. Oil on Canvas, public domain. https://
www.wikiart.org/en/joaqu-n-sorolla/father-jofr%C3%A9-protecting-a-madman-1887.

spoke of the need for protective institutions for people with mental illnesses.
Ten local merchants offered to provide the funding required, and on March 15,
1410, building began for the Hospital of the Lunatics, Insane, and Innocents.
[81] Over time, hospital architecture became more prison-like. Many had
barred windows, reminiscent of jails, and were in an advanced state of disre-
pair. [203] Some have remained and been retrofitted as luxury hotels.* Others
stand empty as testament to an earlier age of psychiatric segregation.

Not only did the architecture of most psychiatric hospitals create a fearful
penal milieu for patients, it also provided a strong and consistent message
to the public, and in places where these buildings still exist, the message remains clear. As the focus of the architecture was on security and segregation,
the public message was that mental patients were dangerous and a risk to
the public. As deinstitutionalization emptied out the majority of patients
from psychiatric hospitals in higher-income countries, those who remained
were the most difficult, further supporting the view that psychiatric hospitals
contained intractably dangerous individuals—so dangerous, in fact, that it

---

* See https://www.architecturaldigest.com/story/former-asylum-hotels for examples.

warranted restrictions on their movement (through locked units and bolted windows) and minimal privacy (through staff surveillance). Lack of resources meant that these buildings were in deplorable condition. In middle- and low-income countries, these structures continue to house the bulk of psychiatric patients. Though large mental hospitals are no longer the norm in high-income countries, contemporary psychiatric units continue to restrict movement with locked doors and characteristically undermine patient privacy. [204]

Fragmentation of Care

In many countries, most people with severe mental disorders do not receive treatment. General healthcare workers and alternative healers are usually not trained to recognize mental disorders when they see them and thus do not identify people in need of treatment or refer them to mental health specialists. [205] International research has demonstrated that the treatment gap for mental disorders is large and varies across countries and health systems [205] owing to factors such as poor economic conditions (particularly in developing countries), low priority attached to mental health services, serious underfunding, and lack of infrastructure. [206] In high-income countries, the majority of people with common mental disorders such as depression or anxiety receive care in the primary health sector from general practitioners who receive little training in the treatment of mental illnesses. In many countries, primary healthcare clinics have no onsite mental healthcare integrated into their practices, with the result that only about one in eight patients receive evidence-based mental health care. [207]

Even in high-income countries, access to psychiatric referrals for their patients is problematic for many primary care physicians. In the United States, for example, it has been estimated that two-thirds of the physicians surveyed could not access mental health services for at least some of their patients—a prevalence that was twice as high as for referrals to other specialists. Fifty-nine percent could not get outpatient mental health referrals because their patients did not have adequate insurance coverage. A similar proportion of physicians identified a lack of service providers, and 51% cited health plan barriers that restricted certain types of mental health services (such as emergency referrals). Limitations in access to services varied by structural factors such as physician practice, health system, and policy. [208]

The situation is different in countries where the majority of the population is covered by some type of health insurance. Referrals to specialists are easily made, though there may be a long wait list. For example, in Canada, where there is universal health coverage, patients can wait approximately 9 weeks from a general practitioner's referral to consultation with a specialist and another 9 weeks from the time of the specialist consultation to the time of treatment. In underserviced areas, people with mental illnesses may not have a general practitioner. [209] The Commonwealth Fund rated access to treatment for mental health services among respondents who wanted or needed to speak with a mental health professional and found significant variation across 11 high-income countries. Top-performing countries across all indicators (access to care, care processes, administrative efficiency, equity, and healthcare outcomes) were Norway, the Netherlands, and Australia. The United States ranked last and Canada ranked second-last. [210]

Since deinstitutionalization, mental health programming has become increasingly complex, such that it is difficult for clients and family members to know how to navigate healthcare systems. Fragmented services are particularly evident for comorbid conditions. Mental and substance use disorders are highly comorbid, with prevalences as high as 40% in adult clinical samples and 60% among adolescent clinical samples. Integrated treatment approaches have demonstrated superior outcomes compared to single-focus treatment. [211] Even so, substance and mental health services are often funded separately, and there appears to be little political will to integrate or coordinate services across these silos of care. People with mental and substance use disorders may receive treatment in one sector only to be denied it in the other. Receiving treatment from some mental health services, particularly pharmacotherapy, can limit eligibility for care in substance use services, which may have a "no drug" policy. [212] In many situations, people with mental illnesses who exhibit disordered behavior or those who are elderly are trans-institutionalized into the criminal justice system or into nursing homes. Those who enter the criminal justice system experience "double stigma" as being criminal and mentally ill. This further solidifies the idea that mental illness and criminality go hand in hand.

PUNITIVE CULTURES OF CARE

There has been a growing interest in shaping healthcare cultures across the full spectrum of healthcare settings in order to improve outcomes. [35] One important challenge has been the lack of consensus on operational definitions on what constitutes a caring culture (over 300 definitions exist). [213] For the most part, however, "caring cultures" are considered to reflect healthcare settings in which high-quality healthcare can flourish based on dimensions such as effective management and leadership; staff engagement and empowerment; teamwork and collaboration; and patient-centeredness. [214] Professionalism is a key component of a caring culture. While there are many definitions of professionalism, increasing it is viewed as delivering services to a high standard, with a technical and scientific knowledge base, and the skills to act in an altruistic manner toward patients. [215] This means being a competent practitioner, respecting patient's rights, knowing the trade, and being ready to help whenever necessary.

The culture of care reflects the entire healthcare experience. This means the taken-for-granted aspects of organizational life—the "way things are done," including the most visible manifestations of the culture (such as the physical layout of services and observable patterns of behavior), beliefs and values of staff (such as respect for patient autonomy and dignity), and shared assumptions about such things such as the nature of the caring role, respect for the knowledge and perspectives of patients and relatives, assumptions about power differentials, and so forth. [213]

In the last two decades there has been increasing interest in cultures of care across the health system, more to explain healthcare failings (such as medication errors or safety concerns) and as a way to implement safety-related performance improvements. Cultures of care have been criticized as task-based when they should be person-based. The priority is to establish cultures that will allow healthcare organizations to provide high-quality care. [216] The management of organizational cultures is increasingly considered to be a key aspect of health system reform. [217] The way care is provided is as important as the specific treatments—some would argue it is more important. For example, studies have demonstrated that the best predictor of positive outcomes in cognitive–behavioral therapy is the quality of the relationship between the patient and the therapist. Meta-analyses have suggested that this, rather than any specific ingredient of the treatment, is up to seven times more influential in promoting change than any specific intervention. Similarly, the placebo effect has been credited with accounting for 60% to 70% of the treatment effect in depression treatment. Factors that have been suggested for this include encouragement and hope brought about by being in treatment. [218]

Rather than cultures of caring, too often people with mental illnesses are confronted with stigma cultures that are punitive, demeaning, dehumanizing, and patronizing. Staff relate to patients not as people but rather as their diagnostic labels, and there is little awareness or expression of recovery principles. Care routines are experienced as invasive, coercive, repetitive, robotic, and more for the convenience of the system than the individual patient or their family members. People with a mental illness may be spoken to as if they are children, assumed to lack capacity for decision-making, not given sufficient information about their condition or treatment options, and presented with veiled threats of coercion if they fail to comply with treatment plans, or outright coercion and seclusion if they become disorganized or aggressive. [1]

Studies have found that fear of being subjected to coercive care is an important determinant of treatment avoidance, particularly among people who have been exposed to historical or current mistreatment by the healthcare system, such as racialized, Indigenous, or immigrant populations. Using leverage to gain treatment compliance and applying excessive rules are among the most stigmatizing experiences. [219]

Inpatient Commitment

Involuntary hospitalization has been used in institutional psychiatry from its beginnings in the 18th century, and it is still widespread. Exactly how widespread is difficult to say because of the lack of monitoring data and the difficulty in obtaining reliable accounts that are comparable within or across countries. Published accounts show wide variation within jurisdictions and between countries, with five-fold to 35-fold differences in involuntary hospitalization rates per 100,000 inhabitants. [220] Cultural differences in processes of care, such as when family members can have a relative admitted against their will, may account for some of these differences. However, large within-region variation also has been noted.

From a human rights perspective, involuntary confinement denies basic freedoms, privacy, and human dignity. The experience of voluntary confinement can be traumatizing, with patients describing their experiences as if they were incarcerated with a basic disregard for their wishes, denial of their rights, and general inhumanity. From a clinical perspective, involuntary commitment is also problematic because it is disempowering and restricts patient autonomy, and can result in a loss of self-esteem, identity, self-control, self-efficacy, and diminished hope in the possibility of recovery. Some research has found that involuntary admission has been associated with less symptom improvement, longer durations of hospitalization, increased likelihood of rehospitalization, and longer-term problems with employment, social functioning, and treatment adherence. It is difficult to know how many of these outcomes are because of the involuntary treatment or because those who were involuntarily admitted had more severe illnesses. However, the opposite also has been noted: Patients have acknowledged that involuntary confinement did help them restore their safety and humanity. Multiple studies (often qualitative) have reported that patients considered that involuntary confinement was ultimately good for them. [221]

It is important to note that quantitative data outlining the frequency and impact of negative, positive, and ambivalent experiences are lacking, making it difficult to know, on balance, if involuntary confinement is predominantly a negative and coercive experience or a positive and recovery-promoting process. Regardless, the World Health Organization (WHO) has called for an elimination of the use of coercive practices such as involuntary admission to become compliant with international legislation such as the Convention on the Rights of Persons with Disabilities (CRPD) and the Sustainable Development Goals. They have also offered detailed guidance on how to accomplish this. [222]

It is also important to note that experiences of punitive care are not restricted to patients who have been involuntarily admitted, though involuntary commitment is a key driver. For example, in a study of a representative cohort of patients admitted to a hospital in Ireland (83 voluntarily admitted and 78 involuntarily admitted), 80% of those admitted involuntarily reported examples of punitive care on a standardized scale. By comparison, 22% of those who were voluntarily admitted reported similar experiences. This means that any recommendations for the improvement of clinical practice for involuntary hospital admissions should be extended to all hospital admissions. Examples include providing information on patient rights, involving families, training staff to manage aggressive behavior, and improving communication across all parties involved. [223]

The United Nations (UN) Convention on the Rights of Persons with Disabilities (Article 14) prohibits the deprivation of an individual's liberty because of a disability. As a result, mental health legislation that provides for involuntary admission for people with a mental disorder does not meet the requirements of the Convention. The Office of the UN High Commissioner for Human Rights has indicated that governments must repeal legislation that authorizes institutionalization of persons with disabilities without their free and informed consent. The CRPD does not entirely exclude involuntary detention, but it must be delinked to the presence of a mental illness. One alternative would be an impaired decision-making approach as a basis for involuntary treatment, as this could be disability-neutral. [129]

Eytan and colleagues assessed the impact of a medico-legal procedural change on the frequency of involuntary admissions in Switzerland (a country with one of the highest rates of compulsory care). [224] Beginning in October 2006, only certified psychiatrists were permitted to admit a patient involuntarily. Prior to this time any physician, including psychiatric residents, had this authority. The study took place in a large university hospital in Geneva with approximately 300 psychiatric beds and approximately 4000 psychiatric admissions per year. In the 4 months prior to the change, 67% of the 1162 hospitalizations were involuntary. This dropped to 60% of 1065 hospitalizations in the 4 months following. When patient characteristics were statistically controlled, patients were 30% less likely to be involuntarily hospitalized following the medico-legal procedural change. While these results are promising in the sense that they showed statistically significant reductions, it should be kept in mind that the proportion of involuntary admissions following the change was still high, suggesting that there may be additional sociocultural factors at play.

Advance directives allow individuals to state their preferences for future care should they become incapacitated to make informed decisions. It is a way to help people retain control over their treatment, support empowerment, and minimize coercion. Creating a plan and developing treatment alternatives actively engages individuals in the decision-making process and so may support their recovery. While psychiatric advance directives could provide a means of meeting the requirements of the CRPD, and despite considerable interest on the part of people with mental illnesses, they are rarely used. A greater understanding of the barriers to their use is needed. [225]

Crisis planning is a form of advance directive that outlines the individual's treatment wishes in the case of a psychiatric crisis. As in the case of any advance directive, crisis planning actively involves the patient and so promotes empowerment and user satisfaction and helps create a working alliance between the therapist and the patient. However, evidence in support of its effectiveness in reducing compulsory admissions is mixed. Lay and coworkers embedded crisis planning into an intensive personalized program involving psychoeducation and 24-month monitoring involving telephone check-ins every 4 weeks. [226] The sample for the randomized trial included 119 patients in the intervention group and 119 patients in the treatment-as-usual group. After 24 months, patients in the intervention group had fewer compulsory admissions (28% of the intervention group vs. 43% of the control group) and spent fewer days in inpatient care. Because this intervention included several approaches, and because of the high dropout rate in the intervention arm, it is difficult to draw definitive conclusions about crisis planning as a tool to prevent compulsory admissions. Also, given the intensity of the intervention, it is unclear whether such an approach could be broadly used in smaller communities and lower-income countries to meet the needs of people with a severe mental illness.

To summarize, coercive care practices are emblematic of the structural stigma brought about by poor funding at organizational and healthcare levels. Despite its widespread use, it is a clear violation of international human rights agreements. A general public that is unwilling to interact with individuals who have a mental illness because they view them as dangerous and unpredictable will support structural mechanisms such as involuntary confinement or treatment because they are so effective in removing "the mentally ill" from public view. Involuntary admission can mark an individual and their family for life. People with a history of involuntary psychiatric hospitalization will have difficulty making social contacts, finding a job, or regaining their self-esteem.

Outpatient Commitment

In the interests of providing care in the least restrictive alternative, many jurisdictions have provisions for outpatient commitment (or a community order) to promote medication adherence, prevent deterioration, and minimize future dangerousness. Proponents of outpatient commitment see it as an important alternative to inpatient commitment in that it promotes self-determination and the ability to remain as a productive member of the community. [227]

Critics of outpatient commitment see it as coercive, ineffective, infringing on civil liberties, and undermining the therapeutic alliance between clinicians and their clients. [228]

Link and colleagues outline two opposing rationales for outpatient commitment. [229] The first is the "coercion to beneficial treatment" perspective that argues that many people with severe mental illnesses lack awareness and insight into their illness, with the result that they avoid treatment and experience social risks such as homelessness, incarceration, violence, and suicide. Outpatient commitment ensures that people who are in this circumstance receive much-needed treatment. From this perspective, stigma is viewed as a consequence of psychiatric deterioration and impaired social functioning, and to the extent that treatment can reduce symptoms, experiences of stigma are also expected to abate. Evidence to support this perspective includes studies showing decreased hospital readmission rates, arrests, and community violence.

Swanson and colleagues studied the effects of outpatient commitment on violence reduction in a sample of involuntarily hospitalized patients who had been ordered to undergo a period of outpatient commitment upon their discharge. [230] Participants who were randomly assigned to the control condition were released by the court from the outpatient commitment requirement and received usual community supports and case management services. When outpatient commitment (6 months or more) was combined with community-based service, the prevalence of violence was statistically lower in the intervention group (24% vs. 48% in the control group). However, neither outpatient commitment nor community-based services alone reduced future violence. In a separate analysis, participants who underwent sustained periods of outpatient commitment had greater subjective quality of life at the end of the study year; this was largely because outpatient commitment improved treatment adherence (and associated receipt of intensive community services) and decreased symptomatology. [231] In the same trial, Swartz and colleagues examined participants' beliefs about the personal benefits of outpatient commitment following their experience of court-ordered treatment. Patients were questioned at the end of 12 months. [232] The majority (72.4%) did not endorse the benefits of outpatient commitment, either because they rejected their need for continued treatment or they did not think it improved treatment adherence. Subjects who experienced positive clinical outcomes were four times more likely to endorse the benefits of outpatient commitment. Male subjects, independent of clinical outcomes, were four times less likely to endorse outpatient commitment.

The second rationale outlined by Link and colleagues is the "coercion to detrimental stigma" perspective, which holds that coercion leads to a broad array of negative and stigmatizing outcomes. [229] Many advocacy groups maintain that services can be effective only when they are not coercive and when the person with a mental illness is a partner in the clinical process. Coerced care is viewed as interfering with recovery and quality of life, potentially intensifying the belief that one has entered a social status that is widely viewed in negative and exclusionary terms. Link and colleagues followed 184 individuals after inpatient treatment in facilities in New York, 76 of whom were assigned to mandated outpatient treatment. [229] A comparison group (n = 108) was composed of outpatients who had been hospitalized in the previous 3 months. All participants were followed for 12 months. Although mandated outpatient treatment was associated with significant improvements in symptoms and social functioning, and marginal improvements in quality of life, reductions in symptoms were not associated with reductions in perceived stigma. Thus, the idea that stigma, quality of life, and perceptions of coercion could be addressed solely by reducing psychotic symptoms was not supported. Perceptions of coercion drove stigma experiences and quality of life. While findings supported the "coercion to stigma" perspective with respect to the pernicious effects of perceived coercion, the ill effects of forced care and perceptions of stigma did not appear to extend to the maintenance of symptoms or impairments in social functioning. These mixed findings highlight the need to better understand the drivers of patients' perceptions of coercion.

Assertive community treatment (ACT) teams try to avoid coercive care by providing community-based supports for seriously ill clients who are not well enough to live independently. However, concerns have been expressed that ACT teams do use coercion with clients to ensure adherence to treatment regimens. This may include friendly persuasion, control of resources, outpatient commitment, threatened hospitalization, and actual hospitalization. More coercive tactics are typically reserved for the most seriously ill clients. It is not clear what proportion of clients perceive coercion in ACT teams, but it may be as low as 5% or as high as 50%. [233] Despite the potential for pressure and coercion, ACT teams remain one of the best-researched treatment models, with a range of positive outcomes including reduced hospital use, improved housing stability, reduced symptoms, and improved quality of life. The assertive outreach components emphasize relationship-building and tangible help, especially with respect to housing and finances. In 88% of 25 randomized controlled clinical trials, patients in ACT programs were more satisfied with services compared to usual care or other treatment alternatives such as brokered care. [234]

Seclusion and Restraint

Coercive care practices such as seclusion and restraint have generated discussions about their justification since the beginning of modern psychiatry, illustrated by the liberation of patients from their chains in the French hospitals of Bicêtre and Salpétrière by Philippe Pinel in 1795 and subsequently famously depicted in Robert-Fleury's 1876 painting *Philippe Pinel à la Salpétrière* (Figure 7.2).

In the second half of the 19th century a "no-restraint" movement emerged calling for the total elimination of compulsory measures in the treatment of people with a mental illness. To date, there are no examples of the complete abolition of seclusion and restraint. There is also no evidence to support their efficacy. While most would agree that it is unlikely that seclusion and restraint could be completely abolished, there is growing recognition of the severe and even fatal side effects that have occurred and calls for reduction in their use. [235] Seclusion and restraint are controversial measures because they infringe on the human and civil rights of service users and contravene international declarations such as the CRPD.

Seclusion and restraint are commonly used to contain inpatients who are considered to pose a risk to staff and other patients because of their disordered or aggressive behavior. Seclusion (sometimes referred to as "time-out") occurs when the individual is placed in a locked room that has minimal or no furniture. The goal is to provide containment, isolation, and reduced sensory stimulation. Restraint involves the manual or chemical restriction of potentially violent behavior. Decisions concerning seclusion and restraint are made by mental health staff who typically assume that they are acting in the interests of the patient and others in the environment who may be at risk. [236] Psychotic behavior, agitation, and disorientation are the most frequent

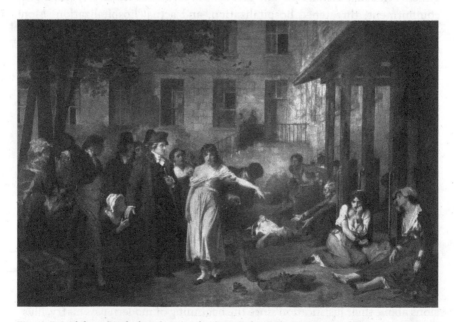

Figure 7.2 *Philippe Pinel à la Salpétrière* by Tony Robert-Fleury (1837–1911)

reasons for using coercive measures, even when clinical indications such as the potential for violence are absent. [237] Forced medication is the most common method of restraint. [238]

The use of seclusion and restraint carries inherent psychological risks to the patient based on previous trauma histories, experiences with coercive interventions, the duration of the seclusion or restraint, the patient's perceived control over early release, and patient preferences. A recent literature review identified a range of adverse psychological effects, including an increased incidence of post-traumatic stress disorder (which ranged from 25% to 46% depending on the study), feelings of punishment, anger, and distress. However, some studies also reported that a minority of patients perceived seclusion to have had beneficial effects. [239] Critics of the use of seclusion and restraint point to its overuse and indicate that psychiatric inpatient units should have the capacity to face emergencies with top levels of preparedness and expertise and should not rely on seclusion and restraint to manage disorganized or aggressive behaviors. These procedures are now widely regarded as signaling failures in care; as a result, the appropriate clinical posture should be to reduce and ultimately end their use altogether, particularly in light of aspirations to create patient-centered systems of care. [240] Increased funding for mental health facilities would allow for improved staff-to-patient ratios and provide for improved training in person-centered and recovery-oriented care so that the need for seclusion and restraint could be prevented.

It has been difficult to know how often seclusion and restraint are used and whether there are large variations between hospitals, regions, or countries—all of which would signal overuse of coercive practices. A large study of seclusion and restraint in 10 European countries did document wide variation in the use of coercive measures among 770 patients who had been involuntarily admitted to a psychiatric unit. [241] The average frequency of coercive measures used in the first 4 weeks of care was 38%, ranging from 21% in Spain to almost 60% in Poland. Forced medication was the most frequently used (56%), followed by restraint (36%) and seclusion (8%). Researchers did not find any influence of the technical characteristics of countries, such as the number of psychiatric hospital beds per 100,000 population, the ratio of staff per bed, or the average beds per room. Thus, they speculated that it was the country's sociocultural traditions and cultures of care in individual psychiatric facilities that played the decisive role. Arguably, it is most likely that the serious understaffing for psychiatric facilities faced by many countries accounts for the lion's share of variation.

Calls to reduce coercive measures have come from many quarters, including mental health advocates, patients, governments, and policymakers. A major challenge is that insufficient research has been done to identify what elements of intervention programs have been successful and how these can be scaled up and replicated elsewhere. Though it is not yet possible to firmly establish evidence-based guidelines to reduce seclusion and restraint, a number of key strategies have been culled from the literature [242]:

1. Policy changes should be made to limit the use of seclusion and restraint at a governmental or service level. Leaders at all levels must demonstrate a commitment to and support for efforts to reduce or eliminate coercive care.
2. External review committees are needed to provide detailed analysis of seclusion or restraint incidents with the purpose of making recommendations for future change.
3. Collection and reporting of seclusion and restraint data should be done to provide staff with feedback, promote benchmarking, and highlight organizational commitment to change.
4. Training strategies should focus on skill development and attitudinal change. Formal training in de-escalation techniques, crisis management, and attitude change is essential.
5. Consumer and family involvement would empower consumers and families with a stronger voice in the collaborative development of reduction strategies.
6. Increased staffing resources would assist in the management of crisis situations and promote greater interaction between staff members and consumers.
7. The therapeutic milieu of the unit could be modified by reducing ambient distress levels, changing unit routines, and providing support to modify interaction styles between staff and patients.

The WHO's QualityRights toolkit is the most recent example of evidence-informed guidelines supporting noncoercive care. It is particularly informative regarding strategies to help staff appreciate the nature of coercive care and provides methods for avoiding this. According to these guidelines, the following seven changes to law and policy are needed to create services free of coercion [222]:

1. Education of service staff about power differentials, hierarchies, and how these can lead to intimidation, fear, and loss of trust
2. Helping staff understand what constitutes coercive practices and the harmful consequences of using them
3. Systematic training for all staff on noncoercive responses to crisis situations, including de-escalation strategies and good communication practices
4. Individualized planning with people using the service, including crisis planning and advance directives

5. Modifying the physical and social environment to create a welcoming atmosphere, including the use of comfort rooms and response teams to avoid or address conflictual or other challenging situations
6. Effective means of hearing and responding to complaints and learning from them, including a systematic debriefing after any use of coercion to avoid future incidents
7. Reflection and change concerning the role of all stakeholders, including the justice system, the police, general healthcare workers, and the community at large.

Despite the importance of these recommendations, it is unlikely that many of them will be realized given the current underfunding of mental health systems worldwide. Significant structural change is required so that healthcare leaders and policymakers give mental health care greater priority and make mental health budgets commensurate with the burden of disability caused by mental disorders. Not only would appropriate funding make it possible to hire and train qualified personnel, but it would also allow for important infrastructure improvements such as repairing buildings and creating welcoming environments. It would also make it possible to provide patients with appropriate food and clothing, something that is lacking in many countries.

Lack of Recovery-Oriented Care

The notion of recovery has dominated mental health policy discussions for some time now and is broadly viewed as a means of achieving person-centered care. [34,35] However, there is still considerable confusion among many clinicians over what "recovery" means in the context of a mental illness because it is often unrelated to the abatement of signs and symptoms. Recovery is used to describe something that individuals with a mental illness experience as they manage their lives, something that mental health services promote, and something that systems facilitate. To help clarify the recovery discourse, Jacobson and Greenley have offered a conceptual model that refers to both internal conditions (such as attitudes, experiences, and processes of change) and external conditions (such as the practices, policies, and circumstances that may facilitate or hinder personal growth). [243] Key conditions for the recovery process to be realized are hope (a belief that recovery is possible), healing (defining the self apart from the illness and gaining control), empowerment (a sense of autonomy, a willingness to take risks, and personal responsibility), and connection (reconnecting with others and developing new meaningful roles in the world). Professionals who view recovery as a return to normal health often resist this notion of recovery because they see it as an unrealistic expectation. They are often not trained in a manner that would have allowed them to learn how to help people with mental illnesses recover their sense of self, self-esteem, and self-respect.

It is worth noting that the term "recovery" has a different origin and evolution in the substance use field. Early debates pitched abstinence as the hallmark of recovery, whereas more recent dialogue understands a range of outcomes, including harm reduction, improved social supports, and improved social integration, as well as abstinence. In 2008, a UK Recovery Consensus Panel defined the process of recovery from problematic substance use as voluntary and sustained control over substance use to maximize health and well-being and social participation. [37] Like recovery in the field of mental health care, recovery in the substance use field is person-focused and addresses wider social factors such as housing, employment, and well-being. For some, abstinence may be an important recovery goal, but for others, smaller incremental steps such as feelings of acceptance, taking responsibility, gaining control, or improving mental health are important. For still others, simply recognizing the need to change may be the most important recovery goal. [38]

Peer support is a key component of recovery-oriented care because it focuses on strengths and recovery—the positive aspects of people and their ability to function effectively in social roles that are meaningful to them. Peer support roles have been introduced into a variety of mental health organizations across the world and peer workers have participated in a broad range of functions within these organizations. What is considered to be distinctive about peer support is a set of values that stands in juxtaposition to the typical mainstream clinical practice that emphasizes medical disability. [41] Peer support workers can be more successful than professionally trained mental health workers in promoting hope, a belief in recovery, empowerment, a positive self-concept, and social inclusion—all of the nonspecific aspects of care. Employment for peer support workers offers the added advantage of promoting their own recovery (through valued social roles) as well as financial benefits. [39] In addition, however, there is evidence that peer support workers teach other staff about recovery and recovery-oriented care [40], so they can be key drivers of cultural change within the health system.

HEALTHCARE PROVIDER BIAS

In the past, mental health professionals led community-based anti-stigma programming. They often had access to organizational resources that grassroots organizations did not, and they considered their advanced education an asset to program planning. Some doubted the competency of laypeople or people who had experienced a mental illness. Many assumed they were exercising power on behalf of their client communities and learned about client needs through community assessment techniques (such as surveys) designed to rise above the clamor of vested interests. Rather than being the first choice for program leads, mental health professionals are increasingly recognized as a worthy target for anti-stigma programming [1]. Both implicit and explicit biases may undermine high-quality care.

Stigma as Implicit Bias

Implicit bias refers to the unconscious stereotypes and prejudices that people may hold toward those with a mental illness. To date most of the research has focused on explicit biases—those consciously reported negative attitudes and beliefs. (Chapter 8 examines how implicit biases originate in early childhood when concept formation is occurring and how they develop over time to influence behaviors.) Robb and Stone conducted a systematic literature review of studies examining implicit bias. [244] Nineteen articles were included in the review, the majority of which (63%) targeted mental illnesses in general rather than specific disorders. Most studies (65%) reported correlations between implicit and explicit biases, particularly with respect to a desire for social distance, which is a proxy measure for behaviors. This suggests that implicit biases could translate into discriminatory behaviors. In their review, Fitzgerald and Hurst also report implicit biases among healthcare professionals with correlations to poor quality of care. [245]

An important part of clinical decision-making rests on intuitive thinking, which is where implicit biases may reside. If unrecognized, they may lead to quality and safety risks such as poor decision-making, role confusion, role conflict, and poor communication. They can interfere with the delivery of integrated physical and mental healthcare and interprofessional collaborative care and may be a key driver of diagnostic and treatment overshadowing. Ungar and colleagues have offered a simple model to assist clinicians manage implicit bias on the assumption that "making the implicit explicit" can result in transformative learning and improve clinical outcomes. [246] They hope that this model also will be used to stimulate conversations about policy to improve quality, though it has not yet been tested against any of these desired outcomes.

Merino and colleagues highlight the importance of understanding and minimizing implicit bias in mental health settings. [247] They view mental health systems as particularly vulnerable to the effects of implicit bias because so much of the clinical care process relies on provider discretion. This becomes a particular problem when dealing with members of other marginalized social groups and may bias the interpretation of symptoms and subsequent treatment management. For example, they noted that even with standardized diagnostic criteria, clinicians are more likely to underdiagnose affective disorders and overdiagnose psychotic disorders among people from marginalized social groups. The incomprehensibility of speech due to social and minority group language differences may be more likely to be interpreted as a strong sign of a serious mental illnesses, such as schizophrenia. In crisis situations, implicit bias may lead a first responder to interpret someone as violent and dangerousness rather than experiencing frustration or fear. This may explain incidents, such as one that occurred in Canada, where a mentally ill man wielding a knife on an empty bus was shot multiple times by police who were on the street outside the bus and not in any obvious danger.

Many educators characterize implicit bias as a problem with awareness—in other words, raise awareness and the problem will take care of itself. However, if implicit bias is a function of stereotypical and prejudicial thinking, it is unlikely that awareness alone will be sufficient to reduce it. Implicit processes are like habits, so they will be difficult to dislodge without repeated, long-term intervention and practice. Byrne and Tanesini describe the typical educational intervention in healthcare settings as encouraging learners to take an implicit association test to measure the extent to which they hold implicit biases, then discussing the nature and possible effects of these biases. [248] Program developers recognize that this approach is likely to provide only modest change and may provoke a backlash from clinicians, who will view this as finger-wagging. Rather, Byrne and Tanesini argue for deliberate habit reformulation as part of the curriculum that would involve multiple small interventions designed to promote egalitarian values, critical reflection on values and value formation, awareness-raising, and multiple encounters to meet members of stereotyped groups until such encounters no longer activate negative stereotypes and affective evaluations. In many parts of the world, the time allotted to teach psychiatry is meager. Consequently, it may be important to help medical educators become aware of their own implicit biases and help infuse more mental health content into their teaching, perhaps even by giving up some of their "real estate" in the medical curriculum for mental health and stigma-related topics.

With respect to curricular change, Boscardin recommends four goals: increase self-awareness; create an inclusive learning environment that approaches learning from a sociocultural perspective; create learning opportunities for positive interaction with members of minority groups and development of cultural competencies; and build empathetic skills to decrease implicit bias. [249] All of these changes are thought to allow students to confront unconscious (and conscious) biases in a safe environment, though none of them have been explicitly tested.

Sukhera and coworkers have noted that, despite an increasing interest in implicit bias recognition and management, many health education programs struggle to integrate these topics into the curricula in a meaningful way because of the difficulty in recruiting faculty champions, perceived lack of relevance, and pressure to focus on medical content. [250] Implicit bias interventions are often implemented as brief interventions that are not well integrated into the curricula and lack systematic evaluation. They have proposed an actionable framework involving six components: creating a safe and nonthreatening learning context; increasing knowledge about the science of implicit bias; emphasizing how implicit bias influences behaviors and patient outcomes; increasing self-awareness of existing implicit biases; improving conscious efforts to overcome implicit bias; and enhancing awareness of how implicit biases influence others. They encourage curriculum designers to first create a logic model to articulate desired outcomes at both organizational and societal levels. Because outcomes may take some time to emerge, they recommend longitudinal strategies involving multiple measurement approaches to capture learner and patient outcomes.

While medical educators increasingly consider implicit biases malleable to curricular change, questions of the stability of that change have not yet been adequately answered. In the short term, implicit biases appear to be changeable, but over time, they seem to regress to their previous levels, making them appear more rigid than previously thought. Vuletich and Payne offer a third explanation—that implicit biases may reflect highly malleable attitudes that are constrained by the stability of social environments. [251] In a re-analysis of study data from 18 U.S. universities (n = 4842 students), they found that individual biases at follow-up were well predicted by the preexisting average score at each university. These results suggest that a person's implicit bias is transient and can change as often as the context changes. These results further suggest that certain contexts encourage discrimination more than others, largely independently of individuals passing through them. This interpretation supports a structural view of stigma and suggests that changing the social environment will be more effective than changing individual attitudes. This might include removing environmental cues to inequality and increasing diversity.

The current focus on individual solutions gives precedence to the role of personal agency in stigma creation rather than the institutional, organizational, and political systems that frame the beliefs and actions of individuals and maintain inequities. Greater attention should be given to the rules, regulations, laws, and cultures that govern the way in which social institutions operate. A structural approach also makes it easier to see the intersecting nature of stigma based on membership in multiple vulnerable groups such as those based on physical disability, gender, or ethnicity. [252] It is likely that a comprehensive approach will be needed to bring about lasting change. Toward this end, it is encouraging to see that there is considerable interest in new curricular models and increasing agreement that implicit bias recognition and management should be integrated into health professions' education. Future research on implicit bias will help to better understand how these new models of training in educational and health environments reduce implicit bias and improve quality-of-care outcomes.

Stigma as Explicit Bias

People with mental disorders report frequent and explicit stigmatized interactions across a range of healthcare settings, including mental health clinics, substance use services, acute care hospitals, emergency services, pharmacies, and dental offices, supporting the view that stigma is a central aspect of the healthcare experience. Negative professional attitudes have been recognized as key driver of stigma within healthcare settings and an important barrier to care. Prevailing stereotypes are that people with mental disorders are manipulative, are to blame for their health issues, overuse and misuse resources, are not vested in their own health, and are undeserving of services. Professionals may have diminished expectations for people with mental disorders, which is experienced by patients as therapeutic nihilism. Patients are assumed to be less likely to follow recommended care plans, make healthy lifestyle changes, succeed in various life domains, or achieve wellness and recovery. Negative attitudes can lead to a number of objectionable care practices, including diagnostic and treatment overshadowing, uncaring and unhelpful behaviors, paternalistic and noncollaborative approaches, withholding of information and services, task-oriented and depersonalized methods, and excluding or rejecting people from services. [253] During the pilot program for the World Psychiatric Association's global program to address stigma associated with schizophrenia, consumers identified that one of the areas that most bothered them was the hospital emergency room. Patients who attended the emergency rooms with psychotic symptoms were typically misidentified and assumed to be experiencing drug overdoses. [69]

Much research has now documented the problem of stigmatization in healthcare settings. However, the evidence base supporting best practices in anti-stigma interventions targeting healthcare providers is still meager. Three types of interventions predominate:

1. Anti-stigma workshop classes that are 1 to 2 hours long and include one or more elements promoting social contact, along with educational or a skills component
2. Half-day multimodal skills training programs that focus on improving communication, diagnostic, and therapeutic skills, with less prominent social contact elements
3. Intensive social contact programs, usually delivered in university settings as part of a larger course. [253]

The Opening Minds anti-stigma initiative of the Mental Health Commission of Canada undertook a grounded theory investigation of 23 key informants (such as program leads, facilitators, instructors, or program coordinators) to better understand the processes involved in delivering a successful anti-stigma program to healthcare providers. [254] Four key stereotypes were identified:

1. Holding pessimistic views about the potential for recovery, with the perception that what health providers do doesn't really matter
2. A tendency to see the illness ahead of the person and engage in behaviors that are interpreted as dismissive and demeaning
3. A lack of competence and confidence in working with patients with mental illnesses
4. Lack of awareness of one's own prejudices and implicit biases.

Figure 7.3 shows the process model developed for designing and delivering successful anti-stigma programs for healthcare providers.

Focusing on 22 interventions delivered to health providers, Patten and coworkers used a grounded theory approach to identify six key program characteristics from the model in Figure 7.3 that were most predictive of positive outcomes. [255] The program should: (1) include social contact in the form of a personal testimony from a trained speaker who has experienced a mental illness; (2) employ multiple forms or points of social contact (e.g., a presentation from a live speaker, a video, multiple points of interaction); (3) focus

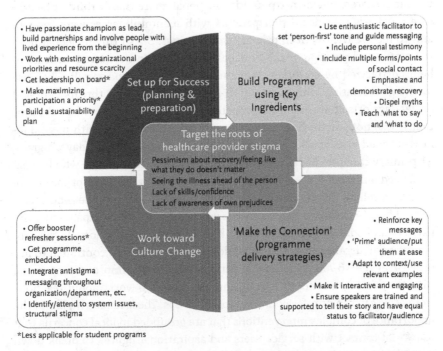

*Less applicable for student programs

Figure 7.3 Process model developed for designing and delivering successful anti-stigma programs for healthcare providers

on behavior change by teaching skills that help healthcare providers know what to say and do; (4) engage in "myth-busting"; (5) use an enthusiastic facilitator or instructor who models a person-centered approach (as opposed to a pathology-first perspective); and (6) emphasize and demonstrate recovery as a key part of its messaging. Programs that included all six elements performed significantly better than those that did not. The two ingredients that emerged as the most predictive of positive outcomes were (1) including an emphasis on and demonstration of recovery and (2) including multiple forms and points for social contact.

Considering what would work best in low-income countries that use primary care systems as a main mechanism of mental health treatment delivery, Kohrt and colleagues adopted a moral experience perspective to target "what matters most" to stigmatizing groups in Nepal. [256] Traditionally, most interventions for provider stigma focus on a knowledge—attitudes—practice framework that erroneously assumes that a more accurate biomedical understanding of mental illnesses will result in improved attitudes and behaviors. A "what matters most" perspective views stigma as a moral phenomenon that threatens the personal and professional identities of people within their local contexts. Using qualitative research, they identified three types of threats—survival threats, social threats, and professional threats—and then developed a program using social contact to address each of these. Survival threats centered on violence potential; in Nepal, more than a third of healthcare providers considered that patients with mental illnesses were too violent to receive treatment in primary care settings. Social threats jeopardized the status and prestige of the healthcare provider and centered on fears of being ostracized by coworkers, community members, and families because of their association with mentally ill people. Professional threats centered on feelings of self-efficacy and competence. Primary care providers thought that it was not worthwhile to provide care because patients with mental illnesses would not follow treatment plans or recover. In the 10-day program, 41 primary care providers heard stories of recovery from people who had experienced a mental illness. Aspirational figures who were local primary care providers talked about their successes in working with people who had a mental illness. Collaborative teamwork was used to help participants identify barriers and solutions and to discuss helpful skills. At the close of the program, social distance scores had significantly decreased and continued to improve over the 16-month follow-up period. Despite this improvement, social threats remained a concern: Participants continued to worry about reactions from others in their professional and social groups. These results highlight the importance of complex interventions that are grounded in local concerns that use social contact with service users and aspirational figures to break down social barriers and convey clinical skills. They are particularly important as they provide an innovative social contact model that could be used across the spectrum of low- to high-income countries to develop anti-stigma programs targeting professional groups. However, it is not clear whether a 10-day program would be feasible in all settings, or whether a shorter program would have similar results.

SUMMARY

This chapter has examined how the structure and culture of healthcare settings promotes interactions that may be experienced as traumatic, coercive, and stigmatizing by people with mental disorders. It traced the origins of stigma among healthcare providers from implicit biases, which are unconscious prejudices and stereotypes, to explicit biases that lead to stigmatizing interactions and poor-quality care. Creating care environments that are person-centered and recovery-oriented will be a significant challenge. However, there is increasing recognition that improving cultures of care, including reducing implicit and explicit biases held by healthcare professionals, should be a priority. Programs that combine social contact with skills-based training seem to hold promise, though much more research is needed to understand how they work, how to take local professional contexts into consideration, and how they may be scaled up to address different target groups in different professional and cultural settings.

CHAPTER 8
Educational Systems

Despite the importance of school settings for anti-stigma education, school officials and teachers are often reluctant to offer mental illness–related programs to students for fear of reprisals from parents or unexpected negative emotional reactions from students who, they fear, may be triggered by the content. In addition to worrying about how mental health content may be received, educators may also lack the confidence to deliver mental health–related programing. [257] This is particularly true when programs target the youngest age groups. For example, Economou and colleagues developed an anti-stigma intervention for high school students that involved both an educational component and a personal contact component. [258] But because of a number of objections from parents, school principals, and teachers, the personal contact component had to be dropped, instead relying on narratives of people who had schizophrenia presented by a mental health professional. In an evaluation of a puppet program targeting young children in grade 3, Pitre and colleagues had considerable difficulty recruiting schools. [259] Time constraints due to a packed curriculum and fear of parental disapproval were among the reasons given for lack of participation. In one case, a teacher who was persuaded to participate by the school principal refused to let the researchers back into the classroom to collect post-test data. Not surprisingly, then, evaluation research is spotty, and studies involving younger students are particularly scarce. In a 2012 meta-analysis of intervention studies, Corrigan and coworkers noted that while the majority of the 79 studies targeted students, the bulk of these were older students attending postsecondary programs. [148] Less than 1% targeted primary or secondary school–aged children. This chapter will review opportunities for anti-stigma programming from preschool to professional education, drawing on evidence-informed practices wherever possible.*

PRESCHOOL (PRE-KINDERGARTEN)

Research has shown that children can distinguish between deviant and normal behavior by the time they reach preschool. [260] Concept formation begins early in life and becomes less intensive as children grow and become adults. Parents, members of the community, other children, and children's media are the first to influence the formation of concepts. Parents, in particular, influence concept formation by what they say and what they do, often unaware of the influence they have. Children remember their parents' comments about other people's behavior, or behaviors around people with disabilities, for example, and use these to develop their own attitudes. [261]

Young children passively store parental and societal attitudes without being able to critically examine or dispute them. Beginning at age 3, children are able to distinguish between socially salient categories, an awareness that is typically accompanied by strong preferences for their own group. This increases until the age of 7 or 8. [262] Once formed, it is difficult for humans to undo concepts, reorder things, or develop new concepts. To do so causes uncertainty, feelings of lesser competence, poorer performance, and a feeling of enhanced danger. Therefore, efforts to reduce mental illness stigma must begin in early childhood in time to prevent the formation of stigmatizing concepts. [261]

Mental health advocates have increasingly considered directing anti-stigma efforts to young children before their attitudes are well-formed and firmly entrenched. [263,264] One approach may be to support and educate parents as to how to prevent stigmatizing concept formation in their children, such as being aware of their language and behaviors and limiting children's access to television shows that denigrate or otherwise stigmatize characters who are emotionally or behaviorally different. [261] In addition to role modeling, childhood educators recommend picture books with accompanying discussions and storytelling as ways to promote social inclusion and diversity. [264] The lack of anti-stigma programs designed to support parents in developing non-stigmatizing attitudes in their children is an important missed opportunity, especially in close-knit nuclear families where there are not multiple generations to participate in early childhood development and provide diversity of beliefs. [261] It is likely that differences in the acceptability of such programs would vary by country depending on a number of factors, including

---

* The age ranges for educational levels given in this chapter are approximate and may vary by country.

normative parenting practices and more general cultural levels of openness and tolerance.

PRIMARY SCHOOL (AGE 5 TO 13)

Children in primary school react negatively to people with a mental illness. Once formed, these attitudes have been demonstrated to remain relatively consistent over time. In 1986, for example, Weiss examined preferences for social distance toward people in seven groups (*normal*, *physically handicapped*, *emotionally disturbed*, *mentally ill*, *mentally retarded*, *crazy*, and *convict*) among 577 children ranging from kindergarten to grade 8. [265] At every grade level a clear preference hierarchy emerged, which remained relatively stable over time. Where the first-ranked group indicated the least amount of social distance (attributed to *normal* people by students in every grade), *mentally ill* was ranked fourth among kindergarten children and was ranked fifth thereafter. *Crazy* was ranked sixth in all grades but grade 8, where it was ranked seventh. These results show that social perspectives about labels such as *mental illness* or *crazy* have developed and become stable by the time children enter kindergarten. As Weiss noted, "crazy people are apparently regarded with the same fear, distrust and dislike and perceived as a threat by young and older children and adults alike" (p. 18). In a subsequent longitudinal study, Weiss was able to contact 34 of the original 65 kindergarten students who were still enrolled in the school district. [266] Comparing social distance from their kindergarten scores to their grade 8 scores, grade-specific hierarchies were again noted, and results were nearly identical to those of the previous study across all groups. By grade 8, those described as *mentally ill* had moved from fourth rank to fifth rank and those labeled as *crazy* had moved from sixth rank to seventh rank. Only *mentally retarded* individuals were viewed with greater tolerance in grade 8 than in kindergarten, perhaps because of an increased emphasis over time on special education and integrated classrooms for children with learning disabilities.

Children's ability to understand more complex topics such as mental illnesses increases with age such that older children (grades 5 through 7) have a more sophisticated understanding than elementary school students (grades 1 through 4). By the age of 7 or 8, children have clear beliefs about the causes of psychological problems and can provide explanations for disordered peer behaviors. [267] This means that younger children may have difficulty relating to or retaining didactic anti-stigma messaging. To overcome this problem, Pitre and colleagues used puppets to engage 324 school children in grades 3 to 6. [259] Three puppet plays depicted characters with schizophrenia, dementia, and depression/anxiety. Each play took approximately 45 minutes to present. Results were promising, indicating positive change on three of the six scales used, including a scale measuring stigmatization. Third-graders displayed a limited knowledge of mental illnesses, asking, for example, whether their dog could get a mental illness.

Ventieri and colleagues evaluated a two-lesson education program for 228 fifth- and sixth-graders (aged 9 to 12) in Victoria, Australia. [267] The intervention had the following main messages:

- Anybody can get a mental illness.
- People with mental illnesses can recover.
- People with mental illnesses are not to blame for their condition.
- Mental illnesses are not caused by being weak or lazy.
- There are treatments that can help people who have a mental illness and alleviate their symptoms.
- Stigmatizing attitudes have an adverse impact on the quality of life of those with a mental illness.
- Negative language can play a role in perpetuating mental illness stigma.
- There is a need to pay attention to the words used when describing people with a mental illness.

Evaluation results showed that children improved their knowledge, attitudes, and social distance scores 1 week following the intervention, and these changes remained at the 4-month follow-up, with only small reductions in effect. These results support the idea that children in primary school are developmentally able to understand and retain information about mental illness and mental illness–related stigma. The authors noted a readiness to learn about sophisticated subjects when the subject matter was tailored to the appropriate developmental level. They also noted the importance of ongoing classroom support and booster sessions to ensure that gains were not lost. Finally, they recommended including significant others, such as parents, and adopting whole-school approaches that would see mental health education included in primary school curricula.

In a study of seventh- and eighth-graders in the United States (N = 193), Wahl and colleagues [268] noted some inconsistencies in their knowledge, particularly about the symptoms associated with specific disorders. With respect to stigma-related constructs, the investigators were surprised that the majority of students recognized that people with a mental illness are often treated unfairly (72%) and shown negatively by the media (66%). Students also endorsed many positive attitudes, such as agreeing that people with a mental illness deserve respect (90%) or disagreeing that people with a mental illness are violent and dangerous (53%). Social distance items were mixed. For example, most students indicated they would be comfortable talking to someone with a mental illness (78%) or making friends with them (71%). However, less than half (42%) would be willing to invite someone with a mental illness to their home or to work on a class project with them (41%). Only 14% indicated they would be willing to go on a date with someone who had a mental illness. While most students reported positive attitudes, a sizeable minority (15% to 31%, depending on the item) reflected stigmatizing responses, suggesting an environment with a substantial undercurrent of negative and socially distancing views.

Most would agree that teachers, indeed entire school systems, are in a pivotal position to influence the attitudes and behaviors of young children through schoolwide programs promoting diversity, tolerance, and after-class social activities; creating accepting class environments; and offering activities that promote awareness and inclusion. [269] Yet, teachers preparing to work in elementary school settings often receive little or no professional training in attitude formation or information about acceptance of children with disabilities. [269] Simple and easy-to-use toolkits and lesson plans for teachers exist, but they have seldom been formally evaluated against stigma-related outcomes. [270] The following are some notable examples of teacher supplements and lesson plans that have been developed to educate primary school children about mental illness–related stigma.

Eliminating the Stigma of Differences

This is a three-module curriculum targeting sixth-graders that is designed to be delivered in the course of a week. Each hour-long module contains a didactic component, a group discussion, and homework exercises. The first module addresses the bases by which others are judged to be different; stigma and ways to end it; and mental illness treatments and barriers to care. Modules 2 and 3 address specific mental disorders such as Attention Deficit Hyperactivity Disorder, anxiety, and depression. The content is intended to stimulate empathy. A video is provided to orient teachers to the content and aims, but the supplement was designed to appeal to teachers who could implement it without specialized training. [271]

Painter and colleagues evaluated the effectiveness of this intervention among 721 sixth-graders in Texas. [270] The curriculum intervention consisted of 3 hours of material delivered by teachers over a 3- to 6-day period. PowerPoint slides were prepared to promote classroom discussion and a teacher's guide provided suggestions for questions, in-class exercises, and homework. The curriculum improved a wide range of knowledge and attitudes such as recognition of mental illnesses, positive orientations to help-seeking, stigma awareness and action, and increased optimism about treatment. The effect on social distance was weak. Measures of avoidance, discomfort, and social distance did not differ from the control group, but items pertaining to less intimate forms of contact, such as being friends or neighbors, or eating lunch with someone with a mental illness, did improve. Additional conditions that were evaluated included a contact-only group, where students received two 10-minute lectures from individuals who had experienced a mental illness and a social marketing group that had informative posters and bookmarks. Neither of these improved the outcomes.

To further test the efficacy of this supplement and its effect over time, Link and colleagues randomized sixth-graders to one of the same three conditions: the curricular supplement, a class where two individuals with bipolar disorder gave a 10-minute in-class presentation, and a class where teachers displayed posters for 2 weeks and provided students with bookmarks that demonstrated the use of person-first language. [271] Data were collected at 6, 12, 18, and 24 months. As in the previous study, neither the contact nor the social marketing interventions were significant for any of the outcome variables. Students who received the curriculum supplement showed statistically improved knowledge and attitudes and a significant decrease in social distance that persisted to the 2-year follow-up. Effect sizes for changes in knowledge and attitudes were moderate, but smaller for social distance. Youth who received the curriculum who had high levels of symptoms at the outset were 3.5 times more likely to seek treatment during the follow-up period, compared to a control condition.

Breaking the Silence: Teaching the Next Generation About Mental Illness

This supplement has been used throughout the United States and elsewhere over the past 10 years and has reached approximately 3200 students. [272] The program is designed for upper elementary, middle, or high school students (roughly grades 6 to 12) and is delivered in three class sessions within a week. What is notable about this toolkit is that it was developed by teachers who were also parents of children with a mental illness. It is a group of teaching packages including lesson plans, games, stories, poems, and posters. Students learn the early warning signs of major mental illnesses, that mental illnesses can be treated, and how to recognize and combat stigma.

Wahl and colleagues evaluated the effectiveness of the lesson plans in seventh- and eighth-graders from four schools in different parts of the United States (N = 193). [272] One class from each school received the instruction and one served as the control. Data were collected immediately before and after the intervention (about 1 week apart) and again at 6 weeks. Students who received the special instruction showed higher knowledge, more positive attitudes, and reduced social distance, and this was relatively unchanged at follow-up. Examining individual items showed more mixed results. For example, only two of the social distance items showed a statistically significant change: willing to have someone with a mental illness as a neighbor (59% to 71% respectively) and willingness to go on a date (15% to 25% respectively). Despite important improvements in specific social distance items, overall social distance remained low. For example, at post-test only about half of the students indicated they would be willing to invite someone with a mental illness into their home or work on a class project. One in four indicated they would be willing to go on a date. Results suggest the social distance content of the curriculum may need to be improved but also demonstrate that content can be delivered by teachers without special training using simple tools such as this supplement.

The Science of Mental Illness

Watson and colleagues evaluated a teacher supplement, *The Science of Mental Illness*, that targets students in grades 6 through 8. [273] It involves five or six 45-minute lesson plans that can be implemented by teachers without special training. This program takes a decidedly biological stance (which the literature subsequently demonstrated to be associated with increased stigma in the general public, among health professionals, and among people with a mental illness). [274] Teachers in 16 U.S. states provided pre- and post-intervention data on 1566 students. Students' knowledge and attitudes improved, but the curriculum was most effective in reducing negative attitudes among the subgroup of students who initially expressed the most stigmatizing views. Social distance was not measured.

These studies demonstrate that elementary school children are developmentally able to absorb mental illness and anti-stigma messages. They also demonstrate that simple curriculum supplements can be successfully implemented by teachers without special training, making them a feasible and cost-effective method of anti-stigma programming in elementary school settings. It is also interesting that two studies demonstrated sustainability of knowledge and attitude change over the short term (6 weeks) and longer term (2 years). Finally, the mixed results with respect to social distance measures suggest that significant work needs to go into the development of elementary curriculum supplements to ensure that they follow best practice principles for anti-stigma programming, particularly in avoiding a heavy emphasis on biological and medical models and ensuring that social contact is provided in the context of an engaging and interactive educational opportunity for students that includes time for discussion, questions and answers, and face-to-face interaction.

Children who are disliked by their school peers are often targets of aggression, rumors, taunting, and rejection. [269,275] Damage to self-esteem and reluctance to seek or accept treatments are among the negative outcomes associated with stigma-related ostracism and rejection. Consequences such as these may be particularly important during preadolescence and adolescence, when children are acutely aware of the judgments of their peers, and when the onset of many psychiatric disorders occurs. [268]

Interventions targeting secondary school students are typically of two types: (1) traditional educational sessions describing mental illnesses and stigma in an effort to help students become more knowledgeable and accepting and (2) contact-based education where individuals who have experienced a mental illness tell their recovery story to students, then engage in interactive discussions with opportunities for questions and answers.

In their meta-analysis, Corrigan and colleagues identified 19 studies that targeted adolescents using either traditional or contact-based educational formats. [148] Both approaches yielded statistically significant effects with respect to improved attitudes and behavioral intentions (typically measured with a social distance scale). However, traditional education had a stronger effect on attitudinal change and contact-based education had a stronger effect on changes in behavioral intentions. Both were in the medium range of effect sizes. In both cases, in-person contact had a stronger effect than video contact. The nature of the interventions provided was often poorly described in the original studies, and there was no evidence that developmental differences were considered. A limitation of meta-analyses is that program content, study designs, and measures are not comparable across studies. Thus, while results such as these can provide us with general guidance, they do not help us understand what specific components to include in anti-stigma programs targeting adolescents. In their literature review of interventions targeting secondary school students, Sakellari and colleagues also noted that while educational interventions tend to be poorly described, most seem to include factual information about the signs, symptoms, and causes of mental illnesses, which is something that may increase social distance. [276]

Koller and Stuart evaluated 21 contact-based interventions targeting 5047 Canadian high school students (grades 9 through 12) using pooled data from across the programs. [277] All of the interventions followed the same study design and used the same standardized instruments, making results directly comparable across studies. Programs contributed data as part of an evaluation network developed under the auspices of the Opening Minds anti-stigma initiative of the Mental Health Commission of Canada. The main outcome was a measure of social acceptance (constructed as a behavioral proxy). Eighteen of the 21 studies showed a statistically significant improvement immediately after the intervention. However, there was statistically significant variation across studies in the magnitude of the outcomes obtained. Several programs adopted intervention approaches that were not supported by best practice evidence and obtained significantly negative results. Programs differed in the amount of time they spent within the classroom and the levels of teacher and school engagement they received. Specific content, such as the extent to which interventions emphasized biological explanations for mental disorders and the ratio of didactic to interactional material, also differed. Overall, males were 40% less likely to pass the threshold for expressing non-stigmatizing views. When males and females were analyzed separately, males who self-reported a mental illness were 60% more likely to be non-stigmatizing; however, self-disclosed mental illness was not significant for females. While these results support the use of contact-based education as an anti-stigma tool in high schools, they also highlight the importance of basing interventions on evidence-based practices.

Programs that are relevant to students' personal experiences and developmental context resonate more broadly. In an effort to address common programmatic shortcomings, Murman and colleagues tested a novel youth-focused intervention entitled Let's Erase the Stigma (LETS). [278] High school students met weekly for a school term in an extracurricular club with a club advisor (typically a teacher) to discuss mental illness–related stigma and anti-stigma activities that they could undertake. The club promoted peer-to-peer interaction and included components of social contact. Students put topics in a suggestion box, and these were used to start weekly discussions. There was no formal educational curriculum, and content was fluid. Students determined the activities that were of interest to them, including meeting with people who had a mental illness, watching videos or movies, organizing speakers, and so forth. Preliminary evaluation of the program was promising. Students who attended the LETS club had more positive attitudes, were less socially distancing, and were more likely to engage in anti-stigma activities. Although not targeted by the program, knowledge also improved. What is interesting about these findings is that the behaviorally oriented measures had larger effect sizes compared to attitudes or knowledge change. While this lends broad support for youth-centered programming, it is impossible to know what specific activities were most influential in bringing about these positive outcomes as there was no standardized content or clearly articulated theory of change. Finally, the students who were most interested in mental illness–related topics were likely the ones who attended the clubs, making it difficult to know if such an approach would be as effective among non-volunteers.

POSTSECONDARY SCHOOL (AGES 18 TO 22)

Because postsecondary school is a time when many students are living independently from their families, stigma has the potential to seriously undermine help-seeking for students who experience a mental illness for the first time. In turn, this can jeopardize their academic outcomes, future career paths, and overall health. Immense pressure to excel academically has been identified as a key source of stress in postsecondary environments. The climate of expectation reinforces beliefs that having mental health problems is an indication of failure. Students with mental health issues are seen as weak, inadequate, and poorly equipped to cope with academic demands. Mental health–related stigma is a barrier to full social engagement for these students and can undermine academic performance. Fearing stigma, students may fail to disclose or reach out for help. [279]

Although the number of intervention studies is growing in this area, it is difficult to draw out best practice guidance from them. Often they target small groups of students, such as psychology students, public health students, or special education students. [280,281,282] In 2013 Yamaguchi and colleagues were able to identify 35 studies targeting students. [283] Almost half targeted future professionals such as medical or nursing students. Most studies were hampered by a lack of methodological rigor, making results difficult to interpret. There was a high level of variability across studies in terms of their measurement approaches and their outcomes. Few interventions were described in sufficient detail to be replicated, and theories of change were noticeably absent. Over 70% of study participants were women, who are known to more easily change their attitudes. [283]

Reviews of the academic and policy literatures have highlighted a growing interest in schoolwide interventions that aim to create campus cultures that promote a sense of belonging for all students, not only those who experience mental health problems. [284,285] To date, however, there are few examples in the literature, so little is known about how to incorporate discrete mental health and anti-stigma programs into a comprehensive campus-wide framework or whether such an approach is effective in reducing stigma. An important exception to this is an intervention and evaluation project created by the advocacy organization Bring Change to Mind. [286] Their intervention targets the college as a community using a peer-to-peer empowerment model of leadership. Students work together in a club to design and implement anti-stigma programs based on best scientific principles and evidence. Student leaders look for opportunities to integrate anti-stigma efforts into the life of the community so that a broad range of students may be impacted, not just those interested in mental health. The approach is flexible and fluid, evolving as ideas grow. The goal is to create "safe and stigma-free zones." The research team followed a cohort of students for 2 years (n = 1193). Main stigma measures were general prejudice, college-specific prejudice, and college-specific social distance. Exposure to anti-stigma activities was measured at two levels: asking students to indicate how many sponsored events they had attended (active engagement) and identifying all of the events that they knew about but did not attend (passive engagement). All of the stigma measures declined over time, with a magnitude of change ranging from 11% to 13%. Active exposure also improved all three stigma measures, but the relationship was nonlinear. Reductions were small if respondents attended three or fewer events and much larger if they attended four or more. Passive exposure was not associated with general or college-specific prejudice. However, it was associated with more positive perceptions of the campus culture pertaining to mental health. This finding is interesting because it suggests that whole-campus approaches can impact not only those who are directly involved in intervention activities but also those in the broader student group. It suggests that the program may shift the larger campus culture surrounding normative attitudes and beliefs pertaining to mental illnesses. Because the interventions are grounded in specific campus communities, such an approach could have broad appeal.

POSTGRADUATE PROGRAMS FOR HEALTH PROFESSIONALS

As noted in Chapter 7, health professionals are often singled out by people with a mental illness as among the most stigmatizing of groups. Postgraduate programs for health professions provide a platform for promoting person-centered and recovery-oriented care to people with mental illnesses. They also can be places where stigmatizing beliefs are "professionalized" and poor-quality practices such as diagnostic or treatment overshadowing are allowed to develop and become entrenched.

Masedo and colleagues conducted a multi-centered study that focused on medicine, nursing, psychology, and occupational therapy students attending their last years in their programs in six universities in Spain and Chile (n = 927). [287] Medical students reported more negative attitudes toward mental health problems and the treatment of people with psychiatric problems. Medical and nursing students were more likely to subscribe to assumptions of dangerousness or lack of possibilities for recovery. They were also less likely to say they would disclose a mental health problem. Psychology students were most likely to minimize physical or medical problems and were more likely to disagree that people with mental health problems should have their physical health assessed. The authors noted that medical and nursing programs are more likely to be based on a biogenetic model with a more pessimistic view about recovery, whereas psychology programs often de-emphasize biogenetic explanations in favor of psychological trauma as a key determinant of psychopathology. These results demonstrate the importance of including anti-stigma programs in professional curricula and suggest that programs directed to medical and nursing students should include a recovery focus. A 5-year follow-up study of 100 medical students in Japan also showed that optimism about the effectiveness of early treatment significantly decreased over time, from 55% to 34%. [288]

Insufficient course content pertaining to mental health is common across many disciplines and likely contributes to professionals' negative attitudes and overall discomfort in dealing with mentally ill clients. Preceptorships, positive mental health placements or rotations, and having diverse opportunities to interact with people who are in recovery could positively influence professional outlooks and behaviors. Critical self-reflection may also raise awareness of the role of explicit and implicit bias in stigma. Finally, greater awareness of the social determinants of health, social justice, and social inequities faced by people with a mental illness would be helpful. [289] All of this would require a major overhaul of current curricula—something that professional educators are often loath to do.

The phrase "hidden curriculum" has been used to refer to the implicit learning that students do by observing their mentors and teachers, which ultimately influences care decisions. Whereas the "formal curriculum" transfers knowledge via traditional mechanisms such as lectures, small group activities, and online learning, the hidden curriculum is a process of acculturation through which students learn what is "good" and "bad" clinical practice. Perceptions of patient worthiness are one aspect of the hidden curriculum that guide actions that ultimately determine the quality and quantity of care provided. In their ethnographic field study examining the qualities of the worthy patient in tertiary-care teaching hospitals, Higashi and colleagues describe less worthy patients as those who cycled in and out of the hospital ("frequent flyers"); patients who had previously left against medical advice or were otherwise deemed to be "frustrating"; drug users and drug seekers who were viewed as exploiting the system for food and housing and not prepared to make changes to their behaviors; nonadherent patients who did not follow treatment plans, including those who refused to refrain from self-harming behaviors; defiant patients who behaved rudely or abusively; and elderly patients, as they were perceived as being too needy. [290] Physicians in training learned that it was acceptable to spend more time with and to devote more energy and resources to nicer, rewarding patients who had medical problems that were more easily "fixable."

Stuart and coworkers studied the opinions of medical teaching faculty in 23 academic teaching sites across 15 countries (Belarus, China, Croatia, India, Indonesia, Iran, Japan, Portugal, Romania, Russia, Scotland, Singapore, Thailand, Turkey, and the Ukraine). [291] Six questions on the survey addressed perceptions of psychiatric patients. The majority of the 1057 respondents indicated highly stigmatizing views such as psychiatric patients are emotionally draining (74%); they are not appreciative of the care they receive (48%); they are often less interesting to work with compared to other patients (48%); and working with psychiatric patients is not rewarding (39%). In addition, 90% thought that psychiatrists were not good role models for medical students and 84% thought that psychiatric patients should be treated in specialized facilities. Further, 57% thought that they should not be treated in general hospitals. However, only 7% thought that psychiatric illnesses do not deserve as much attention as physical illnesses. These results suggest that educators who are responsible for mentoring medical students have the potential to transmit stigmatized views, implicitly through the hidden curriculum or more explicitly through their attitudes and actions.

CONTINUING PROFESSIONAL DEVELOPMENT

Continuing professional education is widely believed to be a major facilitator of change in practitioner behavior. Continuing professional education involves the acquisition of new knowledge, skills, and attitudes to enable competent professionals provide high-quality care. Countries vary in the way in which continuing professional education is provided; however, most involve some sort of credit system for educational hours. Some countries, such as the Netherlands, have legislated recertification systems. Most rely on professional self-regulation, but countries are increasingly moving toward mandatory professional development programs that cover a spectrum of clinical, professional, and managerial activities. [292]

Unfortunately, the evidence base to support the effectiveness of professional development programs in reducing stigma and improving quality of care for people with mental disorders is meager. Intervention studies have typically focused on changing physician behaviors. Though nurses are often identified as a source of stigma, few are researching in this area, and fewer still are testing anti-stigma interventions. [293] Understanding how stigma affects the care provided by healthcare professionals can help determine what types of interventions might be effective in promoting person-centered and recovery-oriented care to people with physical and mental illnesses. The standard model of professional development that relies on conferences or brief workshops is unlikely to bring about desired changes in stigmatizing professional behaviors. [294] More intensive, practice-based approaches are needed—ones that focus on a range of outcomes such as knowledge about treatment and diagnostic overshadowing, attitudes concerning recovery or blame, and skill development to help professionals build a better rapport with their mentally ill clients.

One example of an intensive continuing professional program targeting physicians is provided by the Practice Support Program (PSP) developed in British Columbia, Canada. [295] The PSP targeted family practitioners and office staff to help them provide the best primary care possible for patients with depression and anxiety with comorbid chronic physical diseases. Five trained teams provided support for physicians across the province. Experienced physicians, termed "peer facilitators," taught the learning modules. Medical office assistants received training in mental health first aid to improve their comfort with patients with mental illnesses. A local psychiatrist and a mental health clinician attended training sessions and acted as expert resources. Training consisted of three sessions that were interspersed with two action periods during which physicians implemented their new knowledge and skills in their day-to-day practices. When learners regrouped for the face-to-face training sessions, they shared their experiences, challenges, opportunities, and solutions. A variety of educational materials were used, including videos, role-plays, demonstrations, and the development of action plans. Training took approximately 5 months to complete, and physicians were reimbursed for their training time. Pre- and post-test surveys (at 1 and 3 months) showed significant improvements in all of the outcome measures evaluated, and the changes were sustained over time. For example, 40% of physicians reported a decreased reliance on prescriptions for antidepressant medication and 67% reported increased job satisfaction. Stigmatizing attitudes dropped by 10%. Results suggested that anti-stigma initiatives directed toward clinical personnel, in this case family physicians, will be successful if they provide tools and decrease anxiety around the clinical management of patients with complex health and mental health problems. At the time of publication, 1400 of the province's 3300 family physicians had completed the PSP training. These results are promising as public health agencies and governments are increasingly asking family practitioners to take a principal role in mental healthcare and to improve the quality of care provided to existing mentally ill clients. They also highlight the level of commitment and infrastructure support that must be expended to bring about systemwide change.

As these results suggest, stigmatization by health professionals may be a result of their lack of skills to work effectively with people who have a mental illness. Skill-based training may improve confidence and comfort and, in turn, improve the quality of interpersonal contact between healthcare providers and their patients. Teaching healthcare providers "what to do to help" may be an important perspective to take to diminish clinical distance, improve client experiences, and promote higher quality of care. Also, given that many providers may be unaware of their implicit biases and how these might affect behaviors, it also may be important to consider approaches that take learners' readiness to learn (or readiness to change) into consideration. Ungar and colleagues recommend using a "stages of change model" as a way to assess learners' needs. [296] Using this approach, if health professionals do not recognize or believe their attitudes and behaviors are stigmatizing, then they would be considered to have "unperceived" learning needs and the main educational goal would be to increase awareness. If individuals already feel well attuned to the problem of stigma and consider that they treat people with a mental illness with respect and compassion, a heavier focus on actionable strategies may be more appropriate.

Khenti and colleagues provided a multi-component anti-stigma program to three community health centers in Toronto. [297] Such centers include a wide variety of health practitioners including nurses, nurse practitioners, physicians, social workers, dietitians, counselors, health promoters, and community health workers and provide a broad range of health and mental health services to vulnerable populations. The intervention was developed with input from center staff and clients. The main components included (1) the creation of site-based teams at each center to examine organizational policies and processes and develop anti-stigma action plans; (2) a series of educational workshops using contact-based education, didactic, and interactive components to promote anti-stigma and recovery-oriented competencies; (3) an anti-stigma awareness campaign involving posters aimed at promoting self-reflection and changing behaviors translated into multiple languages; (4) 10 recovery-based arts workshops involving clients and staff; and (5) a review of internal policies and procedures with the goal of identifying points of structural stigma (though only one center completed this). The development and implementation of this intervention took 5 years. Four of the 15 scales used to measure various aspects of professional beliefs and stigma showed statistically significant, albeit mostly small, improvements, ranging from 5.9% (opinions about mental illness), 8.4% (social distance toward heroin users), and 9.4% (recovery assessment for addictions) to 21.0% (stigma toward depression). Five scales showed declines, but only one was statistically significant: Stigma related to people with cocaine dependence dropped by 24.1%. The remaining scales all showed improvements, but none reached statistical significance—perhaps a function of the small sample size, which was as low as 88 for some of the follow-up surveys. Because the intervention was multi-focused, it is not clear which components may have resulted in positive or negative changes or whether the interventions resonated with some disciplines but not others. Because the intervention unfolded over 5 years, staff turnover posed a significant problem for the evaluation. The multiple scales used were time-consuming and resulted in many complaints from staff and supervisors. Refusals to participate and missing data were also problematic.

The optimal duration for anti-stigma interventions targeting healthcare workers has not been established, though longer interventions, such as those described above, appear to be the most promising. Mittal and coworkers compared two brief educational intervention involving 39 healthcare providers: 19 were randomized to receive a contact-based intervention and 20 were assigned to an educational group. [298] Both groups were a mix of physicians and nurses. A "booster shot" was given to each group 1 month after the brief single-session intervention. Neither the contact nor the educational intervention resulted in stigma reductions. While small sample size could have been a problem, the authors speculated that brief interventions alone were not sufficient to reduce stigma among healthcare providers, whom they described as a distinct group given their high levels of medical knowledge and high levels of contact with people with mental illnesses when they are at their worst.

POLICE TRAINING

Police are often overlooked for anti-stigma training, even though encounters between people with mental illnesses have increased as a result of community-based programming. Police are important gatekeepers to the criminal justice and mental health systems and have considerable discretionary powers. Additionally, when incidents occur with someone who is mentally ill, police have been known to overestimate dangerousness and overreact, sometimes with catastrophic consequences. [299]

Silverstone and colleagues have noted that the best methods for educating police officers remain uncertain. [300] Training has often targeted knowledge or attitudinal change without associated changes in behaviors. For example, the most widely used approach has been crisis intervention training, typically a 40-hour course to help officers de-escalate crisis situations and better interact with people who have a mental illness. While some studies have suggested that this approach may reduce hospitalizations, many have found relatively few benefits, with some researchers being highly critical of the approach. The following are two novel examples of programs that have successfully targeted police recruits and police officers in the field, both of which could be successfully replicated in other settings.

Contact-Based Education for Police Recruits

Hansson and colleagues introduced contact-based education into the curriculum for police recruits during their psychiatry training module. [299] It included an introductory lecture on attitudes toward people with a mental illness, including a video with actors who had experienced a mental illness; two 2-hour lectures by people with a serious mental illness describing personal experiences in managing their mental health and recovery; six videotapes containing authentic cases with people who had a mental illness (3 hours);

and advice from two people with a mental illness who were counselors and who provided information on how to best respond to people with a mental illness (4 hours). This was integrated into a 3-week course on psychiatry that was already part of the training. Students who received the intervention had improved attitudes toward people with a mental illness, were more positive about interacting with people with mental illnesses in the future, and had improved mental health literacy. The change in intended behavior is noteworthy and remained the same or better after 6 months.

Scenarios with Discussion

Krameddine and coworkers developed a 1-day program targeting police officers in an effort to improve their interactions with mentally ill individuals by using empathy, better communication, and de-escalation skills. [301] They used six scenarios where interactions were modeled between an actor who was portraying someone with a mental illness and a police officer. The scenarios were chosen with much input to reflect common police encounters with people who have a mental illness. After each scenario there was detailed discussion about the behaviors exhibited, including feedback from the actors indicating how they felt at certain times in the encounter (such as "I felt afraid when you came that close to me"). The main behavioral rating was provided by the officers' supervisor at baseline and at the 6-month follow-up. Officers were rated on their ability to communicate with the public, their ability to verbally de-escalate a situation, and their level of empathy in dealing with the public. There was a 10% improvement in these ratings, which was highly statistically significant. At the same time, there was no improvement in attitudes or understanding of mental illnesses, reinforcing the importance of targeting behaviors. These findings are also important because they underscore the potential effectiveness of brief (1-day) skills-based training for first responder groups.

SUMMARY

This chapter has discussed aspects of stigma-reduction programs in educational settings using selected studies to highlight important and outstanding issues as well as innovative or promising approaches. Despite research demonstrating that preschoolers are already forming stigmatized views, there is a dearth of programming targeting younger children or their parents. Programs and resources aimed at parents of preschool and young children would seem to be particularly useful in preventing stigmatizing attitudes from developing.

While programming exists for primary and secondary school children, there has been a heavy emphasis on teaching about specific mental disorders and their treatments. This approach has been increasingly criticized for promoting biogenetic explanations of mental illnesses, which increases the desire for social distance. [302] Curriculum components that use psychiatric language and labels may account for the common finding that social distance measures are less changeable than measures of knowledge or attitudes. It is important to move beyond literacy-based formats to approaches that fully incorporate contact-based education that include opportunities for students to interact with people who have experienced a mental illness. Research has shown that simple curriculum supplements and toolkits can help primary and secondary school educators enhance their teaching content. These need to be more broadly available for teachers at every level so that they may provide enhanced learning opportunities for their students. More thought needs to be directed to developing age-appropriate content that engages students at each developmental level. In addition, there is a need to change the educational content of teacher training with respect to mental illnesses and stigma.

There is insufficient course content pertaining to mental illnesses and stigma in postgraduate programs for health professionals, with the result that they graduate lacking the confidence and skills to provide care to people with a mental illness. In many settings a "hidden curriculum" may implicitly bias medical students from providing high-quality care to people with mental health problems or their family members. Although evidence is meager, helping medical students and healthcare professionals gain a range of skills, particularly in recovery-oriented care, may be helpful in reducing stigma.

Finally, most interventions are limited to a single session or lecture, and these are unlikely to be potent enough to improve social distance. Ideally, educational settings should adopt a whole-school approach and consider a range of activities that occur throughout the entire school year to improve the culture of the school with respect to mental illnesses and stigma. In addition, anti-stigma programs that omit the education of parents and preschool children are likely to be of limited success in creating lasting cultural change.

CHAPTER 9

Employment Inequity and Workplace Stigma

Despite human rights and employment equity legislation, people with mental illnesses face a number of barriers to employment. Because of stigma, not only is it difficult to get a job, but it is also difficult to keep a job. Yet, employment is a key factor promoting social inclusion and recovery for people with mental illnesses. Employers' knowledge of workplace adjustments (termed accommodations) that could support people with mental illnesses is often limited, and they may be reluctant to adjust the workplace or workflow to allow someone with an impairment to perform their job. This chapter examines workplace programs that target employers and employees, as well as vocational programs that are designed to help people with mental illnesses gain competitive employment.

Figure 9.1 depicts a cycle of employment inequity. [303] In this context, "employment inequity" is used as an umbrella term to refer to situations where someone is a denied a job outright, passed over for advancement, or precariously employed because of a psychiatric impairment without regard to their skills or capabilities. "Precarious employment" refers to work that is poorly paid, lacking in benefits, and insecure. In this figure, a psychiatric impairment triggers a stigmatizing societal response that leads to employment inequity. In turn, employment inequity leads to poverty and marginalization, which can deepen the psychiatric impairment, causing a vicious stigma cycle. Increasing impairments may give rise to system responses such as involuntary hospitalization or criminalization, which only deepen social and self-stigma.

People with mental illnesses identify employment discrimination as one of their most frequent stigma experiences. Historically, finding jobs has not been a priority of the mental health system. The tendency has been to adopt

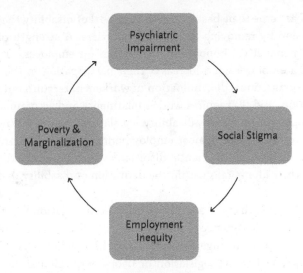

Figure 9.1 The cycle of employment inequity and disability
Adapted from Stuart H. Stigma and work. *Healthcare Papers* 2004;**5**(2):100–11.

minimal expectations and lower standards of achievement. Despite their willingness and ability to work, unemployment rates among people with a mental
illness remain high, some three to five times higher than their non-mentally
ill counterparts. [304]

DISABILITY LEGISLATION

Disability legislation is designed to support equal employment for people with
mental illnesses. Goss and coworkers describe the historical roots of disability
legislation as reflecting two dominant approaches. [305] One is illustrated by
the United States, which emphasizes free enterprise and individual rights.
The Americans with Disabilities Act (ADA) recognizes people with physical or
mental impairments as a minority group whose lack of power has prevented
them from being employed as a result of social prejudices. The other approach
is illustrated by the European tradition of state intervention and regulation,
which emphasizes employment quotas and antidiscrimination measures, such
as the French act of 1987 that required private- and public-sector firms to employ 6% disabled persons (small firms of under 20 workers were exempt). This
approach is also used outside of Europe, such as in Japan, where the Law for
Employment Promotion imposes quotas on employers to hire persons with
disabilities. [306]

   With the enactment of human rights legislation such as the Convention
on the Rights of Persons with Disabilities, most contemporary disability

legislation has come to be based on a social model of disability that promotes social inclusion by removing employment barriers. A strength of disability legislation is that it (1) imposes specific duties on employers to accommodate disabled employees and increases their participation in the workforce; (2) outlaws occupational discrimination of workers in recruitment, retention, and promotion; and (3) requires work adjustments and accommodations for disabled employees. However, disability legislation has not always provided the hoped-for protections against employment discrimination and inequity, particularly for people with mental disorders, who are protected only to the extent that their illness falls within the definition of disability under the legislation. [121]

One challenge is that the success of disability legislation rests on the actions of many people who need to modify rules, policies, procedures, physical spaces, and workplace arrangements. If any of these individuals hold negative attitudes toward disability legislation or people with mental illnesses, then they may not comply, which may have consequences for the system's role as a whole. Colker describes how the American media negatively portrayed plaintiffs under the ADA as receiving special perks and procedural protections for dubious disabilities. [307] She blames the negative and misleading news coverage for the public's negative perceptions of the ADA.

Negative perceptions of disability legislation are not restricted to the United States. For example, Vilchinsky and Findler explored the attitudes of 321 Israeli professionals from five occupational groups (employers, architects, lawyers, teachers, and social workers), all of whom occupy a central role with respect to enacting disability legislation. [308] The survey was conducted 2 years after the new law was approved. Results showed that participants were least in favor of the employment equity themes and that employers held the least positive attitudes. The authors speculated that professional identity was a key ingredient in attitude formation and may account for the more positive attitudes of teachers and social workers. They recommended including issues such as legislation and the rights of people with disabilities into business and health professionals' course curricula.

A second challenge is that employers may have insufficient knowledge concerning their legal obligations to people with mental health challenges. In the United Kingdom, Henderson and colleagues surveyed a random sample of employers in small, medium, and large businesses to determine if their knowledge and attitudes had changed during the time of a large anti-stigma campaign. [309] While there were some improvements in knowledge and certain attitude variables, almost three-quarters of employers indicated that potential employees should disclose mental health problems prior to recruitment, even though this contravened the legal provisions of the Equality Act of 2010, and there was no improvement over the time of the anti-stigma program. The majority reported that they did not know enough about the law regarding mental health in the workplace. These findings suggest that it is necessary for anti-stigma programs to include actions that will help educate employers about their legal obligations under employment equity laws both with respect to employing people with mental health problems and managing employees with mental health challenges.

A third challenge is that without clear incentives for compliance and disincentives for noncompliance, employers simply don't follow through with their obligations under the legislation. Heijbel and colleagues describe a situation where employers, insurance providers, and health systems all failed to respond to their obligations under Swedish legislation designed to reduce workplace absences by ensuring that employees had access to rehabilitation services. [310] The legislation required that individuals be subjected to a rehabilitation investigation after 28 days of sick leave. Only half of employees off work for more than 28 days received a rehabilitation investigation, demonstrating that neither the employers nor the regional social insurance office were fulfilling their statutory obligations.

A final difficulty with disability legislation is that claims of employment discrimination are difficult to make because they must be made by the disabled employee. They are also difficult to win. For example, Colker has described the ADA as a "windfall" for employers based on her analysis showing that defendants win in more than 93% of the cases decided at the trial court level and 84% of cases that are appealed. [307] This is largely the result of a narrow interpretation of disability under the ADA that excludes most mental illnesses. In an attempt to redress these and other problems, the ADA was amended in 2008 to provide a clearer definition of disability. [311]

WORKPLACE CULTURES

Employment equity legislation does not contain provisions that directly address issues of workplace culture or climate. Pervasive inequity is also linked to patterns of exclusion that are embedded in the informal social relations of a workplace. [312] Consequently, employer attitudes play a central role in the success of antidiscrimination legislation. Krupa and colleagues offer a theoretical model depicting the components of stigmatizing workplace cultures. [313] They based their work on a grounded theory analysis of a broad range of publicly accessible Canadian documents published between 1990 and 2003 reflecting the perspectives of diverse stakeholders. The final set of documents included 100 academic, 76 government, 138 popular press, five legal, and 107 from work initiatives across Canada. Examples of the type of documents reviewed included resource guides supporting consumer participation in the workforce from organizations such as the Canadian Mental Health Association, information brochures, government information documents, conference presentations, and academic journal articles. They also completed 19 semi-structured interviews with key informants. Information and interviews were then qualitatively analyzed. Workplace stigma was defined as "a disposition, in the work context, to act in a discriminatory manner towards persons with mental illness" (p. 416). In the workplace, stigma excludes those with a mental illness from full work integration. Workplace stigma is based on a number of assumptions that shape the culture—assumptions that differ from many of those held by the general public. Key among them was that people with a mental illness lack the competence needed to complete work tasks and meet the demands of the workplace environment. Others included that: (1) people with a mental illness are dangerous or unpredictable in the workplace; (2) they will compromise social interactions with colleagues and customers; (3) mental illnesses are not legitimate illnesses and are used as a license for dodging work responsibilities or receiving special privileges; (4) work is not healthy for people with a mental illness; (5) people with a mental illness cannot cope with normal workplace stressors; and (6) providing employment for people with a mental illness is an act of charity inconsistent with productivity goals. The strength of these assumptions and their salience to particular workplaces varied across different types of workplaces.

Tsang and colleagues also show how the nature and salience of stereotypical assumptions differ across workplaces, in part shaped by larger sociocultural forces such as how mental illnesses are understood in a particular society. [314] They compared worker concerns about hiring someone with psychosis in Chicago (to represent U.S. culture), Beijing (to represent traditional Chinese culture), and Hong Kong (to represent a mixture of Chinese and Western cultures). They tested the hypothesis that employer concerns would differ across locations, with the highest prevalence in Beijing, where traditional values that promote negative views of mental illnesses would be the strongest. Employers in each site were randomly recruited from small and medium firms to participate in an interview—40 from Chicago, 30 from Hong Kong, and 30 from Beijing. The two most frequent concerns expressed by Chicago employers were that the mental illness would detract from productivity and job performance (40%) and that there would be a safety threat to fellow employees and customers (33%). In Hong Kong, 87% of employers were worried about a safety threat and 60% were concerned about a potential relapse, whereas productivity concerns were less of a problem (33%). In Beijing, productivity concerns were the most frequent (43%), followed by safety concerns (40%) and the concern that the employee would bother, argue, or lose their temper with coworkers and customers (40%).

While it is largely assumed that negative stereotypes and employment concerns lead to discriminatory practices, workplace discrimination is difficult to document. Because it is illegal in many countries, employers may not admit to direct discrimination on self-report surveys. In addition, employees may not be aware of the full extent to which they have been discriminated against in employment settings. Hipes and colleagues designed a field experiment to assess the number of times a prospective employer showed interest by calling (termed "call-backs") a fictitious candidate received from a job posting bulletin board depending on psychiatric or physical disability status. [315] Despite having highly competitive credentials and claims to be fully recovered, applicants with a prior mental illness were 45% less likely to elicit employer call-backs compared to those with a prior physical illness (15% vs. 22% respectively).

WORKPLACE INTERVENTIONS

As the previous sections have demonstrated, assumptions and behaviors of workplace leaders are key to establishing workplace cultures that are respectful and supportive for all workers, but particularly for those with mental illnesses. In 2018 Gayed and colleagues conducted a systematic review of workplace programs directed to managers to help them improve employee well-being. [316] Ten studies were identified from among the 1332 articles screened, illustrating how little scholarship has been directed to this issue. These studies noted improvements in managers' understanding of mental health issues, their roles and responsibilities, their attitudes, and their self-reported behaviors, but too few studies examined employee outcomes to make any definitive statements about the efficacy of specialized programs in creating a psychologically supportive and inclusive workplace culture.

In 2010 Szeto and Dobson came to a similar conclusion after their review of workplace programs. [317] Programs were few in number, with little evaluation evidence to support their impact. Moreover, many programs had embedded assumptions that may have undermined their effectiveness, such as adopting a biological or disease model, which research has shown does little to ameliorate social distance. They also noted that most of the programs were more generic mental health programs rather than carefully targeted anti-stigma programs; indeed, most had no specific anti-stigma content. They questioned whether general mental health programs could reduce discriminatory behaviors or increase affirming behaviors. None of the studies measured changes in participants' behavioral outcomes, such as reduced social distance.

In 2013 Malachowski and Kirsh conducted a scoping review of interventions specifically targeting stigma reduction in the workplace. [318] Of the 22 studies identified, most had emerged in the previous 4 years and used an educational approach such as workshops, seminars, or internet resources. Interventions targeted different outcomes, typically knowledge and attitude change, and had mixed results such that no definitive conclusions could be reached. None of the interventions included personal contact with someone who had experienced a mental illness. The authors speculated that this may have been because it was considered to be too costly to locate, train, support, retain, and compensate speakers to be regularly involved in face-to-face interventions.

Despite growing calls to improve workers' mental health and the recognition that stigma in workplaces remains a pervasive challenge, examples of evidence-based anti-stigma programs targeting workplaces are still a rarity. [319] The following are examples of evidence-based programs have recently emerged.

The Road to Mental Readiness for First Responders (R2MR)/The Working Mind

R2MR is a 4-hour course designed to increase resilience among first responders and reduce mental illness–related stigma. [320] The program was developed by the Canadian Department of National Defence with the Calgary Police Services and the Opening Minds initiative of the Mental Health Commission of Canada. The program was adapted from the original R2MR program targeting military members to be applicable for police officers, then subsequently adapted for paramedics, fire services personnel, emergency call centers, and correctional officers. The program contains three components: stigma reduction through video contact-based education; information on mental health and illness using a continuum model designed to support self-management strategies; and resiliency skills (e.g., perceived ability to cope with adverse situations; ability to bounce back). An 8-hour version exists for supervisors and leaders with the same components but additional classroom discussion and skill-building tools.

It was implemented in 16 sites across Canada for supervisors and front-line staff in police, fire, corrections, emergency services, and paramedics (N = 4649 matched pre- and post-test surveys). A meta-analysis of the pooled data showed a standardized mean effect of 0.26, representing a weak but statistically significant effect in stigma-related attitudes and no statistically significant variation across studies in effect sizes. [320] The standardized mean effect for resiliency skills was 0.32, also representing a weak but statistically significant relationship, again with low heterogeneity across studies (20%). The lack of variability across programs suggests that it has wide applicability in diverse sites and highlights the importance of the 5-day preparatory training that facilitators received in order to provide the program to participants. At the end of the train-the-trainer program, facilitators received a pass/fail grade. Facilitators were not certified to teach the program if they did not pass. Although the effect sizes were small, the programs were brief, and effects were consistent with outcomes reported in the literature. The gains documented following the intervention were retained after 3 months. The program was subsequently renamed "The Working Mind" and a generic version was created for general workplaces. [321] Across eight replications, the generic program resulted in moderate reductions in stigma and increased self-reported resilience and coping abilities. This study is noteworthy because it used video-based contact of someone with a mental illness, rather than face-to-face contact, which may be more feasible to manage in workplace settings.

Beyond Silence Versus Mental Health First Aid (MHFA)

One of the key reasons for implementing anti-stigma programs in work settings is to promote help-seeking so as to reduce absenteeism, lowered productivity (referred to as "presenteeism"), and short- and long-term disability. Moll and coworkers compared a newly developed contact-based educational program customized for healthcare workers to a widely used mental health literacy training program (MHFA). [322] The literacy program teaches the signs and symptoms of various disorders and approaches to treatment. Beyond Silence used a contact-based educational approach, with programs being co-led by two peer educators (defined as healthcare workers who had previous personal experiences with mental illnesses). This program was designed to promote early intervention and support for workers with mental health issues. Both programs included approximately 12 hours of group-based education. The final sample included 192 participants who were randomized to the interventions. The primary analysis examined behaviors related to reaching out to help others at work and help-seeking behaviors. No change was noted in either of these outcomes in either of the programs. Both programs enhanced knowledge about mental health issues, reduced negative and stereotypical attitudes, and improved attitudes toward help-seeking. Increases in knowledge were significant in both programs at 3 and 6 months. A 3-month follow-up qualitative study with 18 participants identified five key design principles that appealed to program participants [323]:

1. Contact-based education/sharing personal stories. Even though this was not a part of the MHFA training, it was something that participants sought out.
2. Contextually relevant information. Beyond Silence participants valued the opportunity to reflect on and discuss issues and scenarios that were directly relevant to their day-to-day work. MHFA participants liked the structure of reviewing illnesses and saw this as a refresher.

3. The opportunity to explore varied perspectives. Both programs were given to a diverse range of employees and thus provided opportunities to share insights and perspectives from different areas of the organization.
4. Sufficient time to integrate and apply learning. The Beyond Silence participants received 12 hours of training over six 2-hour sessions with five online sessions. They appreciated the time between sessions to integrate and apply the information they were learning. Unfortunately, this also led to a higher dropout rate. MHFA was offered for 12 hours over 2 full days.
5. Organizational readiness and support. Both programs received support from senior executives, front-line managers, union representatives, and health and safety providers.

Based on the qualitative findings, the authors concluded that despite finding no differences in the desired behavioral outcomes, the contact-based approach offered by the Beyond Silence program seemed to add value to participants. This study is interesting because it illustrates the importance of including qualitative data collection in order to better understand potential key ingredients. It is also noteworthy because, despite positive changes in attitudes, neither intervention translated into concrete behaviors.

Mates in Mining (MIM)

The MIM program is interesting because it specifically targets nonprofessional "blue-collar," mostly male employees in the coal mining industry. [324] Developed in Australia, it is a peer-support model that includes three levels of training. All workers participate in a 1-hour general awareness training to improve knowledge of mental illnesses and warning signs, and to encourage workers to offer support to colleagues in need. Volunteer "connectors" are provided with an additional 4 hours of gatekeeper training to provide skills for identifying risk factors and engaging with coworkers. Additional volunteers are provided with a 2-day Applied Suicide Intervention Skills Training (ASIST) to prepare them to support a crisis situation. An onsite peer-support program is complemented by field officers, case management support, and a 24/7 help line. A process evaluation showed the program was feasible and acceptable. [325] With respect to stigma-related items, there was no difference in the number of respondents who felt that an employee experiencing a mental illness would be treated poorly in the workplace if people found out about it or the likelihood of seeking help for a mental health problem. In a follow-up study collecting data at baseline, 6 months, and 18 months, the likelihood of help-seeking improved over the three time points, particularly help from nonprofessional sources. [324] Attitudes towards mental health problems (with items reflecting expectations of stigma) also improved. However, employees with high levels of psychological distress were less likely to indicate they would seek help, suggesting that fear of stigma may have been particularly salient for this subgroup. While the stigma-related content of this program is difficult to gauge, it does illustrate the potential feasibility of targeting anti-stigma activities to male-dominated workforces, who are typically unaccepting of mental health programming.

Looking After Wellbeing at Work (LWW)

LWW is a 2-day mental health intervention targeting firefighters. It was developed with input from local mental health practitioners and service users using a mental health promotion framework. Facilitators used a manual to ensure consistency across offerings. Four key objectives were (1) to promote understanding of the influence on well-being at work; (2) to enable people to look at their own and others' well-being at work; (3) to increase awareness of the experiences of mental health problems; and (4) to promote positive approaches to people with mental health problems. Moffit and colleagues evaluated the effectiveness of the program in improving knowledge and promoting positive attitudes toward mental illness compared to two other interventions (MHFA and an hour-long leaflet session). [326] Participants were randomly allocated to one of the three conditions. Sample sizes were small: 31 for LWW, 41 for MHFA, and 17 for the leaflet session. Both LWW and MHFA were associated with statistically significant improvements in knowledge and attitudes. The leaflet session had no effect. In qualitative interviews participants described improvements in their ability to respond to mental health problems and had changed their attitudes. No behavioral outcome was assessed.

As these courses illustrate, workplace programs tend to focus on general mental health and wellness rather than stigma reduction, though this may be a component, such as in The Working Mind. While knowledge and attitudes are often improved, it is impossible to know if these programs have a similar effect on behavioral outcomes, such as social distance, because none included a behavioral measure. Dewa and Hoch show the importance of targeting behaviors. [327] They explored the cost-effectiveness of a workplace stigma program on short- and long-term disability. In an organization of 1000 employees, a stigma program could break even if it could prevent 2.5 short-term disability claims or reduce the length of short-term disability absences by 7 days. It is likely that programs such as The Working Mind that provide skills so that workers can manage their own mental health and identify and help manage problems experienced by colleagues are likely to lead to a greater reduction in disability days and offer a better return on investment for employers. However, this will need to be confirmed in future research.

WORKPLACE ACCOMMODATIONS

Although workplace accommodations are legally required in many countries, there is little guidance for employers on how to meet these responsibilities in the case of a mentally ill employee. [313] Workplace accommodations are intended to be individualized to meet an employee's particular needs so that the requirements of the job may be fulfilled. However, employees with mental illnesses are less likely to receive accommodations compared to employees with physical disabilities. Accommodations could include assistance from an employment support worker or job coach, flexible scheduling, reduced hours, reduced pace of work, extended training, work from home, or modified job duties. Because workplace accommodations for people with mental illnesses are less tangible compared to those for people with physical disabilities (such as a ramp or modified workspace), employers are often at a loss. In addition, accommodations may be jealously viewed as special and undeserved dispensations by colleagues, particularly in highly competitive environments. If not handled well, they may actually worsen an employee's image and increase stigma. [328]

To be eligible for a workplace accommodation, one must first disclose a mental disorder, the catch-22 being that this may trigger a host of stigmatizing behaviors from supervisors and work colleagues. Consequently, workers are often hesitant to disclose their mental illness in order to negotiate supports. Dewa conducted a large survey of worker attitudes toward mental health and disclosure in Canada (n = 2219). [329] The majority of respondents (61.4%) indicated that they would tell their current manager if they had a mental health problem. Of these, 79.4% said that a good relationship with their manager would be key to their decision; however, a decision to disclose would be based on a combination of other factors, such as having supportive coworkers, organizational policies, and practices. Workers would not disclose if they thought it would jeopardize their careers, if they knew of bad experiences of other workers, or if they feared losing friends. Men, workers over the age of 60, non-white employees, and managers were more likely to express concerns over disclosure. These results show that there is a significant subgroup of workers (some 40%) who would not disclose to their managers if they had a mental health problem and that certain subgroups are at higher risk of struggling silently with their mental illness. They also highlight the importance of management training that imparts skills in creating a supportive, secure, and stigma-free workplace culture as well as organizational policies and practices that are supportive of workers' mental health. It is important to note that willingness to disclose to a manager whom a worker already knows and trusts is quite different than disclosing during a recruitment interview, particularly if a potential employee expects to be stigmatized. These situations are likely to require different approaches for destigmatization.

VOCATIONAL PROGRAMS AND SUPPORTED EMPLOYMENT

A range of vocational programs have been developed to help people with serious mental illnesses acquire employment opportunities. Over time, these have moved away from segregated token economies to placements in competitive jobs. Key outcomes of vocational programs include employment, wages, quality of life, self-esteem, confidence, and reduced future hospitalizations. To date, however, studies have not directly examined the effects of supported employment programs on experiences of stigma and social inclusion. Critics of supported employment have argued that many supported employment approaches still adopt segregation solutions and reinforce assumptions that only noncompetitive work activities are appropriate for those with a mental illness. Therefore, an important benchmark of success is the extent to which supported employment solutions offer people with mental illnesses real-life work opportunities in the competitive labor market. [313] The following is a brief overview of some of the dominant models that have emerged.

Sheltered Workshops

Historically, employment opportunities for people with disabilities have been shaped by policies emphasizing segregation. Sheltered workshops typify this thinking. They included mostly disabled people with little connection to non-disabled people; involved low-skills tasks that were repetitive and monotonous, and undertaken for little or no payment; and were often run out of segregated or protected environments such as psychiatric institutions. The goal of sheltered workshops was to provide basic work skills and habits to individuals with low levels of functioning who were deemed to be unable to enter the competitive workforce. [330]

Sheltered workshops drew criticism because they were insulated from the economies of the competitive labor market and thus allowed program administrators to ignore labor rights and employment contracts, such as offering a minimum wage. Because paid employment is necessary to survive in many modern economies, sheltered workers were denied the right to full citizenship under the pretense that they were being protected. Over time, proponents of the workshop system found it increasingly untenable to mask the charitable and symbolic nature of sheltered work. Sheltered workshops were contested in the context of the growing wave of disability rights activists. Activists and their allies argued that sheltered workshops were the tailings of oppressive regimes that undermined social inclusion by warehousing disabled people out of economic sight. Over time, sheltered workshops gave way to alternative vocational programs such as supported employment (described in more detail below). [331]

An unusual exception to the segregated workshop model can be found in Nanjing, China, where a series of factory-based sheltered workshops have been developed. [332] A unique cultural factor promoting this model is that most urban residents are employed in state-run enterprises where their job is guaranteed for life, regardless of whether or not they become mentally ill— a large incentive for employers to develop programs to support their return to work. Starting in 1973, all of the 34 neighborhood administrative offices began setting up factory-based workshops. In 1988, legislation required all 80 factories in the city with over 3000 workers to establish a sheltered workshop. Psychiatrists from the local hospitals make regular visits to the workstations to examine and treat patients and give mental health training to the medical and administrative staff who are responsible for the day-to-day management of the workshop. Workers do 4 hours of work per day (2 in the morning and 2 in the afternoon) and spend the remainder of their time involved in vocational and rehabilitation activities. They return home at night. This approach gives family members respite and peace of mind as their relative is looked after during the day. An evaluation of the patients who were enrolled in the first four factory workshops was undertaken comparing them to patients diagnosed with schizophrenia receiving outpatient treatment as usual. [332] Although the sheltered workshop group had a longer psychiatric history, more hospital admissions, and a more severe clinical picture at the time of enrollment into the study, those who spent the average of 4 months in the sheltered workshop had significantly better social functioning and less psychopathology as measured by standardized scales. Fewer of the workshop patients relapsed or were admitted to hospital over the 2-year study period. These findings show that "un-sheltered workshops" that are fully integrated into community and factory settings have the potential to remove social and economic marginalization for people with serious mental illnesses. Given the unique situation with respect to workplace obligations to provide a job for life, it is not known whether this specific model could be easily generalized to other cultural settings with different employer obligations.

Transitional Employment

The clubhouse model of psychosocial rehabilitation has been in existence for over 65 years and has an international presence. The earliest clubhouse was developed by discharged patients from Rockland State Hospital, who formed a self-help group in 1948. Clubhouses are open to anyone who has had a mental illness. They are strengths-based and provide opportunities for members to work alongside staff in the day-to-day operation of the clubhouse. They also offer various supported employment programs, key among these being transitional employment. [333]

Transitional employment offers some opportunity for employment in the competitive labor market. The goal is to help clients gain self-confidence and independence that will help them obtain competitive employment in the broader labor market. Vocational staff create close links with local employers who agree to have rotating groups of clients over an extended period of time. The jobs belong to the vocational agency, even if they are located in the community setting. Jobs are typically part-time, can be taught quickly, and require few skills. When individuals experience a relapse, another member is sent in their place, with the result that employees are largely interchangeable. [330]

According to Phillips and Biller, transitional employment is a model that was developed at Fountain House in New York, one of the oldest and largest clubhouse programs for people with serious mental illnesses. [334] Transitional employment is the primary vocational opportunity within Fountain House. It enables members to refine work skills and habits, build confidence and interpersonal skills, determine their ability to work in the competitive job market, establish job references, and assist in seeking independent employment. Over time, members are involved in different job placements, which is considered to be necessary for them to build vocational experience and establish a work history. According to Fountain House's website* 30% of Fountain House members are employed compared to 15% of American adults with serious mental illnesses.

In their systematic review of clubhouse studies, McKay and colleagues were unable to find anything that compared the transitional employment program to other supported employment approaches, such as the widely used Individual Placement and Support (IPS) model (described in more detail below). [333] Although many of the studies reviewed had important methodological limitations, there was some evidence that the clubhouse model was successful in promoting employment, reducing hospitalizations, and improving quality of life. A strength of the clubhouse model is that there are clear guidelines for implementation that can be used to accredit programs. A limitation is that many of the clubhouse services have not been systematically investigated, so it is impossible to know which have the best results. They call for additional research in order to better understand the active ingredients and to ensure that effective programs are not discontinued by funders due to a lack of evidence. Clubhouses such as Fountain House have been widely adopted in both low- and high-income countries, illustrating that this model, if demonstrated to be effective, could be transferable to a variety of cultural settings.

*https://www.fountainhouse.org/get-involved/employment-partners

Social Enterprises

Social enterprises (also called affirmative businesses) have developed to provide employment opportunities for people with disabilities that are more normalized and less segregated from the wider economic community than sheltered workshops or transitional employment programs. Social enterprises use a community development approach to overcome factors such as competition and individualism that perpetuate employment inequities for people with serious mental illnesses. They are entrepreneurial and capitalize on collective strengths. Warner and Mandiberg provide a compelling overview of the social enterprise movement as it has migrated from Europe (where it was first developed) to most countries in the world. [335] Social firms often gravitate to labor-intensive market niches because this allows them to maximize employment and minimize capital investment. Examples include cleaning services, handmade products such as wooden toys, organic food production, or food preparation and catering. The first social enterprise was developed in Italy in 1973 to provide employment for deinstitutionalized patients. By 1994, the annual revenue of the Trieste Cooperative had grown to $5 million; by 2004, it had grown to $14 million. Similar cooperatives have emerged in Germany (with the largest number of social firms outside of Italy), Britain, Ireland, Australia, Japan, Korea, the United States, and Canada. A key to their success is government policies and statutes that favor social enterprises, such as defining them as community interest companies that can access philanthropic investments.

Krupa and colleagues are one of the few teams to have compared outcomes of a traditional sheltered workshop that transitioned into an affirmative business using the sheltered workshop resources. [336] Individuals employed within the traditional sheltered workshop made on average one Canadian dollar per hour. This rose to $6.84 per hour in the affirmative business, which was consistent with the standard minimum wage at the time and well above the standard range for sheltered workshops. Employees in the social business viewed their wages as evidence of their legitimacy. This, and the respect they received in the workplace, their interest in capturing a market share, and their economic well-being contributed to their identity as productive and contributing members of the community. However, disincentives associated with income security policies that limited participation in the workforce caused some distress and restricted the number of hours they could work without having portions of their disability payments clawed back.

Lysaght and colleagues note that social firms can offer employment opportunities for people with serious mental illnesses that are not available otherwise. [337] Although some would view social firms as sheltered work environments, participants view them as competitive businesses that provide real jobs as well as a supportive and therapeutic milieu. Employees gain experience and confidence, and many move on to competitive employment in the community. Thus, social firms can have an important impact on employability and subsequent job retention. However, a wide range of social business models exist, and some may have limited contact with the general public. Nevertheless, this model has the potential to increase engagement in employment for individuals who are otherwise hard to employ.

In order to consider social enterprises as an anti-stigma activity, it is first necessary to consider potential mechanisms of action. In a qualitative study, Krupa and colleagues suggest that social enterprises have the potential to reduce stigma by influencing public perceptions of competency, legitimacy, and value. [338] They also found a range of tensions, such as a medicalized view of competence occurring when administrators interpret problems with products or services as stemming from the mental illness; viewing employees who receive mental health supports as vulnerable patients rather than workers; customers responding in an overly polite manner to business issues in order to protect employees; and greater public negativity toward certain types of products, such as food handling or preparation. In the enterprises they studied, the majority of employees were part time and did not give up government financial assistance. While working in a social enterprise lessened their financial dependence, it did not eliminate it, and few employees moved out of the business to take competitive employment in the community. In this way, workers continued to be associated with disability and stigma, creating a public image of the working poor.

Supported Employment

Supported employment programs provide individual placements in community jobs that pay at least minimum wage and allow any person to apply for them. They facilitate job acquisition and often send staff to accompany clients on interviews and provide support if the client is employed. Programs differ in the extent to which vocational and rehabilitation staff are integrated into the program. Clients obtain real-world jobs, which promote their social inclusion and work against stigma. The most studied and evidence-based model is the IPS model. [330] Supported employment has become the standard of care within psychiatric rehabilitation, with nearly two-thirds of people enrolled in supported employment programs obtaining competitive employment compared to less than a third of those in other vocational programs. However, program successes have ranged from as low as 25% to as high as 75%, depending on fidelity to the program and employment specialists' training and skills. [339]

Mueser summarizes the IPS model according to eight principles, which, when implemented with fidelity, result in superior employment outcomes [340]:

1. Eligibility to participate is based on client choice with no exclusion criteria.
2. Vocational and clinical services are integrated and regular meetings are held to coordinate services.
3. The focus is on competitive employment as opposed to sheltered or partially sheltered types of work. This means that jobs must pay a competitive wage and must occur in community settings, and the pay is owned by the person, not the vocational program.
4. The search for work begins almost immediately after the client joins the program. Based on a place-train approach, lengthy prevocational training to get the client ready for work is not required.
5. Client preferences for type of job placement (e.g., work setting, location, schedule, total hours, distance from work, and amount and type of social interactions required) are respected.
6. Employment specialists develop relationships with a network of employers to facilitate optimal job matches, as research shows that clients who have to manage their job search on their own often give up.
7. Once a job has been obtained, individualized job supports are provided by the employment specialist and mental health treatment team. This may be to help workers solve problems at work, access their clinical treatment team, get directions regarding how to perform new job tasks, or obtain suggestions regarding workplace accommodations. If a job ends, the employment specialist helps the client plan for the next job experience.
8. Counseling is provided on the effects of work income on government disability and health benefits.

SUMMARY

There is a growing awareness that people with mental illnesses have the desire and ability to work in competitive jobs, particularly when work cultures are supportive and accommodations are made. Unfortunately, many workplace cultures are toxic for people with mental illnesses and employers don't know or are unwilling to make accommodations, arguing that they cause undue hardship. Colleagues may be unsupportive and view workplace accommodations as special and undeserved perks. Charges of workplace discrimination under disability legislation have been difficult to win, largely due to the overly restrictive interpretations of "disability" that exclude many people with mental illnesses. Workplace mental health programs are relatively new on the scene, so more research is needed to demonstrate their effectiveness as anti-stigma tools. More often they target general wellness rather than stigma reduction, and results have varied widely across studies. While some have demonstrated changes in knowledge or improved attitudes, none have demonstrated improved social equity.

This chapter has presented vocational programs that promote employment for people with a mental illness as a potentially powerful anti-stigma tool. Such programs continue the treatment and recovery process beyond clinically based mental health programs, which are themselves stigmatized; help people normalize their lives and integrate into their communities; boost self-confidence and self-esteem; provide marketable skills; and improve quality of life. Some vocational programs, such as transitional employment or affirmative businesses, have demonstrated good outcomes with respect to employment, quality of life, and feelings of self-worth. However, restrictive disability legislation has often limited the hours that employees can work without benefit clawbacks, with the result that they have been less than successful in creating financial independence for their workers. Future development of anti-stigma programs that target employers, supervisors, and employees would be useful. In addition, it would be important to create tools that could be used by progressive companies to identify and eliminate stigma that may be embedded in organizational policies and practices.

CHAPTER 10
Using Technology to Fight Stigma

Anti-stigma advocates have made good use of "older" technologies such as television, movies, radio, theater, and printed materials, to name a few. Newer digital technologies are increasingly viewed as a panacea for mental health promotion and stigma reduction. Not only can they reach vast audiences, but they are also cost-effective, relatively easy to produce, and feasible to implement in today's technological age. Interventions specifically focusing on stigma reduction are relatively new and largely untested. Theories of change explaining why certain interventions might reduce stigma are lacking and the extant literature is relatively silent on evidence-informed approaches. Because the field is so new, with few intervention studies, technology should be viewed as an emerging practice that still requires evidence. This chapter reviews some examples of the approaches that are experimenting with technologies to reduce stigma and promote prosocial behaviors.

VIDEO-BASED CONTACT

In Chapter 6 we outlined how films can demonize or humanize people with mental illnesses. Films also have been a powerful medium for educating healthcare students and members of the public about different aspects of mental illnesses and their treatments. For example, *A Beautiful Mind* shows the horrors of schizophrenia and the challenges associated with treatment and rehabilitation. It also shows the fears of the public as it portrays the impact of schizophrenia on Nash's friends and colleagues, some of whom were nervous and hypervigilant around him and others (students) who taunt him. Others, like *Rain Man* or *Forrest Gump*, depict what it is like to have autism spectrum disorder or a learning disability. [341]

Given the power of film, there has been considerable interest in the effectiveness of video-based interventions as a surrogate for face-to-face contact-based education. Videos are cost-effective to create and are scalable to broad geographic areas. They may be incorporated as part of a formal, didactic educational effort, or they may be accessed independently online. Once posted, they can remain available for extended periods of time; thus, large libraries of contact-based videos can be created and easily accessed by interested viewers. For all of these reasons, video-based interventions are enticing for anti-stigma advocates. What is not yet clear, however, is whether they work or what formats should be followed to maximize success. Systematic reviews have been helpful in pulling the available evidence together, but they have been limited in their ability to draw definitive conclusions. Even considering differences in study designs, the outcomes measured, and the quality of evidence, video content is often poorly described, and videos are compared to a wide range of alternative conditions, including face-to-face testimonials, didactic education, and no video conditions. At times, videos are embedded in more complex interventions, making it all the more difficult to tease apart the various effects. For example, the national anti-stigma programs described in Chapter 5 have created numerous videos to educate, promote health, encourage help-seeking, and reduce stigma. Examples of the emerging evidence base for video contact follow.

Corrigan and colleagues conducted a randomized experiment to compare the discrete effects of a 10-minute contact-based educational video containing a personal narrative from someone who had a mental illness to a 10-minute didactic educational video addressing myths and facts. [342] The same person was used in each video, the only difference being that mental health status was not disclosed in the didactic educational video. They measured stereotyped attributions immediately before, after, and 1 week following the program in 244 college students. The contact video led to positive changes in four of the 10 dimensions measured (pity, empowerment, avoidance, and segregation), and effects were still evident after 1 week. Two of the dimensions showing positive change were proxies for discriminatory behaviors (avoidance and segregation). The only significant change for the didactic education video was in beliefs about responsibility for the illness. In addition, education also led to a significant drop in the belief that power is important for people with a serious mental illness. These results cast doubt on the use of video-taped didactic education and provide some support for the use of contact-based education using video formats.

Tergesen and colleagues [343] also evaluated the effects of didactic and contact-based videos on stigma among medical students in Nepal. Two randomized trials were conducted. In the first (n = 94), the video focused on depression. The didactic video used content for depression education as recommended by the World Health Organization. The testimonial was from a person who experienced depression. The control condition was no video. In the second study (n = 213), the contact-based videos included depression and psychosis. Interventions were given in a single 1-hour session. In the first study, both the didactic and contact-based groups had similar, significantly lower social distance scores compared to control subjects. In the second study, neither intervention had an impact on social distance. The authors speculated that the greater stigma associated with psychosis may have elicited more social distance, and pairing psychosis and depression may have led to increases in negative stereotypes about depression. These results are interesting because they support the view that mental illnesses should not be bundled when developing anti-stigma interventions as each disorder may be stigmatized in different ways.

Short videos have been used successfully to improve attitudes among nursing students in the Czech Republic. In their study of 499 nursing students from 21 schools, Winkler and colleagues randomized students to receive a short video, a seminar, and a leaflet (control condition). [344] The 45-minute seminar described the state of the art with respect to the stigmatization of mental illnesses. The video intervention contained three short (2 to 3 minutes) clips of people who had experienced a mental illness. At post-test, all three conditions showed improvements in attitudes. The flyer and the video showed small improvements (d = 0.25 and 0.49 respectively). The seminar had a medium effect (d = 0.61). These effects were diminished across all interventions at 3 months; however, the seminar intervention retained the strongest effect. Regarding intended behaviors, effects were smaller: negligible for the flyer (0.04 at post-test), small for the video (0.35), and medium for the seminar (0.58). By 3 months, these had all significantly weakened (0.04 flyer, 0.21 video, 0.26 seminar), suggesting the need for regular booster sessions.

Whitley and colleagues describe a method known as Participatory Video. Using this approach, a group of marginalized people jointly script, film, and produce an educational video. [345] Videos can be documentary style or can be a digital story of someone's experiences. Once completed, community screenings are organized to educate viewers and catalyze change. Because the videos are rooted in local community experiences, they are thought to be more engaging and resonate better with local audiences compared to more generic offerings. Whitley and coworkers developed and tested a participatory action video that they named RADAR (Recovery Advocacy Documentary Action Research). Three working groups produced 26 videos (double the original target) ranging in length from 2:20 to 22:05 minutes. They showed their videos to local audiences and assessed their impact on knowledge, attitudes, and behaviors with a brief, five-item questionnaire. Screenings were attended by 1,542 people, 1,104 of whom completed the brief survey. The item most endorsed was a behavioral item ("My behavior to people with severe mental illness will change for the better in light of this video"). On a 5-point agreement scale, the average score was 4.03. The next most endorsed item pertained to changing attitudes toward people with severe mental illness (mean = 3.94). In subsequent focus groups with a small number of viewers, the videos were described as relatable, providing a well-rounded normative portrayal of people, and having moved beyond the label to show individuals as active citizens. These results show that participatory videos are a feasible and potentially effective anti-stigma strategy that can benefit the individuals creating them as well as those who screen them. The researchers have packaged the RADAR model so that it can be implemented by people with mental illnesses elsewhere.

Another participatory model that holds promise is Photovoice. Tippin and Maranzan used Photovoice to create video content to convey the experience of living with a mental illness and its associated stigma. [346] In a randomized controlled trial of 303 undergraduate psychology students enrolled at a Canadian university, they demonstrated that empathic concern elicited by the video photos was associated with decreased stereotypes (dangerousness) and decreased desire for social distance. As many anti-stigma interventions use cognitive strategies, these results underscore the importance of eliciting a positive emotional response from viewers.

Janoušková and colleagues conducted a systematic review to determine whether video-based interventions could be used to destigmatize mental illnesses among young people. [347] Of the 1426 articles initially identified in their search strategy, 23 studies were included for the final analysis. Eleven of the interventions focused on people with schizophrenia. Of the 51 outcome measures used, only four studies examined social distance and two studies measured actual behavior, with mixed results. All the studies were conducted in high-income countries. Some aspects that were associated with successful video interventions were not dissimilar to those for face-to-face contact-based interventions, as follows:

1. The most effective videos included an element of social contact, such as a narrative of a person who had experienced a mental illness, accompanied by expert information provided by a mental health worker such as a psychiatrist.
2. The majority of effective videos emphasized recovery and the potential to lead a good life despite having a mental illness.
3. High and moderate levels of stereotype disconfirmation were more effective than videos with low levels of disconfirmation.
4. Videos that were entertaining were popular, and repeated exposure improved attitudes.

Most often, video content is generic and designed for members of large groups, such as students or the general public. However, it can be tailored to meet the interests and needs of specific groups. For example, Hamblen and coworkers developed a unique web-based gallery of 77 veterans who have experienced Post Traumatic Stress Disorder and received treatment, entitled AboutFace. [348] Viewers can hear the stories of individual veterans to learn about how PTSD and stigma has affected their lives. Stories are unscripted and filmed in natural settings, with storytellers looking directly at the camera to create an intimate and authentic peer-to-peer experience. There is a section where viewers can receive advice from peers or clinicians (e.g., about seeking help or the effects of PTSD on family members). This is a new program that has not yet been rigorously tested, but it does illustrate the power of the web to host multiple peer-based educational experiences designed to reduce stigma. Preliminary investigation has shown that the website is feasible and usable by veterans, suggesting that tailored peer-to-peer contact-based education may offer a more nuanced approach.

A key outstanding question is whether well-designed videos can produce a lasting effect, as most studies have follow-up periods of 6 months or less. Research has pointed out the limited effects of one-time interventions and the need for booster sessions, but it has not been clear how often these sessions should be provided. To begin to address this question, Yamaguchi and colleagues [349] conducted a randomized controlled trial that examined the effects of contact-based videos. Stigma outcomes were measured at baseline, immediately after the intervention, and at 1 month, 12 months, and 24 months. Participants (n = 249) were undergraduate and graduate students from 20 colleges and universities in Tokyo. Students in health-related programs such as psychology or medicine were excluded. For the contact-based intervention, participants watched a 30-minute film containing interviews with two men with schizophrenia, a woman with obsessive–compulsive disorder, educational lecture slides with an audio explanation of mental illness, and information on resources. An internet self-study group provided the first comparison. Participants were given instructions to search the web for information using two keywords, "schizophrenia" and "mental illness." The control group played computer games for 30 minutes. At 24 months, both the social-contact group and the internet self-study group showed statistically greater knowledge compared to the control group. Behavioral intentions were also significantly better in the social-contact group compared to the control group at 24 months. There was no difference in previous contact with someone with a mental illness. These results suggest that a well-designed social-contact intervention may be effective in improving behavioral intentions over the long term.

ENTERTAINMENT EDUCATION

Entertainment education has been a popular strategy for promoting health messaging in order to improve awareness, increase knowledge. and change behaviors. Entertainment education occurs when prosocial messages are embedded into plots for dramatic appeal or to deliberately influence health behaviors. [350] For example, in Chapter 6 we described how SANE Australia worked with producers and scriptwriters of a popular teen soap opera to create a storyline where one of the main characters experienced schizophrenia. Non-stigmatizing behaviors and recovery messages were modeled by the character's friends and family. Another example is viewing an accurate and empathetic movie followed by educational trailers. [351]

Entertainment education is considered to be superior to other forms of persuasive media communication, which can cause a boomerang effect, because it overcomes psychological resistance. Viewers are drawn into the story and thus don't feel forced. When they identify with and like the central characters, they are less likely to counterargue or discount the message. Less engaging forms of persuasive communication, such as media campaigns, may be perceived as a threat to one's freedom, even if the message is in the best interest of the individual, and it may cause the individual to engage in more of the discouraged behaviors in order to assert independence. This is why some persuasive messages fail to produce the desired changes and may result in an increase in unhealthy behaviors. [350]

DIGITAL GAME PLAYING

It has been estimated that more than 1.8 billion people worldwide play video games, and for many, it is a daily activity. A recent review of video games showed that the dominant mental illness stereotypes normally identified in the news and entertainment media also appear in the gaming world. [352] However, there is a growing realization that video games may also be used to transmit positive and prosocial messages. For example, digital game playing has been used to prevent and treat various psychological disorders, such as depression or anxiety. So far, however, their use in addressing stigma has been limited. Proponents of digital game playing identify several advantages, such as providing immediate feedback that can further motivate the user. They are thought to improve the learning process and are easy to use. Once developed, they can be widely disseminated.

As one example, Cangas and colleagues developed a video game called *Stigma-Stop* to familiarize young people with selected mental disorders (depression, agoraphobia, schizophrenia, and bipolar disorder) and demonstrate how to actively help people with these disorders in different situations. [353] Students were able to choose the gender of their preferred avatar. The game requires the player to visit each one of four young people with a disorder to interact with the characters and indicate which reactions they consider most appropriate in given situations. At various points in time options appear regarding the interaction, and the player must choose the correct interaction to continue with the game. A number of mini-games embedded in the program allow the player to learn specific information about the illnesses. The game was tested on 552 students aged 14 to 18 in Almería, Spain. Participants were randomly assigned to the game or a control group with video games unrelated to mental health. The game group showed statistical improvements in stereotyped views of people with a mental illness, particularly with respect to dangerousness, though behavioral outcomes such as social distance were not measured. Nevertheless, the authors considered that the *Stigma-Stop* game could be a useful component of a more fulsome anti-stigma strategy including personal contact with people who have experienced a mental illness.

Ferchaud and coworkers compared the effects of playing a video game to watching the same video game on stereotypical attitudes and social distance. [354] What is interesting about this experiment is that the avatar in the game has psychosis, so the player experiences some of what it is like to have this mental illness. The game uses 3D microphones to give the illusion that the protagonist is hearing voices. The videogame tested was *Hellblade: Senua's Sacrifice*, which is set in the age of the Vikings. Senua is on a quest for the soul of her dead lover. This game was designed with mental health experts and people who had psychosis. It was widely acclaimed for its accurate and respectful depiction of psychosis, winning several important gaming awards. It was tested on 198 university students, aged 18 to 35, from Florida State University. Participants played or viewed the first 45 minutes of the game. Results showed significantly reduced social distance (corresponding to a weak effect) but no significant difference in stereotyping—an interesting finding given that social distance is usually harder to change. The analysis showed that the effects were mediated by the extent to which players were transported into the game and the extent to which they identified with the main character. In a subsequent study Mullor and colleagues showed the video game had effects on stigma attributions that were similar to contact-based education and a talk from a professional. [355]

Research focusing on college or university students, particularly psychology students, is limited in its usefulness as it tells us little about whether digital games would be of use more broadly. Hanish and coworkers developed a digital game-based training program to help managers in the United Kingdom promote employee mental health and reduce workplace stigma. [356] They depicted warning signs and recommended actions along a mental health continuum ranging from health, acute stress, chronic stress, and illness. At several points in the training the manager had to assess the employee's mental state along the phases of the continuum. Afterward the player was given feedback. The training occurred in a single 1.5- to 2-hour session. Data were collected before, after, and at 3 months on 48 managers working at a single site. Knowledge, self-efficacy to deal with a work situation, and overall stereotypical attitudes all improved over time, and effects were sustained over 3 months. However, the item-specific questions pertaining to work-related stereotypes—workability and competency—did not change. Also, attitudes related to helping an employee if they got behind in their work remained relatively negative. Neither did managers express any intentions to promote employee mental health. These findings suggest that digital games may not be broadly applicable as an anti-stigma tool, though more research on diverse groups is needed.

INTERNET INTERVENTIONS

Like other forms of technology, internet sites are appreciated for their ability to attract wide audiences and offer cost-effective interventions. Griffiths and colleagues examined the destigmatizing effects of two depression internet sites on personal stigma and expectations that others would stigmatize someone with depression among Australian adults. [357] Participants (N = 525) were people with high levels of depression measured by standardized scales. They were randomized to a depression literacy site (BluePages), a cognitive behavioral program site (MoodGYM), and a control condition. For both of the internet sites, participants were directed to read different specified sections over a 5-week period. All participants were contacted weekly by an interviewer. For the control condition, participants were asked questions about their perceptions of depression. Both internet sites showed small but statistically significant reductions in personal stigma. The depression literacy site had no effect on the extent to which participants considered that others hold stigmatizing views, and the web-based therapy condition showed increased perceived stigma relative to the control group. As neither intervention specifically addressed stigma, the mechanism of action for reduced personal stigma or increased perceived stigma is unknowable. The authors speculated that messages of treatability contained in both sites may have decreased the extent to which participants self-stigmatized and increased the perceived controllability of people with depression to others, particularly for those in the cognitive–behavioral therapy site.

Shann and colleagues provide an example of an online intervention targeting workplaces. [358] Their goal was to create an online intervention that would reduce leaders' depression-related stigma and develop their skills to manage depression in the workplace. The intervention was developed by Beyond Blue in Australia with input from industry and employer associations, unions, and mental health professionals. Information was provided using a variety of techniques, including an introductory video of a manager talking about mental health in the workplace, short segments of information to be read, and interactive exercises. They measured affective stigma (emotional response), cognitive stigma (to capture beliefs about employees with depression), and behavioral stigma (intentions to exhibit relevant behaviors). Both affective and behavioral Stigma improved but showed small effect sizes. There was less emphasis on traditional psychoeducation in this intervention, possibly explaining the lack of change in the cognitive stigma component. Qualitative data captured as part of the study highlighted a number of barriers preventing leaders from taking appropriate actions to create a mentally healthy workplace. These included a lack of organizational readiness for changing political priorities, a lack of commitment from senior leaders, and levels of stigma in the workplace. As a result, organizations that most needed the program—those that were the most stigmatizing—were the least likely to promote mentally healthy workplaces.

An illustration of a computer-assisted anti-stigma educational intervention is provided by Finkelstein and colleagues. [282] They enrolled 193 graduate students (99% female) studying to be teachers of children with special needs from a university in St. Petersburg, Russia. Students were randomized to one of three conditions: a computer-assisted education program, a reading group, and a control condition. The computer-assisted education provided a series of short messages followed by a multiple-choice question. The curriculum was provided in three sections, with each section being followed by a quiz. Three components of stigma were addressed: lack of knowledge or misconceptions about mental illnesses (a cognitive dimension), feelings toward people with a mental illness and treatments (emotional dimension), and behavior toward people with a mental illness (behavioral dimension). The reading group received printed materials containing similar content. Students had two study visits with a follow-up interval of 6 months. Attitudes and social distance improved in both computer and reading groups immediately after the intervention. These gains largely disappeared after 6 months in the reading group but remained significant in the computer group. With respect to social distance, significant improvements were noted in both groups that persisted over the follow-up period.

SOCIAL MEDIA

Social media are internet-based applications that allow users to create and exchange user-generated content. Estimates from the United Kingdom suggest that 67% of the adult population and 69% of children aged 12 to 15 years use social media.[*] In the United States, 70% of Americans use social media, and this number has been steadily increasing over time.[†] Social media use is

[*] https://cybercrew.uk/blog/social-media-statistics-uk/
[†] https://www.pewresearch.org/internet/fact-sheet/social-media/

dramatically less in many low-income countries such as Tanzania (20%), India (20%), or Indonesia (26%). However, it is on the rise in low-income countries, with many approaching levels of use typical of high-income countries. [359]

Social media, particularly social networks, are promising vehicles for health information for a number of reasons. They can reach vast audiences with little difficulty. Messages can be delivered via existing contacts, likely making them more influential than if they were sent as part of a traditional marketing strategy. Unlike other web-based interventions, social media often have high levels of user engagement and retention, and they allow users to actively engage and generate content. [360]

As yet, social media have not been well studied as an anti-stigma force, but they do show promise. As Betton and colleagues point out, many individuals have brought mental health conversations to social media, and what is interesting about these is that personal narratives are often at their core. [199] Social media platforms such as Twitter also have been used to successfully launch anti-stigma protests. One example is when thousands of people took offense at a "mental patient" Halloween costume advertised on a national supermarket's website. The topic went viral and tweets were passed across networks. The story was picked up by the national media and was the lead story. The offending retailer, and others who carried the costume, removed them from sale, apologized, and made donations to England's Time to Change anti-stigma initiative. The sharing of tweets by thousands of people created a sense of solidarity. People with lived experience of a mental illness posted selfies with text indicating what a "real mental patient looks like" (p. 443). This illustrates the ability of social media platforms to be the launch site for bursts of protest that can be initiated by one individual and then widely shared. As demonstrated in this example, collective action has the potential to influence mainstream media and policy. For all of these reasons, large anti-stigma programs such as New Zealand's Like Minds, Like Mine or Australia's Beyond Blue have incorporated social media into their programming.

Livingston and colleagues describe a social media campaign that targeted youth in British Colombia, Canada. [361,362] The intervention, In One Voice, was a brief social media intervention to (1) increase activity on a youth-focused website and (2) improve attitudes and behaviors toward mental health issues. The campaign included a 2-minute public service announcement featuring a popular local hockey player who was speaking in support of a teammate who had announced that he had experienced depression. The campaign ran for 3 months, during which time it was featured in a variety of hockey-related venues (e.g., the National Hockey League's all-star game, the Canucks for Kids telethon) and forums (sports and news media). It was deliberately designed to reach youth through social media (e.g., listservs, Facebook, Twitter, and YouTube). For the initial evaluation, a marketing research firm developed two survey samples, before and 2 months after the campaign was initiated, each composed of 403 youth. Results showed that use of the website increased, but there was no effect on attitudes or social distance. Additional funding was secured to conduct a second evaluation 1 year after the campaign. The third sample consisted of 438 youth who did not complete the prior surveys. The proportion of the sample that remembered the campaign grew from 25% at time 2 to 49% at time 3, and the elevated activity on the website noted in the first evaluation was sustained. Small but statistically significant reductions in negative attitudes and social distance were now noted, which had not been present at time 2. Self-rated abilities to help others with a mental health problem or engage in positive behaviors (such as seeking information) did not change. These findings are interesting because they suggest that interventions using social media have the ability to accumulate in their effects over time, perhaps because, once posted, they remain available for viewing; there is no real end date. These results confirm previous research showing the difficulty of changing behavioral outcomes with brief marketing campaigns, but also point to the importance of conducing follow-up research beyond the usual 3 or 6 months.

E-CONTACT

E-talk or E-contact is a computer-mediated form of communication involving members of different groups who interact online, either face to face or through text chatting in real time. It is considered to be a bridge between direct and indirect forms of contact. E-talk may be a more feasible strategy than direct contact, particularly when groups are physically or psychologically divided. Since the onset of the pandemic, many people have become used to computer-based meetings using platforms such as Zoom. Maudner and colleagues experimentally evaluated text-based E-contact for reducing stereotyped attitudes and social distance toward people with schizophrenia in Australian psychology undergraduate students. [363] Participants (N = 133) were randomly assigned to one of three groups: intergroup E-contact, intragroup E-contact, or no contact. Students were informed that they were participating in an online, text-only chat with an interaction partner under the supervision of a moderator. They were to develop a chat program to be delivered to university students. Their interaction partner and moderator were not live, and their responses were standardized and preprogrammed. The interaction was divided into two stages: introduction, during which time the interaction partner disclosed having experiencing schizophrenia, and cooperation, when they worked together on their collaborative task. Results showed that the intergroup contact condition was significantly related to reduced fear, anger, pity, stereotyping, and social distancing compared to the other groups.

Rodríguez-Rivas and colleagues incorporated E-talk into a multicomponent program to reduce the stigma of mental illnesses. [364] It included project-based learning, clinical simulations with standardized patients, and E-talk with real patients. Forty university students in Santiago, Chile, were randomly allocated to the intervention program or an online educational program on cardiovascular health. Both interventions lasted about 14 hours and occurred over 2 days. Large reductions in stereotypes and attributions were noted ranging from standardized effect sizes of 0.83 to 2.33, indicating exceedingly large differences of one to two standard deviations between pre- and post-test scores. No differences were noted for students in the control condition. Unfortunately, the components of the intervention were not evaluated separately, making it difficult to judge the specific effects of the E-talk portion. Also, it is not known how the intervention would have influenced social distance as this was not measured. Nevertheless, this is a promising example of how E-talk, if effective, could be used in the context of a multicomponent stigma-reduction program.

White and coworkers think there may be some advantage to using text as opposed to face-to-face E-contact. [365] They suggest there may be less anxiety when communicating with stigmatized people through text rather than through face-to-face communication. Texts remove visual cues and allow respondents greater control over their responses and self-presentation. When using text, participants have time to think, type, and edit their responses before sending. Text may also be less threatening when interacting with people who elicit fear or are viewed as dangerous, such as individuals with schizophrenia. Finally, text may encourage greater self-disclosure because participants remain more anonymous than if they were talking face to face. As E-contact has been found to reduce stereotypes and improve attitudes in a wide range of religious and cultural groups, it stands out as a promising new practice for stigma-reduction programs.

SIMULATIONS

It has become popular to use simulated experiences to help individuals better understand and increase their empathy for people with disabilities. Because these interventions are thought to promote empathy, they have been assumed to be effective in reducing mental illness–related stigma. For example, a number of interventions have been developed to simulate hallucinatory experiences. Ando and colleagues have conducted a systematic review to determine the anti-stigma properties of such simulations. [366] Ten studies were included in their analysis, eight of which were conducted in the United States, one in Australia, and one in Canada. Auditory hallucinations most often used audio recordings and headphones. Participants were asked to do routine tasks while hearing negative or derogatory voices. All but one used the "Hearing Voices that Are Distressing" training package, though only one used the full package that included a pre-simulation DVD with filmed social contact. None of the studies included members of the general public. Most often participants were healthcare students, typically undergraduate psychology students, but also nursing students, medical students, and correctional officers. Two randomized trials measured social distance, and both found that social distance increased following the simulation. Two randomized trials examined empathy, and both found that empathy increased. Effects on attitudes were mixed. Qualitative studies suggested that the simulated experiences did provide participants with the experience of cognitive impairment, emotional and physical discomfort, and poor task functioning. Yet, results showed that improved empathy did not lead to reduced social distance—opposite to the working hypothesis. Instead, they showed that simulated hallucinations increased desire for distance, thereby increasing stigma.

By way of a more detailed illustration, Brown randomly assigned 127 participants to a 16-minute portion of the Hearing Voices simulation in the lab or walking around campus. [367] The simulation contained sounds (a faint rhythmic sound) and voices such as repeated phrases, whispering, or laughing. Phrases contained a mix of material: benevolent neutral (you are the one); derogatory (you suck, loser); paranoid statements (everyone is laughing at you); and commands (stop it). Those on campus were told to walk around, purchase a pack of gum at a store, then pick up a map at the library. Those in the lab condition listened to the simulation while being monitored by a research assistant for signs of distress (of which there were none). Results showed a decreased willingness to interact with individuals with a psychotic disorder. No differences between the members of the two groups were noted for the fear/dangerous scale or the negative emotions scale.

Avatars have emerged as a novel therapy to reduce auditory hallucinations in people with schizophrenia. [368] They allow face-to-face interaction with a digital representation whose speech matches the pitch and tone of the persecutory voice. The voice becomes increasingly conciliatory, allowing the person hearing the voice to gradually gain control over the relationship. Another approach to simulation uses embodied conversational agents (ECAs) or avatars who have online conversations with users. They are designed to simulate face-to-face interactions. They have been used in a variety of different contexts, but rarely to address mental health–related stigma. A strength is that they can be easily applied to different contexts simply by changing dialogue scripts, looks, or behaviors to better resonate with the target audience. One study evaluated whether ECAs could be effective in reducing stigma related to anorexia nervosa among 245 undergraduate psychology students in Australia. [369] Participants were randomized to receive two short (4 minutes) videos featuring two actresses discussing their experiences with anorexia (a contact video) or a similarly timed ECA group with two segments (an individual describing personal experiences and a doctor discussing causal factors). Two attitude scales were developed to assess the extent to which participants saw anorexia as normative or a beneficial behavioral choice (termed positive volitional stigma) and the extent to which it was trivialized and viewed as unimportant or not serious (termed negative volitional stigma). Both the video and the ECA intervention aided in the recognition of anorexia and improved both positive and negative volitional stigma. No difference was noted with respect to social distance. According to the authors, this study was the first to demonstrate that video contact and ECA education can be effective in improving aspects of stigma among university students, thus opening new opportunities for stigma research using simulated people to deliver "personal" stories.

Kirschner and colleagues tested avatars in a 30-minute online intervention directed to college students where users entered a virtual environment and were involved in a series of interactive exercises. [370] This included simulated conversations with the student avatars who gave individualized feedback on how to discuss mental health issues and connect users with resources. Users were provided with information on the importance of supporting peers and offered potential gatekeeper options to guide an individual to resources. In the control condition, participants acted as a convenience store clerk and interacted with a virtual customer who wanted to buy tobacco products. They measured personal and public attitudes toward seeking help, and self-stigma (measured as the extent to which seeking help would alter one's perception of oneself). A total of 85 college students were randomly assigned to each arm. Personal and public attitudes toward help-seeking improved in the intervention group but not in the control condition. Unexpectedly, perceptions of self-stigma did not change in the intervention group but became more negative in the control condition, particularly for those with a mental health problem. It is not clear why those in the control condition would develop a harsher view of themselves if they were to seek mental health treatment, but it serves to highlight the potential to create paradoxical effects, particularly when strong theories of change do not undergird the intervention.

E-THERAPIES

The pandemic has prompted a surge in E-health tools and widespread acceptance of E-therapies among professionals and patients alike. [371] Certain types of E-therapies have the potential to reduce stigma, particularly if the user remains anonymous and invisible. In their literature review, Dowling and Rickwood outline four types of E-therapy [372]:

1. Online counseling and therapy: These involve a patient (or group of patients) and a therapist using various types of communication, including email exchanges, forums, instant messaging audio, and webcams. They can be synchronous (occur in real time) or asynchronous (with a lag between communication).
2. Web-based interventions: These are primarily self-guided and can include educational interventions, self-help therapies, and therapist-supported interventions.
3. Internet-operated therapeutic software: These interventions go beyond web-based programs by using advanced computer programming such as artificial intelligence and language recognition software. This includes computer simulations of therapeutic conversations where the client inputs text or key terms for analysis and a "therapeutic" response. Responses use algorithms that are based on scripts of therapeutic conversations.
4. Other: These include online support groups, mental health assessments, and smartphone applications.

While E-therapy programs are abundant and growing, most have not been formally evaluated. One exception is MoodGYM, an E-therapy program that is freely available and targets people with mood and anxiety disorders. It has been available for over 15 years (perhaps the longest of any) and has been evaluated. It has five sessions that are based on cognitive–behavioral principles consisting of written information, animations, interactive exercises, and quizzes. Users also have a choice of whether they want guidance from a clinician. It is estimated to have more than 850,000 registered users. Twomey and O'Reilly conducted a meta-analysis of randomized trials of MoodGYM with mixed results. [373] Small to no effects were noted for depression, medium effects were found for anxiety, and there was no significant effect for general psychological distress. Adherence rates were also problematic, falling below 10%. These results suggest that MoodGYM will benefit a minority of users with anxiety but is not effective for general distress.

While E-therapies hold considerable future promise for making mental health interventions widely available, much more research is needed to demonstrate not only their utility and efficacy but also their destigmatizing properties.

SUMMARY

Using E-technologies is quickly emerging as a method of fighting stigma. However, the development and implementation of E-techniques have vastly outstripped the development of a corresponding evidence base. Nevertheless, certain E-techniques offer considerable promise. If effective, they could be widely disseminated for little cost. A growing body of research is showing that video-based contact has the potential to bring about desired changes in behavioral intentions that last over time (measured up to 2 years). However, information on the pertinent design elements that promote effectiveness is not yet available. Video content that is developed using participatory models appears to be a particularly effective approach, with benefits to both the developers and the viewers. There is sufficient evidence that simulated hallucinations create social distance to abandon them as an anti-stigma strategy or altogether, but other simulations may hold more promise. Because E-technology progress is so recent and the techniques so new, we can only speculate as to how they will complement, fit into, or replace existing anti-stigma strategies. In addition, as much of the current research uses convenience samples of psychology or other undergraduate students (which should now be avoided), much work remains to be done to understand how existing methods might, or might not, be used in larger and more diverse groups.

CHAPTER 11
Research

The public health importance of mental disorders with respect to their associated burden of disease has been known for some time. Since the early 1970s, epidemiological studies have consistently documented a high prevalence of mental illnesses in the population. But it was not until the development of the disability-adjusted life-year (DALY) that the full public health burden of mental illnesses became known. Indeed, the first Global Burden of Disease study, conducted in 1990, catapulted mental disability onto the world stage. Five of the top 10 leading causes of disability worldwide were from mental illnesses, accounting for almost a quarter of the total years lived with a disability. [374] More recent estimates show the disease burden for mental illnesses growing. For example, unipolar depression was ranked fourth in DALYs in 2002 but is projected to rise to second by 2030. [375]

Previously, we have described stigma as a key driver of mental health program inequities. In this chapter we show how stigma is also a key driver of research inequities. We also describe approaches to the measurement of stigma and highlight important and innovative measurement tools that focus on high-priority evaluation outcomes such as behavioral change or self-stigma.

INEQUITABLE FUNDING FOR MENTAL HEALTH RESEARCH

It is now well recognized that pervasive structural discrimination has slowed the production of evidence in the field of mental health relative to other equally disabling conditions. With fewer prospects for significant and sustained career funding, many promising young researchers gravitate to other areas, leaving the field with less capacity to produce the high-quality evidence needed to compete for program funding. [376]

In setting funding levels, policymakers directly influence the nature and scope of research. In 2020, the International Alliance of Mental Health Research Funders analyzed over 75,000 research grants awarded by 350 funders from 35 countries. [377] Their report provides a comprehensive view of the nature and extent of mental health research funding and funding inequities. Findings show that worldwide, approximately US$3.7 billion is spent on mental health research each year. This translates into approximately 50 cents per person. Not surprisingly, most research funding (99%) is spent in high-income countries, largely because most funders (96%) come from there.

Compared to research on physical disorders, research into mental health is underfunded. For example, cancer research and infectious disease research received more than twice as much global funding as mental health research (19% and 18%, compared to 7%, respectively). Over half (56%) of mental health research was on basic research. We can speculate that basic research has received more funding not because it is related to mental disorders, but because it has implications for a wide range of health and illness states. Also, it fits better within a biologically driven investigative paradigm. The report also noted that substance use and depression were comparatively better funded than other conditions such as suicide and eating, conduct, obsessive–compulsive, and personality disorders. Of particular concern is the lack of research funding allotted to prevention, which accounted for less than 7% of the total investments in mental health research, and comorbid mental and physical conditions, which accounted for only 14%. The lack of investment in research involving comorbid mental and physical conditions is particularly problematic given the high physical comorbidities among people with mental health conditions, the complexity of their care, and their high premature mortality. For example, Chang and colleagues report a substantially lower life expectancy for people with a mental disorder: by 8 to 16 years for men and by 10 to 18 years for women. [54] The report called for increased transparency in the distribution of funding and greater equity for the mental health field; see Woelbert and colleagues for more details on the methods used. [378] It is also important to note that although we have gained considerable knowledge about the primary prevention of mental disorders, a great deal has not been translated into practice.

Hoagwood and coworkers examined trends in funding for child and adolescent mental health services by the National Institute of Mental Health (NIMH) in the United States from 2005 to 2015. [379] NIMH is the largest federal source of research funding in the United States for psychiatric disorders, treatments, and delivery systems, including community-based programs (such as supported housing, illness self-management, and assertive community treatments) designed to promote greater inclusion for people with mental illnesses. Whereas funding for children's mental health research tripled between 1991 and 2005, it dropped by 42% between 2005 and 2015 from

US$52,218,771 (indexed to 2015 dollars) to US$30,219,846—only about 2% of the total 2015 NIMH budget. This drop came at a time when U.S. healthcare systems were undergoing dramatic change, thereby undercutting the evidence base needed by policymakers to make key programming decisions. They also noted that funding was overly skewed to neuroscience research. These results highlight the precariousness of mental health research and how it can wax and wane without consideration for the underlying needs of the population.

Figure 11.1 compares the annual funding for the U.S. National Cancer Institute (NCI) with the NIMH between 1987 and 2020. While funding for both institutes increased, the baseline level of funding for NIMH was significantly less than the NCI, and the funding gap increased considerably over time.

An analysis based on all grants provided in the United Kingdom to children and adults found that research funding for mental health remained stable over a 5-year period (2015 to 2019) with an average of US$3.7 billion each year (indexed to U.S. dollars). Government funding provided the lion's share (72%). Only about 10% of research dollars were from fundraising by charitable organizations. The remainder (18%) came from philanthropic organizations. Mental health–related research made up approximately 4% of all research funding. [378]

Christensen and colleagues assessed mental health research funding in Australia relative to disease burden. [380] Diabetes, asthma, cancer, arthritis, and cardiovascular disease all received proportionately more research dollars per DALY compared to mental health. Until 2008, mental health funding was at the lowest of the seven National Health Priority Areas. In 2009, funding

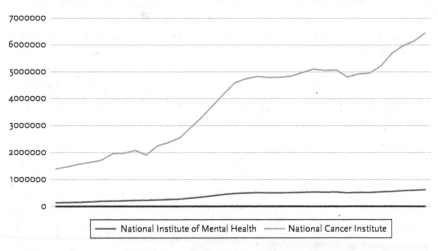

Figure 11.1 Annual funding, 1987 to 2020, for the NIMH and the NCI (in thousands of U.S. dollars)

Source: https://www.nih.gov/about-nih/what-we-do/nih-almanac/appropriations-section-1. Accessed October 4, 2021.

increased slightly to place mental health at the second-lowest rank, above cardiovascular disease. Diabetes received the highest amount of research dollars per DALY. Within mental health, substance misuse and autism fared proportionately better than eating disorders, attention-deficit/hyperactivity disorder, anxiety, depression, and schizophrenia. While funding for mental health had increased slightly between 2001 and 2009, there was no "narrowing of the gap" between mental health and other research areas. The largest increases in funding were in the areas of diabetes and asthma.

Table 11.1 compares the annual research investment in mental health and other selected disorders worldwide per year lived with a disability and year of life lost. These demonstrated inequities raise the important policy question of whether research funding should be redistributed to better match the burden of illness.

Larivière and colleagues compared the number of scientific publications produced by researchers in 18 countries between 1980 and 2010. [382] To the extent that scientific publications are a proxy indicator for research funding, their results highlight significant differences by country, and over time, in infrastructure and support for mental health research. In some areas, such as the United States and the United Kingdom, where funding increased during the study period, publications also increased. Canadian research remained at 1980 levels, with a significant drop during the 1990s. Brazil, Russia, India, and China (reflecting 40% of the world's population) contributed only 8% of the research publications, with a small increase over time. Overall, the volume of mental health research grew four-fold over the period, from 5810 papers in 1980 to 27,866 in 2010. The frequency of mental health research papers as a share of all clinical and health-related papers rose from 29% to 54%.

Perhaps as governments and other funders begin to accept the public health importance of mental illnesses and the lack of evidence base relative to

Table 11.1 RATIO OF ANNUAL RESEARCH INVESTMENTS TO YEARS LIVED WITH A DISABILITY (YLD) AND YEARS OF LIFE LOST (YLL)

Illness category	US$ per YLD	US$ per YLL
Cancer and neoplasms	$755	$26
Infections (including HIV/AIDS)	$161	$22
Cardiovascular, blood and stroke	$77	$8
Neurological	$56	$108
Mental health	$15	$49
Metabolic and endocrine	$14	$24
Respiratory	$13	$3

Adapted from the International Alliance of Research Funders, The Inequities of Mental Health Research Funding ([381], p. 19)

other disabling conditions such as diabetes or cancer, additional funding may be directed to mental health research, though this is likely to take considerable advocacy on the part of the mental health community. In this context, epidemiological evidence such as that coming from the Global Burden of Disease Study will be an important advocacy tool.

MENTAL HEALTH FUNDING AGENCIES

Outside of pharmaceutical companies, few countries have granting agencies that are specific to mental health, with the result that there is often no dedicated funding for mental health–related research. Perhaps the largest agency that is entirely dedicated to funding mental health research is the NIMH, which funds more than 3000 research grants and contracts annually. Since 2017, its budget has risen from $1.5 billion to over $2 billion. The Wellcome Trust in England has holdings of almost $40 billion.* However, it funds a range of research across all branches of medicine. It is noteworthy that as of 2019, the Wellcome Trust has made mental health a priority area for funding. [383] The European Union's Horizon 2020 fund holds more than €80 billion.† What is interesting about this program is that research funding is not segregated into disorder categories. The fund is open to everyone, with reduced red tape and time to get innovative projects off the ground more quickly. This means that mental health researchers can compete on par with researchers in other fields.

Twenty-six funding partners worldwide make up the International Alliance of Mental Health Research Funders, who describe themselves as the world's largest funders of mental health research. They are in Australia (four), Austria (one), Canada (five), Denmark (two), India (two), Ireland (one), The Netherlands (one), and the United States (three). An additional funder is in multiple sites (Israel, France, and Switzerland), and one, a large pharmaceutical company, has global reach. Only two funders are situated in a lower-income country. [377]

BUILDING AN EVIDENCE BASE FOR ANTI-STIGMA PROGRAMMING

A key driver for building a better evidence base for anti-stigma programming comes from the rise of evidence-based practice in general. Clinicians and

*https://www.nimh.nih.gov/about/budget/fy-2022-budget-congressional-justification
†https://ec.europa.eu/programmes/horizon2020/what-horizon-2020

program administrators face unprecedented pressure to support their interventions with evidence, as well as to develop the research and evaluation skills necessary to critically appraise research reports. One of the major claims of the evidence-based approach is that it provides objective data about the impact of interventions by eliminating subjective decision-making and practitioner bias, thereby creating a more equitable distribution of resources. [376] However, a close look at the nature of the evidence required and the methods used to generate it highlight significant challenges for mental health and anti-stigma researchers, primarily because the evidence-based paradigm ignores the social and cultural forces that influence both the funding and production of evidence. [384]

In health sciences, evidence is rank ordered according to the methodological strength of the study, meaning the ability of study designs to provide unbiased estimates. The gold standard of evidence is a review (or meta-analysis) of high-quality randomized controlled trials. Study designs that use non-experimental observational methods are considered to be weaker because they are more open to bias from unmeasured variables. While randomized controlled trials are increasing in stigma research, most of the evidence is still produced from "lesser" study designs that are seen as being fundamentally flawed by conventional evidence-based standards. In the case of large population-based interventions, or interventions that target an entire organization, randomized controlled trials are logistically difficult, if not impossible. In some cases, a specific law, policy, or organizational practice is the target or agent of change, and these are best studied using case studies or other qualitative designs. A more pragmatic approach would recognize that there is no single way to identify programs and interventions that work. Such questions can only be answered with ongoing, extensive, longitudinal, and multifaceted evaluations. Many factors other than a program's efficacy (such as feasibility or acceptability) can impact its success. [385]

Scholarly interest in anti-stigma programming and evaluation is increasing. The World Psychiatric Association (WPA)'s Scientific Section on Stigma and Mental Disorders, inaugurated in 2005, includes almost 40 clinical researchers, scientists, and advocates from across the world (Figure 11.2). Through this network of international researchers and practitioners, the Section engages in scholarly, scientific, and public health activities to reduce prejudice and discrimination and improve social inclusion for people with mental illnesses and their families. More specifically, the Stigma Section (1) disseminates information about prejudice and discrimination because of mental disorders through academic and technical publications, symposia, and workshops offered at international and regional conferences and meetings; (2) advances scientific knowledge about stigma through collaborative research and evaluation; and (3) provides training opportunities to support the development of effective programs to fight

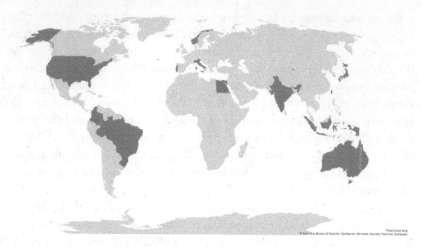

Figure 11.2 Stigma Section members

prejudice and discrimination because of mental disorders. A bibliography of members' recent publications is contained in the Appendix.

The members of the Committee of the Section work with partners from around the world to mount an international conference entitled Together Against Stigma. The conference is held every 2 to 3 years. Figure 11.3 highlights the locations of past conferences and their attendance. To date there have been nine international congresses hosting more than 4,000 delegates. The 2021 conference was virtual and hosted by colleagues in Prague.

The conference is unique in that it grew out of a global network of anti-stigma initiatives undertaken by the WPA involving researchers and advocates in low-, medium-, and high-income countries: Austria, Brazil, Canada, Chile, Egypt, India, Italy, Germany, Greece, Japan, Morocco, Poland, Romania, Slovakia, Spain, Turkey, the United Kingdom, and the United States. The first conferences were created to provide a forum for the partners to discuss activities in their respective countries and share promising practices. [69] Delegates are now from various walks of life, including people with lived experience of a mental illness, family members, representatives of advocacy organizations, policymakers, clinicians, and scientists. In this way, the Together Against Stigma conferences foster multidisciplinary interest in developing better and best practices in stigma reduction. They break down the silos that often occur between disciplines and sectors and drive efforts to bridge the gap between evidence and practice. During the conference in Ottawa in 2012, members of national advocacy organizations formed a global alliance, which meets at each conference to share insights, approaches, and tools.

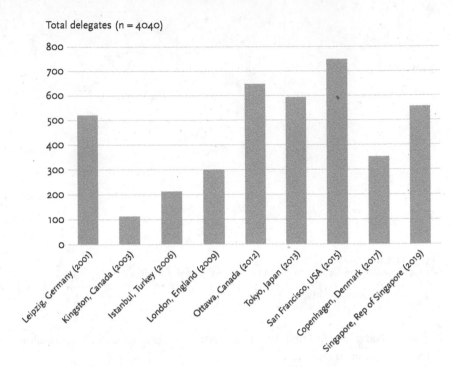

Total delegates (n = 4040)

Figure 11.3 Together Against Stigma meetings

RESEARCH NETWORKS

Over the past 15 years, several large international research networks have been formed to highlight the scope and magnitude of stigma and strengthen the evidence base for stigma-reduction strategies. These networks are notable because they span both high- and lower-income countries. One example is the International Study of Discrimination and Stigma Outcomes (INDIGO) network, which originated in 2006, led by Professor Sir Graham Thornicroft, Professor Diana Rose, and Professor Norman Sartorius.[†] It has grown to a collaboration of research colleagues in over 40 countries (Figure 11.4).

The first two studies that were conducted examined the nature and severity of stigma experienced and anticipated by people with a mental illness. Since then, the INDIGO Partnership program has developed to test new methods to reduce stigma through culturally adapted multi-level interventions in China, Ethiopia, India, Tunisia, and Nepal. This program uses locally validated tools and is done in partnership with people who have experienced a mental illness. Also, nested within the INDIGO network is the Anti-Stigma Programme

[†] https://indigo-group.org/indigo-projects/

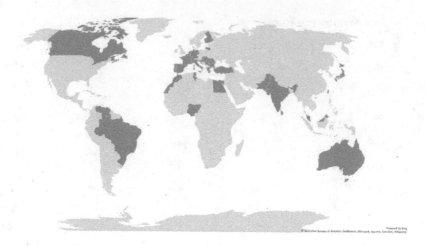

Figure 11.4 INDIGO partners
Adapted from Lasalvia A, Zoppei S, Van Bortel T et al. Global pattern of experienced and anticipated discrimination reported by people with major depressive disorder: A cross-sectional survey. *Lancet* 2013;381, DOI: 10.1016/S0140-6736(12)61379-8.

European Network (ASPEN), which focuses on stigma related to depression across 34 European sites. [118]

Networks such as these are important in that they build global capacity for research and provide a forum for international mentorship opportunities. Participants have offered a number of lessons learned to make a research network successful, productive, and sustainable [386]:

1. Clear descriptions of the roles and responsibilities of all partners are required.
2. A learning collaborative must be established so that members actively support each other, particularly those who have a similar language or resource level.
3. Members must take a long-term view for sustainability and purposively support early- and mid-career academic staff.
4. Shared leadership, responsibilities, and cooperation are necessary, such as translating specific roles into discrete work packages, then assigning them to task teams.
5. Partners must be free to work within a framework that jointly sets milestones and timelines.
6. Multidisciplinary research approaches bring researchers from various disciplines together.
7. Regular communication is needed to build a sense of belonging to a valued group of colleagues and to celebrate successes.

The Global Alliance of Mental Illness Advocacy Networks—Europe (GAMIAN-Europe), which was registered in Switzerland in 1998, provides an example of a network composed of people with lived experience of mental illnesses.§ GAMIAN-Europe is a user-driven organization that involves advocacy organizations from over 50 European countries. The group represents the interests of people impacted by a mental illness and advocates for their rights. Full members are those organizations that are active in mental health and ensure full participation of service users on their boards and in their activities. If organizations cannot meet these criteria, they can become associate members. In addition to the group's broad advocacy goals (many centering on reducing discrimination), members also conduct research. Since 2014, GAMIAN-Europe has been actively involved in European Union-funded research and organizes meetings of its members to provide feedback to these projects, thus ensuring their relevance to service users. A key aspect of GAMIAN-Europe's research work has been to conduct surveys to highlight the lived experiences of people with mental illnesses. Data from these surveys are used to raise awareness and promote advocacy goals. One example of a survey conducted by the group involved 1732 members of 12 European advocacy groups from 11 countries focusing on mood disorders. [387] Results showed a need for more information about mood disorders and their treatments. They also highlighted the impact of public stigma and stigma from family members.

A third model for a research network is provided by the Opening Minds anti-stigma initiative in Canada, in which university researchers from across the country were paired with anti-stigma programs to jointly conduct evaluations. [119] Most programs had never been evaluated, so their effectiveness was unknown. Program members, while interested in having evaluation results to "prove" the effectiveness of their programs, had neither the funding nor the expertise to conduct evaluation research. Therefore, Opening Minds funded a series of evaluation projects as the first phase of a nationwide anti-stigma strategy. The goal was to identify the most effective programs, then replicate them in other locations. To identify candidate programs, a "request for interest" was widely disseminated. To be selected, program leaders had to agree to work with researchers to conduct evaluations using standardized measurement tools rather than their own home-grown measures. Initially, 233 submissions were received from programs targeting healthcare providers (n = 130) or youth (n = 103), the first two groups to be targeted. An international committee reviewed program submissions and selected those that used the most promising approaches (specifically contact-based education), had stable funding (so they would be sustainable during the evaluation), and had the potential to be widely disseminated if found to be effective. In the youth network, for example, researchers and student trainees developed and psychometrically tested a new measure based on the various types of questionnaires

§ https://www.gamian.eu/about-us/gamian-europe/

that had been used by program staff. When psychometrically tested, program staff completed the standardized survey and data were sent to the researchers for analysis and reporting. Researchers spent considerable time (1 to 1.5 hours per program) developing report formats that were easily understandable to lay readers and talked program staff through their respective reports, drawing out implications for improvement. Research team meetings with all researchers, trainees, and Opening Minds staff ensured that approaches were as consistent as possible across various target groups and the knowledge gained from the evaluations was made available for full discussion and use.

APPROACHES USED IN STIGMA SURVEY RESEARCH

Researchers have been interested in measuring stigma since the 1950s, when Cumming and Cumming used a variety of measures to assess the effects of a multilevel anti-stigma intervention in a small Canadian town. [388] Measurement of stigma is typically approached using direct measures that elicit a belief or attitude from a respondent based on their own self-report. Two types of prompts have figured prominently. Labeling theory predicts that labels such as "mental illness" trigger stereotypical views, which in turn lead to status loss and disadvantage. Researchers subscribing to this view typically provide one or more diagnostic labels for the respondent to react to. A second approach has been to provide a vignette describing someone's appearance or behavior. The vignette uses the behavioral cues of someone with a mental illness to trigger a response. In each case the respondent answers questions about the person so labeled or depicted in the story. [389]

Whether a question or a vignette is used, one of the most common ways of measuring responses is a Likert scale. Once respondents are provided with a series of statements designed to tap an attitude or stereotype, they indicate their degree of agreement, typically on a 5-point scale (strongly agree; agree; neither agree nor disagree; disagree; strongly disagree). Responses may be averaged across each item or summed across all items. In some cases, the middle category is omitted as it may be difficult to interpret, or to force an opinion as people who don't want to share a negative opinion may gravitate to the center. [390]

SELECTING THE RIGHT OUTCOME MEASURE

Today, researchers and program staff conducting evaluations have a much broader range of measurement tools available to them than they did 15 years ago. Also, there has been considerable work done with several newly developed scales. Many of these are becoming widely used, making meta-analyses and literature syntheses more meaningful. A key challenge is that most scales are based on self-report. Over the years, anti-stigma efforts may have sensitized the public that it is improper to reject someone because of a disability status. When asked directly about their views, respondents may not want to appear prejudiced and so may mask their true feelings, leaning toward answers that are socially desirable. Social desirability bias can result in underestimates of the extent of stigma and create a false picture of change following anti-stigma interventions. [389] However, it is interesting to note that Kassam and colleagues included a social desirability measure in their development and assessment of a scale to measure stigma among healthcare providers and found a weak correlation (0.10), suggesting that social desirability may not be as significant a problem as originally thought. [391] It would be helpful if more researchers would include a measure of social desirability so that we could better understand how self-reports may be biased (see Loo and Thorpe for psychometric data on the full and short versions of the Marlowe-Crown Social Desirability Scale [392]).

Global or Specific Stigma Content

A central issue in stigma research has been the extent to which an overall uniform construct of *mental illness* or *mental disorder* exists in the social conscience, or whether this is stereotypical and stigmatizing. Angermeyer and Dietrich have questioned whether the assessment of stereotypes associated with generic constructs is of any value at all. [64] There are more than 300 discrete diagnostic categories, and research has demonstrated marked differences in public perceptions across several disorder categories, making generic categorizations problematic. For example, Pescosolido and colleagues found significant differences in expectations of dangerousness across categories such as schizophrenia, major depression, alcohol dependence, drug dependence, and a person who was described as "troubled." [393] When categories are generic, it is not clear what image respondents have of someone with a "mental illness" or whether their images are uniform within the sample. In addition, respondents typically stereotype symptoms and behaviors, such as dangerousness or incompetency in addition to labels (making vignettes helpful). For these reasons, it is best to ensure that any measure used is disorder-specific. This fits with previous advice to target anti-stigma programs.

Reliability

Internal Consistency

Many of the scales used in the stigma literature have not been psychometrically tested or validated or do not have strong properties. Stigma scales are designed to measure an underlying attribute that cannot be measured directly, such as discriminatory intentions. Items (questions) are chosen to measure different aspects of the attribute and, to the extent that they do, the item scores will be highly correlated. Items that aren't correlated with the scale score are problematic as they are likely measuring something else. Internal consistency is typically measured using the Cronbach's alpha statistic (named after the developer). Alphas test how intercorrelated scale items are. An alpha of 0.7 or above is considered acceptable. Extremely high alphas, such as 0.9 or above, suggest that the scale could be shortened as some of the items are redundant. The assumption underlying the use of alpha is that the scale items assess a single unidimensional construct. When subscales are involved, then alphas should be assessed for each subscale, not the aggregated score. An alpha for the entire scale should not be reported, and items should never be summed across the entire scale to measure a program's outcome; individual subscales should be used instead. A difficulty in the literature is that many psychometric analyses fail to provide the scale scores, and, in many evaluations, scales are aggregated across their subscales to provide a single measure. This is especially problematic as subscales could behave in different ways, depending on the nature of the intervention. When reporting evaluation results, it is useful to present the alpha statistics for the measures used. If a scale is unreliable, it will be difficult to accurately measure an outcome. A true change may be masked because there is too much noise in the measurement. This means that useful and effective programs may be misinterpreted to be unhelpful and ineffective. [394]

Test–Retest Reliability

Test–retest reliability refers to the consistency of scores across two separate measurement times, and it is often considered to be more important than internal reliability. A challenge in evaluating test–retest reliability is that a true change in the underlying attribute may have occurred, particularly if the tests are far apart. A short interval, such as 1 or 2 weeks, lowers the possibility that a real change has occurred, but it may also increase the likelihood that respondents remember how they answered the time 1 questions. Some respondents interpret the second measure as a test of their memory or their ability to be consistent. Typically, scores at the first administration are statistically correlated with scores at the second administration, though mean differences also have been used. As with Cronbach's alpha, any correlation above 0.7 is considered to be acceptable. [395]

Inter-rater Reliability

At times, it will be necessary to collect data using individuals who interview and code answers or observations. In this situation, it is essential that coders are provided with training on the instruments to be used and that any two coders give the same ratings consistently. Inter-rater reliability is the extent to which two coders will agree. To assess this, some or all of the study subjects must be rated by two or more coders. Often a subset of respondents is used for feasibility. Several approaches can be used to calculate inter-rater reliability depending on the nature of the data (e.g., categorical, numerical) and the study design, all of which will require someone to have specialized knowledge and access to statistical software—a situation that could be addressed with a strong partnership with local researchers. [396] A frequently used measure is the kappa statistic. Kappas of less than 0 indicate poor agreement; 0 to 0.2, slight agreement; 0.21 to 0.40, fair agreement, 0.41 to 0.60, moderate agreement; 0.61 to 0.80 substantial agreement; and 0.81 to 1.0 almost perfect agreement. [397] Because inter-rater agreement is study-specific and dependent on the training and preparation provided to the raters, it is not particularly helpful to know the kappa statistics from other studies. They must be computed for each study and, if low, additional training must be provided to the raters until they are able to achieve at least substantial agreement. Inter-rater reliability may drop over time, so it is important to assess it at different points during data collection, providing additional training to coders if reliability drops.

Factor Structure

It is never enough to assess a scale using only Cronbach's alpha. This is because scales with more than 15 items could be multi-dimensional and have a high alpha simply because of the large number of items. [394] Therefore, the factor structure of the scale must always be confirmed (such as from existing literature). For a completely new scale, there may be no predetermined idea about how the items will group, or not group. In exploratory factor analysis the goal is to find out whether items load onto a single factor or multiple factors. In confirmatory factor analysis (often done using structural equation modeling), the researcher has a predetermined structure for the data and may, for example, postulate a series of subscales represented by different factors. Factor loadings are the correlation of the item score with the remaining variables making up the factor. Typically, loadings of 0.4 or above are considered acceptable. Then, the job is to confirm that the items fall as they were intended on each subscale. In addition to revealing the underlying structure of scale scores, factor analysis also can be used to reduce the number of items on a scale to create a shorter version (e.g., when alphas are more than 0.9). Items that are the least strongly loaded can be removed. When choosing a scale for evaluating anti-stigma programs, it is important to determine if researchers have assessed the factor structure—whether there is a single underlying factor (in which case the data are summed across all the items) or if there are subscales (which must be used individually).

Sensitivity to Change

When choosing a scale, it is important to determine whether it is sensitive to change, meaning it can pick up any difference that may have been caused by the program. A good indication that a scale is sensitive to change is that previous evaluations were able to capture differences. A cautionary note is that ineffective programs would not produce differences, so it is important to locate scales that have been used in multiple settings and locations.

Cultural Sensitivity

In Chapter 2 we described how concepts of mental illness differ across cultures. To date, cultural concepts have been infrequently incorporated into measurement approaches. Typically, measures are developed and validated in a Western culture, then translated into another cultural context and re-evaluated for their psychometric properties. A second approach is to develop a measure across multiple contexts to represent the universal aspects of stigma. Yang and colleagues conducted a literature review of 196 articles to identify new, culturally relevant constructs. [113] Most studies (77%) used adaptations of existing stigma measures developed in Western countries to new cultural groups. Instead, they recommended developing culturally specific measures of stigma using a "what matters most" framework. This framework allows researchers to identify and measure aspects of stigma that block meaningful social participation in day-to-day life—for example, losing face or family status among Asian groups. Because culturally specific measures cannot be directly compared across different cultural groups, their further recommendation was to include both a generic and a culturally specific measure. Much work must be done to develop culturally specific measures.

Procedures for translating an instrument into another language and cultural setting are available. For example, Tsang and colleagues suggest forming an expert committee including researchers who are familiar with the construct you are trying to measure and, most importantly, collaborators from the target culture who speak both languages fluently. [398] The first step is to make the initial translation (termed "forward translation"). Ideally, this should be done by at least two independent translators. The next step is to "back translate" the instrument into the original language. Misunderstandings and unclear wording will be revealed. Members of the expert committee will review all translations, resolve any discrepancies, and ensure that both versions are conceptually (rather than literally) equivalent. Then the translated version should be pilot tested on a small sample of potential respondents to make sure that all items are easily understood and have the expected meaning. Cognitive interviewing techniques may be used to help the respondents verbalize their thoughts as they are completing the survey items. The interviewer may ask the respondents to think aloud when they are completing the items or may ask direct questions regarding the basis for their responses. This will highlight any misconceptions or unclear wording (see Beatty and Willis for more detail). [399]

MEASUREMENT OPTIONS

There is no shortage of measures that examine public stigma. Many of these measure stereotypical attitudes. As we have pointed out earlier, it is not clear that attitudinal change corresponds to behavioral change or greater social inclusion, which should be the ultimate goals of anti-stigma work. This section highlights selected measures that focus on aspects of behavioral change and reports their psychometric properties.

Social Distance Scales

Social distance measures are one of the most used to assess behavioral intention, both of the public and among subgroups such as students or employees. Though not a direct measure of behaviors, desire for social distance is used as a proxy for how willing or unwilling people are to interact with someone who has had a mental illness. Items typically span a range of closeness, such as living on the same street, working alongside them, or having them marry into the family. Social distance scales have versatility and may range in items from a few (e.g., four) to more than a dozen. They are robust and show good reliability and construct validity in different samples and settings and over time. [389]

Alexander and Link used a social distance scale to compare the extent to which members of the public who had prior contact with someone with a mental illness were as socially distancing as those who had no prior contact. [400] This study is noteworthy because they used a brief four-item social distance scale. Their contact measure was made up of four types of contact: family, friend, public, and work. A total contact score was created by summing the number of contacts reported. The alpha for this scale was good (0.81). The social distance scale contained questions about how willing the respondent would be to have someone with a mental illness as part of their workplace, community, schools, or social networks. The alpha for this scale also was good (0.84). They found that people who had prior contact with someone with a mental illness were less likely to endorse the dangerousness stereotype and were less socially distancing.

Reported and Intended Behavior Scale (RIBS)

The RIBS was developed by the INDIGO network to provide a short, population-level measure of reported and intended stigma-related behaviors. [401] Items were culled from an earlier longer social distance measure and reviewed for content validity by service users and international stigma researchers. Items ask about reported and intended behaviors in different contexts: living with, working with, living nearby, and continuing a relationship with someone with a mental health problem. The first four items are scored on a yes/no/don't know basis and assess the prevalence of behaviors in each of these domains. The next four items ask about future intentions and are scored on a 5-point agreement scale. The RIBS was piloted and then tested in three different samples. The internal consistency across the four scale items was 0.85, with good test–retest reliability (0.75). Factor analysis was not undertaken, but social distance items tend to group on a single factor. A strength of this instrument is its brevity, taking only about a minute to complete. It has been widely used and translated into a number of different languages, such as Italian, Portuguese, and Japanese. [402,403,404]

In addition to the RIBS, the INDIGO network has developed scales to assess factual knowledge (Mental Health Knowledge Schedule), clinicians' attitudes (Mental Illness: Clinicians' Attitudes), expectations of discrimination among people with a mental illness (Questionnaire of Anticipated Discrimination), barriers to accessing treatments (Barriers to Care Scale), costs of discrimination (Costs of Discrimination Assessment), and the Discrimination and Stigma Scale long version. These scales have been translated into 31 languages and have been used in 67 countries. All scales are available on request through the INDIGO network." [386]

** http://indigo-group.org/indigo-projects/project-1-developing-a-short-version-of-the-discrmination-and-stigma-scale-lead-dr-sara-evans-lacko/

Social Acceptance Scale for Youth

Recognizing that youth have become an important target for anti-stigma efforts, Koller and Stuart [405] modified traditional social distance items to be applicable to this subpopulation. The resulting Social Acceptance Scale for youth contained 11 items reflecting different aspects of social distance and social acceptance (e.g., "I would be upset if someone with a mental illness always sat next to me in class"; "I would tutor a classmate who got behind in their studies because of their mental illness"). The scale was worded at the sixth-grade level using the Flesch–Kincaid reading-level score. Items were scored on a 5-point agreement scale ranging from strongly disagree to strongly agree. The scale was tested in three samples of students—one for exploratory factor analysis (N = 1352), one for confirmatory factor analysis (N = 576), and one for test–retest reliability (N = 190). Confirmatory factor analysis demonstrated a single factor with strong factor loadings above 0.5. Cronbach's alpha of 0.85 showed high internal reliability. Test–retest reliability over a 2-week period also was strong, with a correlation of 0.82.

Perceived Devaluation and Discrimination Scale

In 1987 Link developed a 12-item scale to measure cultural expressions of devaluation and discrimination toward, at that time, "mental patients." [406] The scale is noteworthy because it measures community-level attitudes through respondents' perceptions of the extent to which "most people" would devalue and discriminate against someone with a mental illness. Responses are measured on a 6-point Likert-type agreement scale. The scale was initially tested using five groups who varied in their level of pathology and treatment contact in New York City: psychiatric patients having their first contact (N = 67), current psychiatric patients with multiple treatment contacts (N = 117); community residents who had been treated in the past (N = 96); community residents who were untreated but had symptoms (N = 143); and community residents with no evidence of pathology and no treatment (N = 171). Internal consistency was strong in each group: 0.78, 0.79, 0.82, 0.73, and 0.73 respectively. Scores did not differ across the groups, and group membership predicted only 1.2% of the variation in the scale scores. These results showed that people who differed widely in their mental health experiences held common beliefs about community-level stigma, confirming that the Devaluation and Discrimination Scale was a community-level indicator, not an indicator of respondents' own personal prejudices. It has been used extensively and is robust to modifications. It is important to note that, because it is a community-level indicator, it may not be sensitive to change for targeted anti-stigma interventions. Nevertheless, it could be used to track population change over time.

Mental Health Experiences Scale (MHE)

The MHE was developed and tested by Statistics Canada[††] for use in large population-based surveys to assess stigma impact over time. [407] The scale asks people with lived experience of a mental illness (in this case depression) if others have expressed negative opinions about them or treated them unfairly because of a past or current mental or emotional health problem. The original scale included the following domains: family relationships, romantic life, school or work life, financial situation, housing situation, self-confidence or self-esteem, social contacts, overall physical health, overall mental health, peace of mind, and sense of belonging to the community. Responses are on a 5-point agreement scale. Initial testing showed high alphas (0.94), with all items loading on a single factor, and strong factor loadings (between 0.64 and 0.89). Both the English version and the French version had strong alphas (0.94 and 0.96 respectively). The high alphas suggested that a shorter version could be used—an important consideration for a large national survey. Statistics Canada used the first five items, which took less than 3 minutes to complete. A longer scale may be useful if specific items, such as feelings of social belonging, are targeted by anti-stigma programs. The same scale items can be used to assess the impact of stigma on the family. Psychometric testing of the family version showed a single factor with strong alphas (0.88).

The MHE has been used in two population surveys conducted by Statistics Canada using identical methods and has demonstrated sensitivity to change. In the first survey (conducted in 2010), 38% of those who had received treatment for a mental or emotional problem in the prior year reported having been stigmatized, compared to 25% in the second survey (conducted in 2012). [408] This change occurred at a time when there were active national anti-stigma activities ongoing, though it is difficult to attribute cause. Nevertheless, the MHE appears to be a useful tool that can be easily incorporated into national survey questionnaires or used in smaller program evaluations.

Discrimination and Stigma Scale (DISC)

The DISC was developed to rate the degree to which people with a mental illness have experienced discrimination in various areas of life such as work, relationships, parenting, housing, leisure, and religious activities. [409] It contains a quantitative component to rate these experiences and a qualitative component to provide specific examples. A preliminary version of the scale was developed in 2009 for use in the INDIGO study (described earlier

[††] https://www23.statcan.gc.ca/imdb/p3Instr.pl?Function=assembleInstr&Item_Id=119788&wbdisable=true. Accessed September 17, 2021.

in this chapter). In 2013, more extensive psychometric work was undertaken. A unique feature of this scale is that it has been developed and tested with respondents across multiple countries. The original scale was composed of 35 items. Following psychometric assessment, a 22-item version was recommended that focused on discrimination experiences and unfair treatment in social relationships. The shortened version was found to be reliable, acceptable, feasible, precise, and valid. However, because of the small sample size (under 100), the factor structure of the scale could not be assessed. The scale has continued to be refined, with the most recent version being version 12 (DISC-12). [410]

In subsequent work, the developers of the DISC considered the length (22 items) to be a disadvantage, particularly in large studies requiring multiple measures. A shorter scale was preferable in low- and middle-income countries. To address this, researchers developed and validated a shortened version, named DISCUS. [410] The sample included 1087 people with major depressive disorders and 732 people with schizophrenia across 42 countries. Using factor analysis, 11 items with the strongest factor loadings were retained to form a short version of experienced discrimination in personal and social relationships. Cronbach's coefficients were good, ranging from 0.70 to 0.86 across seven geographic regions. The scale was associated with other related measures in expected ways, supporting its construct validity. Based on the strong psychometric results, it has been recommended for use.

Self-Stigma

The scales highlighted to this point have all focused on self-reported behavioral intentions or experiences of discrimination. As we have discussed previously, programs are emerging that target the self-stigma experienced by people with a mental illness. Self-stigma scales are a newer development. In this section, two promising self-stigma scales are reviewed.

Internalized Stigma of Mental Illness (ISMI)

The ISMI scale was developed in 2003 by Ritsher and colleagues to measure the psychosocial impact of negative and discriminatory experiences on individuals with mental illness. [411] This measure is interesting because it was developed with significant input from people who had experienced a mental illness and it is one of the most frequently used measures. Items were kept short and simple and focused on the respondent's own identity and experiences. Initial testing was performed on 127 outpatients in a Veterans Administration medical center in the United States. The original scale comprised 55 items, but this was shortened to 29. Five subscales were covered: alienation (feeling out of place); stereotype endorsement (thinking that stereotypes about the mentally ill apply personally); discrimination experiences (experiences of discrimination or social distance); social withdrawal (not talking about oneself); and stigma resistance (reverse-coded items such as feeling comfortable being seen with someone with a mental illness). The five subscales showed the following reliability coefficients: alienation, 0.79; stereotype endorsement, 0.72; discrimination experience, 0.75; withdrawal, 0.80; and stigma resistance, 0.58. Because of the low reliability of the stigma resistance subscale, these items were dropped for the factor analysis, giving 24 items. To date, this scale has been used widely and has been translated into several different languages (see below). Scale scores have been associated with other stigma-related measures, providing evidence of construct validity. Most researchers continue to use the original 29-item scale with similar weak results for the stigma resistance subscale. [412] Individuals using the ISMI for program evaluation may consider dropping the stigma resistance subscale as it may be too unreliable to capture change. Alternatively, they may reword it so that it does not need to be reverse-coded, as this may impact internal consistency.

In 2014, Boyd and colleagues searched the international literature for translations of the ISMI. [413] These included English (the original), English (brief), English (South African), Arabic, Armenian, Bengali, Bulgarian, Chinese Simplified (Mainland), Chinese Traditional (Taiwan), Chinese (Hong Kong), Croatian, Dutch (Belgium), Estonian, Farsi, Finnish, French, German, Greek, Hebrew, Hindi, Japanese, Khmer, Korean, Lithuanian, Luganda, Maltese, Polish, Portuguese (Brazil), Portuguese (Portugal), Romanian, Russian, Samoan, Slovenian, Spanish (Spain), Swahili, Swedish, Tongan, Turkish, Urdu, and Yoruba. In addition, the ISMI has been adapted in English for substance abuse, eating disorders, epilepsy, inflammatory bowel disease, leprosy, smoking, ethnicity, caregivers, and parents of people with a mental illness. See Boyd and coworkers for full citations for each version. [413] Undoubtedly there have been additional translations since this 2014 paper was published, making the ISMI one of the most versatile multinational scales available.

Self-Stigma of Mental Illness Scale (SSMIS)

The SSMIS examines self-stigma across four dimensions, three of which are similar to the ISMI:

1. Stereotype awareness, where the person is aware of the negative and prejudicial beliefs held by the public
2. Stereotype agreement, or the extent to which the individual endorses the same public stereotypes

3. Self-concurrence, or the extent to which they believe public views apply to them
4. Self-esteem decrement, or the extent to which people's self-esteem is diminished due to their concurrence with the negative beliefs.

Initially, 60 items were generated, 15 for each domain. These were reviewed by a focus group of 12 people with a mental illness and their families, who recommended 15 additional items. Items were scored on a 9-point agreement scale. Initially, 54 people with a psychiatric disability completed the measure twice, 1 week apart. Preliminary analysis of internal consistency resulted in the elimination of five items from each subscale. Cronbach's alphas were moderate to high (ranging from 0.72 to 0.91) for the revised subscales. The stereotype agreement subscale showed the weakest reliability (alpha = 0.72). Test–retest reliability was moderate to good (ranging from 0.68 to 0.82).

Subsequent research demonstrated two problems with the measure. Some of the stereotypes were considered offensive because of their harsh tone (e.g., people with mental illnesses are disgusting or below average in intelligence). Also, it was too long. In response, the developers substantially revised the SSMIS to address these problems. [414] Thirteen mental health consumers rated the 10 stereotypes reflected in the measure. The five stereotypes rated least offensive were retained, leaving five items per subscale (20 items total). Using the data from three prior studies, the psychometric properties of the shortened scales were assessed: stereotype awareness (0.73 to 0.87); stereotype agreement (0.72 to 0.79); self-concurrence (0.22 to 0.74); and self-esteem (0.76 to 0.82). Examination of the relationships between the shortened scale supported construct validity. The subscales of the SSMIS-SF are recommended for use in evaluation studies, recognizing that (1) the subscale measuring stereotype awareness may be insensitive to change as it is measuring public stigma, and (2) the subscale measuring self-concurrence may be problematic due to the low alpha obtained in the original study.

Structural Stigma

Literature reviews of stigma measures have not identified any measure deliberately designed to measure structural stigma. [389,415] Link and colleagues note that this form of discrimination is "almost entirely unaddressed" in the literature. [389] Topics such as insurance parity or resource inequity are discussed, but they have not been integrated into the measurement literature on stigma.

As we have noted in previous chapters, considerable stigma is entrenched in healthcare systems, in their cultures, processes of care, and professional attitudes and behaviors. In a recent qualitative study of stigma experienced in healthcare settings (preparatory to measurement development), focus group participants emphasized the importance of having input from people with lived experience in the development and testing of new measurement tools. [416] In the context of structural stigma in healthcare settings, the characteristics of an ideal measurement tool were described as:

1. Grounded: Measures should be developed and tested based on meaningful input from clients and family members so that scale items are important to service users.
2. Client-directed: Service users and family members, rather than health professionals, should complete the measures so that care experiences are assessed from the perspective of the person with a mental illness.
3. Comprehensive: The tools should capture the client's experience of their overall care, rather than individual care processes.
4. Person-centered: The tool should address the extent to which care environments meet clients' needs and are empowering, affirming, and recovery-oriented.
5. Generalizable: The tool should be applicable to a broad range of health and mental health settings to ensure that physical, social, and mental health needs of clients are met in supportive environments across the full spectrum of the healthcare system, ranging from primary care practices, to emergency rooms, to tertiary mental health services.
6. Psychometrically sound: Tools must have undergone rigorous psychometric testing to ensure their reliability, validity, and sensitivity to change.

A number of measurement instruments are available to assess caring cultures, person-centered care, and recovery-oriented care—all characteristics of non-stigmatizing environments—though these have not been conceptualized as stigma measures. However, to date, most measurement tools in these areas have been developed by researchers, for researchers, with little input from people with lived experience of a mental illness. [417] Measures that focus on client perceptions of their healthcare experiences are few and, when available, typically focus on a single provider–patient relationship (such as doctor–patient), a single location in the health system (such as a family practice clinic), or a specific clientele (such as cancer patients or elderly people in nursing homes). Evidence in support of their reliability and validity is largely lacking. In a recent review of instruments in this area, none has emerged that meet all the criteria outlined above. Therefore, the lack of tools that could be used to assess structural stigma in health environments, and elsewhere, stands out as the single most significant gap in the stigma-measurement field. [416]

SUMMARY

Given the lack of funding for mental health research, building an evidence base for anti-stigma programming has been a challenge. Without evidence, funding for anti-stigma initiatives may remain out of reach. Also, although many instruments are available, the bulk of them examine knowledge or attitudes; few address discriminatory behaviors expressed by members of the public or experienced by people with a mental illness. If the goal is to make a difference in the lives of people who have a mental illness, then instruments that assess their experiences must remain paramount to evaluation efforts.

As outlined in Table 11.2, all the behaviorally oriented measures reviewed in this chapter are relatively brief, unidimensional, and internally consistent.

Table 11.2 SUMMARY OF MEASURES

Scale name	Attribute measured	Length	Internal consistency (alpha)
Social Distance Scales	Behavioral intentions	4	0.84
Reported and Intended Behavior Scale	Behaviors Behavioral intentions	8	Reported behavior (N/A) Intended behavior (0.85)
Social Acceptance Scale for Youth	Behavioral intentions	11	0.85
Perceived Devaluation and Discrimination Scale	Community-level attitudes	12	0.73 to 0.82
Mental Health Experiences Scale	Personal experiences with discrimination	11	English (0.94) French (0.96)
DISCUS	Personal experiences with discrimination	11	0.70–0.86
Internalized Stigma of Mental Illness	Self-stigma	29	Alienation (0.79) Stereotype endorsement (0.72) Discrimination experiences (0.75) Social withdrawal (0.80) **Stigma resistance (0.58)**
Self-Stigma of Mental Illness Scale, Short Version	Self-stigma	20	Stereotype awareness (0.73–0.87) Stereotype agreement (0.72–0.79) **Self-concurrence (0.22–0.74)** Self-esteem (0.76–0.82)

Note: Subscales that may be problematic are **bolded**.

Apart from the Perceived Devaluation and Discrimination Scale, all are appropriate for use in evaluating interventions. The Perceived Devaluation and Discrimination scale may not be appropriate for program evaluations because it measures broad community-level attitudes, which are slow to change. The measures of self-stigma are more complex as developers have tried to capture the various elements in the process of internalizing stigma. Both are multifactorial, with certain subscales that may be problematic for evaluation research. Given that internal consistency varies across samples, as is reflected in Table 11.2, it is important to understand both the factor structure and the reliability of each measure used.

Finally, though structural stigma has been one of the key drivers of stigma experienced by people with a mental illness, and one that created significant resource inequities, no measures of structural stigma were identified. This remains an important gap and an area for future research. A framework that systematically reviews laws and other organizational documents for systematic bias may be a useful approach and one that is consistent with the protection of human rights outlined in the Convention of the Rights of Disabled People.

CHAPTER 12

Stigma and Substance Abuse

A wide range of substances have been stigmatized, including tobacco, alcohol, prescription drugs (such as opioids), and illicit drugs. With the rise of public health professionals in the 19th century, the stigmatization of particular groups was regularly used as a public health tool to avoid infectious diseases such as smallpox, typhus, or tuberculosis, raising a serious moral conflict. Public health officials want to stigmatize substances to limit their use, while at the same time they work to destigmatize people with drug dependencies to promote help-seeking and greater social acceptance. Immigrant groups have often been identified as being the culprits for contagion and heavily penalized. Infectious diseases were portrayed as a penalty for transgressing moral rules. Particularly in the case of tobacco use, public health officials wielded a heavy hand in marginalizing and de-normalizing smoking. [418] This chapter considers the stigma surrounding drug use, including opioid use and alcohol use. Because substances are stigmatized differentially, we have not collapsed alcohol and other substances into a single group, as many studies do. We also consider stigma of substance use in non-Western cultures, substances used in religious ceremonies, and substance use among women, as they are typically judged more harshly. We also consider access to treatment and stigma as a public health tool. The chapter closes with approaches to stigma reduction.

DRUG-RELATED STIGMA

Considerable research has shown that the public holds negative and stereotypical views of people who use illicit drugs. In the United Kingdom for example, the Royal College of Psychiatrists commissioned a survey to form the basis of an anti-stigma campaign. [419] Of the 2679 subjects identified, 66.8% were interviewed. Opinions were solicited about eight stereotypes often ascribed to people with mental and substance use disorders: dangerous to others; unpredictability; hard to talk to; feel different; selves to blame; pull self together; not improved if treated; and will never recover. Seven disorder groups were presented: severe depression; panic attacks; schizophrenia; dementia; eating disorder; "alcohol addiction"*; and "drug addiction." Drug addiction, alcohol addiction, and schizophrenia elicited the most negative responses, particularly for items pertaining to dangerousness and unpredictability. For example, 74% of the sample considered people with drug addictions to be a danger to others, compared to 71% for schizophrenia and 65% for alcohol addiction. Drug addiction was also the most stigmatized disorder for unpredictability (78%) and being hard to talk to (65%). People with drug and alcohol problems were frequently rated as blameworthy for their illnesses (68% and 60% respectively). In a follow-up study conducted in 2003, 74% expressed a negative attitude toward "drug addiction." [420] In the same two studies, "alcoholism" was viewed negatively by 69% and 66% respectively. There were no differences in the percentage of the sample holding positive opinions (4% and 5% for "drug addiction," and 6% for "alcoholism"). In a similar U.S. survey of 815 respondents, the highest level of social intolerance was expressed toward people with a "drug dependency." U.S. research shows that the American public also consider people who use drugs to be more responsible for their condition, less often worthy of help, and less often deserving of assistance finding a job. [60]

Lloyd reviewed 185 papers assessing public stigma toward people who use substances, confirming that substance users are consistently more stigmatized than people with a mental illness. [421] He found a sizeable body of research showing the stigmatizing attitudes of health professionals towards people who use drugs. Stigma from healthcare providers not only prevents people from seeking help for general health problems but may also prevent people from revealing their drug use to health professionals, potentially putting them at risk. Stigmatizing attitudes also have been experienced from pharmacy staff by those on methadone maintenance therapy. In qualitative studies methadone clinics have been described as environments filled with stigmatized identities where staff sit behind bulletproof glass. [422] Relationships between clinic staff and care recipients may be paternalistic and one-sided, with excessive rules, restrictive dispensing policies (e.g., 2 hours a day), and a lack of privacy—all reinforcing feelings of disempowerment. Clients also felt that they were "outed" in some pharmacies where the reason for their visit seemed obvious to others—drinking green liquid from a small cup or exchanging syringes in full view.

---

*The terms "addiction" or "addict" are now considered to be stigmatizing. In this section, we will use the terms used in the original publication so that the reader may understand what survey respondents were responding to.

Using data from the 1996 U.S. General Social Survey (N = 1444, 76.1% response rate), Martin and coworkers examined the role of five factors thought to influence the public's willingness to interact with people who have a mental or substance use disorder: the extent to which they would move next door, make friends, spend an evening socializing, work closely on the job, have a group home in the neighborhood, or have them marry into the family. [61] Five vignettes describing major depression, alcohol dependency, drug dependency, schizophrenia, and a person with normal troubles were used to elicit responses. The highest level of social distance was toward people with drug (77.8%) and alcohol (55.7%) dependencies. In addition, few Americans defined substance disorders as formal mental illnesses (10.9% for alcohol dependency and 13.3% for drug dependency).

Corrigan and colleagues found that public stigma was worse for people with drug disorders compared to those with a mental illness or a physical disability requiring a wheelchair. [60] They recruited a sample of 815 Americans using random-digit dialing from a national sampling frame of all telephone numbers available in an online panel. The sample was stratified to be representative of the American, English-speaking adult population and represented a 71.4% response rate. Respondents were randomly assigned to read one of three vignettes with the themes of mental illness, drug addiction, or physical disorder requiring a wheelchair. Respondents were then asked a series of questions to measure two stereotypes often associated with mental disabilities: attributions of dangerousness and responsibility for the condition. People with a drug use disorder were viewed as significantly more responsible for their disorder, less likely to overcome the problems associated with their condition, less often considered worthy of help, and less often deserving of assistance in finding a job.

The prevailing social norm has been to view drug use as a moral and criminal issue under the person's control rather than a public health concern, making it unique from other stigmatized health conditions and more subject to stigma. [423] Room talks about the "heavy load of symbolism" and "moralization" that surrounds drug use. [424] Despite attempts to adopt a public health model, drug use disorder (and, more generally, substance use disorders) continue to be rooted in a moral model, making them among the most highly stigmatized conditions. Room reports the degree of social disapproval associated with 18 disabilities in 14 countries. All countries reported to the World Health Organization through key informants. "Drug addiction" ranked among the lowest, reflecting the greatest stigma, with eight countries ranking it 18 out of 18, four countries ranking it 17, and the remainder ranking it 15 or 16 (for an average rank of 17). By comparison, "alcoholism" received an average rank of 14 and "chronic mental disorder" received an average rank of 12.

Studies of opioid use and its associated stigma are infrequent and largely from North America. Consequently, little is known about opioid stigma in low- and middle-income countries. In addition, research has been largely descriptive, meaning that it has not closely examined differences in expressions of stigma by factors such as culture, social class, gender, or age. Unfortunately, we know far less about opioid-related stigma (and substance use–related stigma in general) than mental health–related stigma.

Historically, opium was not stigmatized as it is now. [425] For example, in China opium was imported as early as 618 B.C. During the period 1368 to 1644, opium was quite reputable and used for a wide range of afflictions (from cholera to stomach pains), and as a general tonic, as it was in many parts of the world. Opium was widely available and was used extensively as a recreational or medicinal drug in many countries. By the early 18th century, eating opium was regarded as invaluable for its medicinal properties and by the 19th century it was a mark of hospitality. By the turn of the 19th century, opium became the scapegoat for political and economic problems experienced in China and was demonized for its association with the West. [426] In 1680 in England, the apothecary Thomas Sydenham created Sydenham's Laudanum, which was a compound of opium, sherry, and herbs. His compound became popular as a remedy for many ailments. In 1803, the active ingredient in opium was discovered by a German scientist, and the resulting morphine was widely lauded by physicians as "God's own medicine."[†] Opium came to the United States through Chinese workers who immigrated to help with the country's westward expansion. Difficult working conditions drove the workers to opium dens for gambling, prostitution, and drugs. It became associated with crime and underworld activities, with the result that it was ultimately criminalized. [426]

Today, opioid stigma carries all the moral connotations of the stigma related to other substance use disorders, with some important differences. One factor that sets opioid use disorder apart from most other substance use disorders is that medication maintenance treatment (a best practice in the treatment of opioid dependence) is also highly stigmatized and judged to be morally wrong. The common misperception is that one legal medication is being substituted for an illegal one. This widely held view has been attributed to the slow response rate of governments and health agencies to promote harm-reduction and treatment strategies. [421]

The extent to which stigma undermines access to care has emerged as an important but understudied issue. According to a 2016 editorial in the *American*

[†] https://www.pbs.org/wgbh/pages/frontline/shows/heroin/etc/history.html. Accessed October 16, 2021.

Journal of Medicine, over the past 50 years, strong evidence has supported medication maintenance therapy (such as with methadone or buprenorphine), such that the World Health Organization has added these drugs to the list of essential medications. [427] Yet less than one in 10 (8%) opioid users worldwide currently receive this treatment. In the United States, Pearlman reported that fewer than 12% of Americans with an opioid use disorder in 2014 received treatment. [428] In Canada, approximately 25% of people with an opioid use disorder receive methadone treatment. [429]

A second difference is that a proportion of opioid users became addicted because of prescriptions provided by their physician, though this is probably only true of high-income countries where doctors and prescriptions are easily accessible. Indeed, fentanyl was introduced as a prescription medication used in medical settings for pain control following surgery, unfortunately with little conversation with doctors on how to be careful prescribing this drug. Aggressive marketing by drug manufacturers and poor post-marketing surveillance contributed to this problem. [430] According to the U.S. National Institute on Drug Abuse, 21% to 29% of patients who are prescribed opioids for chronic pain will misuse them and 8% to 12% will develop an opioid use disorder. Approximately 80% of Americans who use heroin first misused prescription opioids, making them a gateway drug.‡

In 2017, Kennedy-Hendricks and colleagues [431] conducted a nationally representative web panel survey of the U.S. population (n = 1071, 17% recruitment to the survey, response 75%) to understand public attitudes and beliefs toward persons affected by prescription opioid use disorder. Respondents also rated their support for punitive and public health–oriented policies. A third of the sample reported having had personal experience either through a family member, close friend, or themselves. Unlike stigma associated with non-substance-related mental illnesses, there was no evidence that personal experience reduced prescription opioid stigma. Instead, respondents with personal experiences expressed higher levels of stigma on several of the measures used. As expected, higher levels of stigma were associated with greater public support for punitive policies and lower support for public health–oriented policies. Even though respondents were rating prescription-based opioid use disorder (and not illicit opioid use), a large majority (78%) considered that individuals with prescription opioid use disorder were to blame for their problem. They also considered that some people lacked the self-discipline to use prescription opioids without becoming addicted (72%). They were unwilling to have a person with a prescription opioid disorder marry into their family (68%), were unwilling to work closely with them (58%), and thought

‡ National Institute on Drug Abuse. Opioid overdose crisis. [Online]. 2018. Available at: https://www.drugabuse.gov

that they were more dangerous than the general population (56%). Further, they considered that employers should be allowed to deny employment (55%) and landlords should be allowed to deny housing (39%) to someone with a prescription opioid disorder.

Recent data released by Statistics Canada[§] shows that most Canadians (77%) aged 18 and over are "very" or "somewhat" aware of the opioid issue. Almost a third of Canadians (29%) reported using some form of opioid in the 5 years prior to the survey and one-quarter of these reported that they kept their leftover opioids in their homes. Over a third (36%) of Canadians reported that they would not want their family or friends to know if they were using opioids without a prescription, or even with a prescription (14%). Qualitative research conducted in the United Kingdom with people who used over-the-counter codeine reported feeling "dirty," "guilty," or "addicted" as "much as a heroin addict." As a result, people often hid their opioid use for fear of reactions from family and friends [432] These studies demonstrate that the public stigma and self-stigma associated with illicit drug use have transferred to individuals who use opioids that have been prescribed for pain management.

The news media have fueled existing public fears of people who use drugs by recrafting worst-case scenarios into "typical" cases. News stories often use stigmatizing language such as "junkie" or "addict," fostering a stigmatized identity that is closely associated with crime and criminality. McGinty and colleagues [433] analyzed national and regional news sources in the United States to understand how opioid use was being framed. Between 1998 and 2012, the news media were more likely to frame opioid use as a criminal justice issue than a treatable health condition, which undoubtedly has important implications for the public's and policymakers' preferred solutions to the problem. Law enforcement interventions targeting illicit drug dealing were often reported as a solution rather than other prevention or treatment approaches. Public health approaches were rarely mentioned, and expanding substance use treatment was mentioned in less than 3% of the stories.

News media (and others, including health professionals) commonly use stigmatizing language when referring to prescription and other opioid use. For example, people who are dependent on prescription opioids are portrayed as "junkies" or "druggies"; drug test results are reported as "clean" or "dirty." As described in an earlier chapter, stigmatizing language maintains the us– them dichotomy and reinforces the "addict" identity through self-stigma. [432] We could find no similar references to stigmatizing language used in other cultures, though undoubtedly these words exist.

According to a report from the Executive Council on Addictions, opioid stigma affects everything from clients' choices to start maintenance treatment,

§ https://www150.statcan.gc.ca/n1/daily-uotidien/180109/dq180109a-eng.htm

to physicians' prescribing behaviors, to decisions by governments and regulatory bodies to establish policies and funding for maintenance therapy. [32] Opioid stigma has also had a significant impact on health systems' abilities to enlist physicians and pharmacists to provide methadone maintenance therapy.

STIGMA AND ALCOHOL

Schomerus and colleagues conducted a systematic review of all population-based surveys capturing public beliefs about alcohol misuse. [434] They surveyed both the academic and gray literature and identified 17 studies from Europe (seven), North America (five), New Zealand (three), Ethiopia (one), and Brazil (one). Beliefs about whether alcoholism was a mental illness and whether people who were alcohol-dependent were responsible for their illness differed across studies, but social distance was relatively consistent. Ten of the 17 studies reported high social distance scores. Results indicated that people with alcohol dependence were more severely stigmatized compared to people with other mental illnesses such as depression or schizophrenia. They were less often regarded as being mentally ill, were more frequently held responsible for their condition, and elicited greater social rejection. Two of the studies examined trends in public attitudes, finding little change over time. Only in Ethiopia were people with leprosy, schizophrenia, and tuberculosis rejected more strongly, again highlighting the importance of cultural contexts in shaping stigma and the need for more multicultural research.

Because of persistent stigmatization, people who have an alcohol use disorder who are in recovery face difficult choices with respect to disclosure, particularly at work. Human resource personnel view substance misuse as a serious problem with important implications for workplace productivity and safety. The human resource literature contains little information about recovery, which is itself a consequence of stigma. As a result, people in recovery face considerable challenges in their career development. [435] As an anecdote, in some countries, such as Istria, people with psychotic symptoms were more accepted by their communities if they were also perceived to be "drunkards." Their alcohol use explained their odd behavior, making them more understandable and acceptable.

STIGMA AND OTHER "NON-ADDICTIVE" SUBSTANCES

Several other substances, such as prescription or over-the-counter medications, attract stigma, even when they are unlikely to produce an addiction or do so in a small proportion of misusers. Almost no research could be found relating to these substances. Anabolic steroids are one exception. The media portray anabolic steroid users in overwhelmingly negative ways, often connecting steroid use with cheating in sports ("doping") and even aggression and criminality. Steroid users who disclose this to health professionals have reported feeling stigmatized and, at times, openly ridiculed. Griffiths and colleagues studied anabolic steroid use in a sample of 304 Australian psychology students. [436] Respondents expressed significantly more stigma toward steroid users than marijuana users. For example, almost half of the sample (45%) agreed or strongly agreed that using anabolic steroids was morally wrong, compared to 23% for marijuana use. Previous exposure to people who had used anabolic steroids was not associated with decreased stigma.

Benzodiazepines are often associated with addiction and psychomotor impairment. In a meta-analysis, Rapoport and colleagues found an association between benzodiazepine use and motor vehicle accidents. [437] Because of the large number people driving under the influence of benzodiazepines in the United States, they made the policy recommendation to introduce legislation to limit prescriptions. In a letter to the editor, Freeman described this as based on a stigmatized view that did not recognize the efficacy of benzodiazepines in treating conditions such as panic or anxiety disorders. [438] He argued that although they should be prescribed with caution, legislative action and limitations on prescriptions are not warranted and are overly zealous (it is important to note that Freeman disclosed that he has received multiple grants and research support from big pharmaceutical firms, and these may have influenced his views).

Another example concerns anti-obesity drugs. Halpern and Halpern focus on the under-prescription and under-development of new anti-obesity drugs in the United States, where the prevalence of obesity is high. [439] They point to several stereotypes surrounding drug use for weight loss such as the failure of patients, the media, and many health professionals to accept that successful treatment of obesity requires long-term, even lifelong management. There is resistance to using obesity drugs except in the short term, when weight is usually gained back. They point out that many known metabolic diseases, including diabetes, hypertension, and hypercholesterolemia, require long-term medication management, and morbid obesity is no different. They attribute this situation to an "obesity bias" that exists in primary care, where practitioners are unwilling to prescribe long-term anti-obesity agents. However, another explanation is that obesity drugs may be stigmatized because obese people are stigmatized: They are assumed to be impulsive and to lack willpower, motivation, and personal control. [440]

Several "normal" medications are also frequently misused. Ones that immediately come to mind include cough syrup, melatonin and other sleeping medications, over-the-counter analgesics, and energy drinks. The research literature is silent on whether there is a stigma attached to these; however, we might speculate that there is none, precisely because they are viewed as part of the usual tools people employ to address their everyday health and wellness. In addition to these, it is important to point out that there are several other dependencies that are not rooted in drugs, including "addictions" to gambling, sex, and physical exercise, to name a few. Gambling and sexual addictions are highly stigmatized. Physical exercise is not stigmatized, perhaps again because it is viewed as a health and wellness tool and so is "good for you."

STIGMA IN NON-WESTERN COUNTRIES

As with most stigma research, little is known about drug-related stigma in non-Western countries. One exception is a study conducted by Mattoo and colleagues, who examined stigma experienced by men who were seeking treatment for alcohol dependence (n = 50) or opioid dependence (n = 50) at a multispecialty teaching hospital in India. [441] Those in the alcohol group were significantly more likely to be married and older. Their average duration of dependence was 11 years, compared to 6 years for the opioid group. Unlike Western countries such as the United States, the alcohol group reported significantly higher discrimination on the Stigma Scale. There were no differences with respect to perceived stigma of substance abuse. Being employed, longer duration of substance use, and being abstinent were associated with greater stigma.

Gunn and Guarino studied stigma experiences in a qualitative sample of 26 young people from the former Soviet Union living in New York City. [442] Their views were particularly harsh, having been shaped by Soviet-era drug policies that severely criminalized drug use. Women who used drugs were judged more harshly than men. Drug use among women was associated with sexual promiscuity and sex work. Drug users avoided contact with treatment and community outreach services to avoid their drug use, or a child's drug use, becoming known in their immigrant community. Family members were particularly stigmatizing because they expected their children to be upwardly mobile. These findings echo the messages from earlier chapters that stigma must be understood within a cultural context and point to the importance of developing culturally appropriate services—in this case, services that would preserve individuals' anonymity within their community.

Ronzani and colleagues studied stigma expressed by 609 healthcare professionals in Brazil. [443] This study is interesting because it compared judgments across several different health conditions. The health conditions that elicited the greatest moral judgment from participants were tobacco use (78%), marijuana/cocaine dependence (73%), and alcoholism (61%). Schizophrenia, Hansen's disease, and depression elicited the least at 5%, 8%, and 12% respectively. HIV/

AIDS and obesity both ranked higher than the serious mental illnesses (45% and 41% respectively). With respect to cannabis/cocaine dependence, nurses were the group that showed the highest percentage of moral judgments (84%). Physicians were the lowest, though still highly moralizing (64%). The views captured were mostly based on ideas of attribution of responsibility for the health condition rather than social disapproval. This may be why tobacco outranked substance and alcohol use. These findings underscore the need to change professionals' views of people who use substances.

SUBSTANCES USED IN RELIGIOUS CEREMONIES

Historically, psychoactive substances have been used in religious ceremonies without shame or stigma. For example, shamans and priests have regularly taken substances to induce dissociative trances and promote spiritual reflection or connectedness. The *Amanita muscaria* mushroom (the beautiful white-spotted red mushroom depicted in Figure 12.1) has been at the center of religious rituals in Central Asia for more than 4000 years. It has also been featured in fairy tales and Christmas cards, making it highly recognizable to children. [233]

According to an article posted on Recovery.org, a website sponsored by American Addiction Centers, several religions have used psychoactive

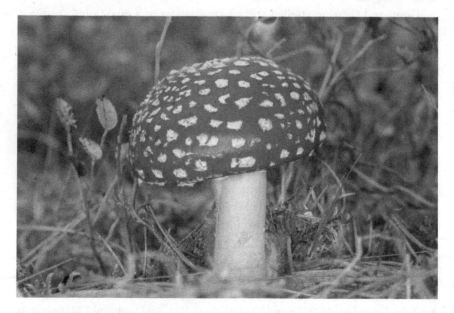

Figure 12.1 The *Amanita muscaria* mushroom
Source: Mikhail Kochiev / Shutterstock.com.

substances as part of religious ceremonies, such as the Native American Church (peyote), Rastafarianism (cannabis), Hinduism (a cannabis-derived drink called Soma), and the Bwiti religion of the Babongo people of West Africa (iboga, a hallucinogenic drug). [444] A wide range of drugs have been used, such as peyote (producing mescaline), Ayahuasca (derived from Amazonian plants), psilocybin (also known as magic mushrooms), cannabis and the *Salvia divinorum* plant of south Mexico and South America, kava (made from the *Piper methysticum* plant native to the Pacific Islands), Ibogaine (from the bark of the *Tabernanthe iboga* plant in Africa), and the *Amanita muscaria* mushroom (featured above), which is the oldest hallucinogenic mushroom used by man. It is important to note that substance use has not been accepted by all religions. Religions that have opposed substance use include Islam (both alcohol and drug use unless medically indicated), the Seventh-Day Adventist Church (all substances, including alcohol and tobacco), the Mormon Church (all drugs, including alcohol and caffeine), and Jehovah's Witnesses (any drugs, including tobacco).

The use of wine in religious ceremonies dates back more than 6000 years. [445] While expressly forbidden by some religions (as described above), in a number of faiths wine has played an important role. In ancient civilizations, the use of wine was part of the worship of certain gods, such as Renenutet, the Egyptian goddess of the harvest. In Greece, Dionysus was the god of wine and theater and was celebrated in religious ceremonies such as the festival of winemaking. Romans celebrated Bacchus by drinking wine to the point of intoxication, which was considered normal. In Christianity, wine is noted in many places in the Bible with reference to festivals, the liberation of Lot, and Noah, who planted a vineyard following the flood. In the New Testament, Jesus turned water into wine and, since then, it has played an important role in Christian ritual either literally or symbolically. In the ritual of Communion, it represents the blood of Christ. However, in 1830 in the United States a movement from within Protestant churches redefined wine drinking as evil, and this became a key part of the temperance movement. Even then, winemakers were permitted to make sacramental and Kosher wines for religious ceremonies.

WOMEN AND DRUG DEPENDENCE

Drug dependence is typically viewed as a male issue, but historically drug use has increased more rapidly among women. Kandall reports that by the end of the 19th century in the United States, women made up three-quarters of the people who were dependent on opium as well as a significant number of cocaine, chloroform, and cannabis users. [426] One reason for this increase was the rise in prescription opiates by physicians and pharmacists for just about anything that was considered to be a "female problem." From 1969 to 2005, women represented approximately 35% of patients treated in methadone maintenance programs. Women were also liberally prescribed psychoactive drugs and, by the late 1960s, made up two-thirds of psychoactive prescription users. During the 1980s female drug users became the object of significant public prejudice and were demonized for giving birth to babies who were exposed to drugs. These mothers were forced to avoid the healthcare system for fear their children would be removed from them—which they typically were, as they were universally viewed as unfit mothers. Rising awareness of drug-related infant mortality and low-birthweight babies continued to stoke the anger and stigmatization expressed by the public toward drug-dependent women.

There have been fewer treatment options for women than for men. In addition, women who enter recovery programs often face co-occurring problems such as child custody, domestic violence, history of sexual abuse, incest, and low self-efficacy. [446] Despite data indicating that women's needs are different, programs tailored to women and their outcomes are not widely reported in the literature. As a result, treatment professionals have limited evidence on which to base their practice.

SUBSTANCE USE AMONG NURSES

Substance use is a major problem within the nursing profession. While not all nurses are women, nursing has been a traditionally female profession. In a survey of 242 nurses in Tennessee by Grower and Floyd, participants estimated that 15% of their colleagues currently had a problem involving substance abuse and 15% were estimated to have had a past substance use problem that impaired their ability to practice. [447]

The "feminine" nature of nursing may account for the greater stigma associated with nurses who abuse substances and the tougher sanctions that are applied to them compared to other helping professions. Historically, the reaction to nursing impairment has been immediate dismissal or discipline, thereby contributing to the stigma surrounding substance use by nurses. As a result, impaired nurses tried to hide their addiction by avoiding treatment. Because it remains a taboo subject, healthcare organizations have typically turned a blind eye to substance misuse among nurses, claiming not to have the problem. More recently, organizations have begun to identify impaired nurses, divert them to treatment programs, and support their workplace reentry, but this is still uncommon. [448] In one program in Florida, since the program's start in 1983, 80% of nurses who have received services have successfully returned to nursing practice. [449]

There is also a serious lack of understanding of recovery within the nursing profession. In at least one province in Canada, for example, impaired nurses' names are entered into a public database managed by the nursing association. The database can be searched by prospective employers and members of the public. Though diagnoses are not entered, practice restrictions such as "unable to work around narcotics" clearly indicate which nurses have abused substances. Even when nurses have been in recovery for over a decade, their name remains in the database, making it virtually impossible for them to change jobs. Lack of prognostic optimism is a major factor underlying these discriminatory policies. Brewer and Nelms have noted that chemically dependent nurses who are in recovery continue to be deemed impaired and thus experience considerable rejection and a lack of support from their colleagues. [450]

ACCESS TO TREATMENT

Stigma from healthcare providers and expectations of being stigmatized are important barriers to care. People with drug use problems may avoid seeking help or may hide their substance use problem from their healthcare providers. Stigma can undermine both the physical and mental health of people who use drugs. [451]

Harm-reduction strategies take a middle position between the moral model and the disease model of addiction and thus have the potential to reduce stigma. As Marlatt describes, harm-reduction strategies were initiated by grassroots advocates who were looking for a pragmatic, compassionate, and public health–oriented set of principles and procedures to reduce the harmful consequences of substance dependence. [452] Harm reduction does not necessarily mean use reduction, though this would be ideal; for example, shifting someone to a less dangerous substance may be the goal. Harms are conceptualized as being a detriment to the substance user and to the larger society. Instead of focusing only on abstinence as a moral imperative, harm-reduction strategies offer a variety of options. They also apply to a wide range of substances, from tobacco, to alcohol, to drugs. Because the focus is switched from labeling the addiction as deviance, people are more likely to come for help. Street outreach services, typical of harm-reduction approaches, also build trusting relationships and promote help-seeking.

Critics of harm-reduction approaches often argue that they will encourage drug use and keep people stuck within a pattern of substance misuse, or that the underlying ulterior motive is to legalize drug use. [453] While there will always be naysayers, increasing numbers of countries are adopting harm-reduction approaches. For example, during the 1990s virtually all of the EU countries had needle and syringe exchange programs in place. Methadone treatments are also available throughout the EU. [454]

Ashton and colleagues reviewed the evidence supporting harm-reduction strategies. [453] Almost immediate reductions in the transmission of viral diseases such as HIV or hepatitis were associated with the implementation of needle exchange programs, making a strong argument for their public health effectiveness. Community-based outreach programs that provide literature about HIV and risk reduction and that distribute condoms and bleach to disinfect needles and syringes also have been associated with a number of benefits, including cessation of injecting, reduced injecting frequency, and cessation or reduction in reuse of needles and syringes. So far, the emphasis in this body of literature has been on the physical outcomes of harm-reduction strategies rather than the social ones. When stigma has been studied, it has been from the perspective of the negative views held by others toward harm-reduction strategies. Consequently, little is known about the effects of harm-reduction strategies on stigma reduction experienced by substance users. However, because they have the ability to guide people into treatment and reduce harms, harm-reduction strategies have the capacity to redress some of the health inequities often experienced by substance users. It is important to note, however, that harm-reduction strategies are not a comprehensive "fix" to the problem of social inequity. Pauly [455] argues that harm-reduction strategies are not sufficient to redress the inequities in health and access to healthcare that are caused by social structural factors. The focus needs to expand from one that emphasizes distribution of existing resources to disadvantaged groups to the social structures that are at the root of these imbalances, factors that harm-reduction strategies cannot ameliorate.

STIGMA AS A PUBLIC HEALTH TOOL

Phelan and colleagues have conceptualized a number of grounds for stigmatizing people. [456] With respect to substance use, it is to produce social conformity or to clarify for members the bounds of conformity with norms. This type of stigma applies to behaviors that are deemed to be under the individual's control; in other words, it is directed toward people who are deemed to be voluntarily "deviant." Examples of behaviors that are stigmatized on these grounds include non-normative sexual behavior identities, various forms of criminal behavior, substance abuse, obesity, and smoking.

The public health community has been sharply divided with respect to its stance on stigma. On the one hand, public health educators have deliberately used stigma to reduce substance misuse. [457] From this perspective, stigma is a necessary form of social control and a key public health tool. Proponents of the "stigma as social control" strategy argue that stigmatizing measures are an acceptable deterrent and are adopted as a means of reducing harmful behaviors, such as substance misuse. The short-term erosion of individual rights is considered to be an acceptable tradeoff for better population health. Policies that constrain liberties are justified because of the broad-based benefits they can produce. As one example, legislation in Minnesota and Ohio required drivers convicted of drinking and driving to display license plates publicizing their offense to shame and blame them. However, not only did this publicly shame the driver, but it also shamed family members or anyone else who may use the "marked" vehicle.

The "international war on drugs" waged in the United States clearly linked drug use with criminal activity, further stigmatizing users. Stigmatizing substance users has the effect of eroding their social capital, which is an important factor in recovery. Stigma can lock people into deviant roles and entrench inequalities. For example, with respect to smoking, Ritchie and colleagues noted that legislation requiring smoke-free environments and the creation of segregated smoking areas has resulted in smokers feeling as if they were "lepers" and "outcasts" and concentrated smoking among the working poor. [458]

Despite evidence that they don't work, public health communicators have increasingly adopted marketing methods that include "fear appeals" by providing vivid images to gain attention and arouse motivation. For example, advertisements admonishing excessive alcohol consumption regularly show young people covered in vomit or being made to recall embarrassing incidents. Guttman and Salmon describe these tactics as being of dubious morality and call for increased attention to the ethics of public health strategies that may stigmatize, victimize, and raise issues of culpability for socially undesirable health behaviors. [459] Messages that raise the issue of culpability place importance on personal responsibility and ignore the broader social and structural determinants of public health problems. They also promote the perspective that people should be held morally and, in the case of substance use, legally accountable for their behaviors. "Blaming and shaming" the victims leads them to experience a range of negative psychosocial consequences, raising further ethical concerns. They call for greater consideration of ethical issues as an essential component in the development and implementation of public health communications.

Our view is that it is fundamentally wrong and unethical to stigmatize people under any circumstance. Research has shown that there are serious long-term ramifications for individuals and groups who, once stigmatized, become locked into roles and identities that can further marginalize and exacerbate inequalities in health and social outcomes. [457] Sartorius and Schulze have argued that the stigmatizing mental illnesses is one of the greatest barriers to social equity. [69] They adopt a public health model that identifies cycles of stigmatization that interact to affect people who have a mental illness, their family members, and professional caregivers. At the individual level, a mark or characteristic allows an individual to be differentiated, and this becomes negatively loaded. Once negatively loaded, anyone displaying this characteristic will become stigmatized, with the result that they will experience numerous disadvantages, including inequitable access to care, poorer quality of care, frequent setbacks that can damage their self-esteem, and additional stresses that may amplify the original mark and make it more likely that the individual will be further stigmatized.

APPROACHES TO STIGMA REDUCTION

In 2012, Livingston and colleagues conducted a systematic review of the effectiveness of interventions designed to reduce the stigma of substance disorders. [460] Only 13 studies were identified, highlighting the lack of research in this area. Seven of them were conducted in the United States, with the remaining being conducted in the United Kingdom (three), Canada (two), and Australia (one). Three of the interventions focused on self-stigma, three targeted social stigma, and seven addressed structural stigmas. Of the 13 studies, seven reported positive results on all stigma-related outcomes. Six reported mixed results and one did not show any improvement. With respect to internalized stigma, group-based assertive community treatment (ACT) significantly reduced shame and internalized stigma, though scores on perceived stigma and experiences of rejection remained unchanged. An employment skills–based training improved participants' view of society and decreased their feelings of alienation but did not result in an improved self-image. An observational study that involved surgically removing "track marks" from injection drug users in recovery seemed to have had beneficial outcomes. With respect to social stigma, three studies conducted by the same study team showed that didactic educational fact sheets were not effective in changing public perceptions, though educational leaflets with positive depictions and motivational interviews were. Finally, with respect to structural stigma, changes to medical students' training reduced negative perceptions and increased a sense of responsibility toward people with substance use problems. Several studies targeted changes in medical students' views of pregnant women who abused substances, with mixed results. Instructive and interactive crisis intervention skills training programs for police significantly reduced officers' desire to maintain social distance. ACT produced significantly reduced negative thoughts held by substance use counselors about their clients. Finally, substance use counselors who participated in multicultural training had significantly reduced negative thoughts. The authors concluded that, among people with substance use disorders, therapeutic interventions such as group-based ACT and vocational counseling were the most likely to produce positive results. Communication strategies that promote positive imagery are best for changing public attitudes. Fact sheets are ineffective. Finally, educating medical students about substance use problems and promoting contact with people who use substances is likely to have positive effects. These results are not too dissimilar to those found in programs targeting stigma related to mental disorders such as depression or schizophrenia, suggesting that the substance use field could transfer knowledge of promising and best practices from the mental health field.

An interesting example of a structural intervention is illustrated by Massachusetts's response to the opioid epidemic. [428] Governor Baker introduced a bill that, among other things:

1. Limited first-time opioid prescriptions to a 3-day supply (though the final bill that passed in the House increased this to 7 days, subject to exceptions for those experiencing chronic pain)
2. Required hospitals to evaluate those who were admitted for an overdose within 1 day and expand on the training guidelines required for physicians prescribing opioids
3. Required physicians to use a prescription monitoring program to avoid prescribing opioids to those who were prone to misuse
4. Mandated public schools to verbally screen students who may be prone to becoming addicted.

To support these activities, an additional $250 million was provided in the Massachusetts budget.

Pearlman recommended increasing awareness of and access to voluntary treatment programs and launching even more mandatory education programs for medical professionals so that they could better identify the signs of addiction and monitor prescription drug use. [428] In 2013, the Boston University School of Medicine launched a Safe and Competent Opioid Prescribing Education (SCOPE of Pain) program targeting physicians and other healthcare providers.** It is offered online and live. The curricula use a clinical case at three time points: the initial visit assessing chronic pain and opioid misuse risk; 1 week later to study initiating or continuing opioid therapy safely; and months later to assess and manage aberrant medication taking. After taking the program, 87% of participants indicated they were planning to make at least one change in their practice. The most frequent changes were improving opioid prescription documentation (56%), implementing or improving opioid prescription patient education or communication (53%), and instituting or improving patient–provider agreements (47%). Two months following the program, two-thirds of participants reported increased confidence in opioid-prescribing practices and 86% had improved how they prescribed opioids and monitored patients for benefits or harms. While the program seems to have improved clinicians' opioid-prescribing outcomes, it is not known if it also reduced the number of opioid deaths or addictions.

** https://www.bumc.bu.edu/busm/2015/09/03/education-positively-impacts-safe-opioid-prescribing-among-clinicians/

DECRIMINALIZATION OF SUBSTANCES

Decriminalization of drugs has been widely discussed in the literature as a solution to substance use epidemics and to stigma. Some countries have decriminalized all drugs for personal use, and some have decriminalized only cannabis use. Cultivation and trafficking of drugs are not decriminalized. By delinking personal substance use with criminality, decriminalization has the potential to destigmatize people who use substances. It has been estimated that the criminalization of drugs costs $100 billion annually worldwide, with 83% of all drug-related offenses being for simple possession. [461]

Criminalization causes social marginalization and inequities (e.g., employment decline, housing insecurity, and public health harms). As a result, a number of governments have passed legislation legalizing drugs for personal use. As an example, in 2009, Argentina's Supreme Court stated: "Criminalising an individual [for drug use] is undeniably inhumane, subjecting the person to a criminal process that will stigmatise him for the rest of his life and subject him, in some cases, to prison time." [461, p. 13]

Several prominent United Nations agencies, including UNAIDS, the World Health Organization, the United Nations Development Programme, and the Office of the United Nations High Commissioner for Human Rights, have all supported decriminalization of drug possession for personal use. When implemented correctly, decriminalization has a number of positive outcomes, including directing more people into treatment, reducing criminal justice costs, improving public health outcomes (such as a reduction in HIV/AIDS transmission), and shielding people who use drugs from social stigmatization and marginalization. [461]

The total number of countries that have decriminalized drugs in some form or another is hard to determine. Using web-based reports and personal knowledge (such as recent changes to Canada's drug policy), Figure 12.2 highlights some of the countries that have decriminalized drugs in one form or another.

In two cases, the United States and Australia, only certain states have moved to decriminalize drugs. In the remainder of the countries, drug decriminalization for personal use was implemented on a national level. Four countries have decriminalized cannabis only (Canada, Belize, Jamaica, and the Virgin Islands).[††] Decriminalization may be particularly effective in reducing stigmatization if countries were to reinvest the funds saved into public health solutions such as harm-reduction and treatment strategies.

[††] Sources: https://www.worldatlas.com/articles/countries-that-have-decriminalized-drugs.html and https://www.citywide.ie/decriminalisation/countries.html. Accessed October 14, 2021.

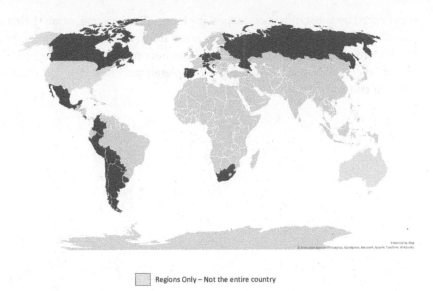

Regions Only – Not the entire country

Figure 12.2 Countries that have decriminalized drugs

SUMMARY

Although the stigma associated with substance use has not been compre-hensively studied, it is clear that people who are dependent on substances are among the most stigmatized of any mental health group. Women have been particularly demonized and penalized for substance dependence. Governments have actively pursued strategies that criminalize, stigmatize, and socially exclude people who use substances from mainstream society at tremendous social and economic costs. In an effort to curb substance misuse, the public health community has adopted a moral stance and deliberately used stigma as a deterrent. In Canada, more people have died of opioid overdoses than COVID-19, but the public health responses could not be more dissimilar. A massive outpouring of resources has been directed to reduce the pandemic, but much less (some would say little) has been done to curb the opioid epi-demic. Perhaps this is in part because the opioid epidemic is not seen as infec-tious, but it is also because policymakers have not prioritized stemming the huge toll in opioid deaths in this marginalized group.

There is a lack of research on approaches that could be used to destigma-tize substance use disorders in most parts of the world. Nevertheless, several approaches look promising but need more evaluation. Harm-reduction strat-egies deliberately take a nonjudgmental stance, and there is a growing body of evidence showing that they have beneficial outcomes for both the individual and the broader society. Yet, little is yet known about their effects on stigma experienced by substance users, especially internalized stigma, or on their social inclusion—an important research agenda for future scientists to address. Much more work needs to be done by researchers to understand the process of substance use stigmatization more completely and how it is manifest in different cultural settings.

CHAPTER 13
Summary and Reflections

When we wrote the first *Paradigms* book (*Paradigms Lost*), we were driven by our desire to provide guidance to budding anti-stigma efforts based on our many years of working with the World Psychiatric Association's Global Program to Fight the Stigma of Schizophrenia. [1] In working with colleagues in approximately 25 countries, including lower- and middle-income countries, we developed the view that much could be done on a shoestring budget with a cadre of well-intentioned volunteers. While many substantially funded national programs have come (and some have gone) in the interim, we remain convinced that everyone can contribute in some small or large way to removing the stigma associated with mental illnesses and substance use disorders. We described key elements in successful anti-stigma programming that reflected novel ways of operating. We tried to identify what we considered to be outmoded paradigms and replace them with approaches better situated to generate new thinking about anti-stigma programming.

In many ways, the most important lesson we learned from our work was that conventional programmatic approaches based on linear thinking (moving from a goal to implementation to outcome) and research evidence were hampering our abilities to jump on important opportunities when they arose. We had to be lean, to be able to pivot quickly, and to go where evidence didn't exist using our best judgment and incorporating evaluation activities to produce evidence. We also learned that program planners and researchers did not know what is best for people who are experiencing stigma, even though they thought they did. When people were asked, we were often surprised that what was most upsetting was something that could be readily addressed. This was particularly the case in lower- and middle- income countries, where the solution was something as simple as setting up a parent support group or making sure that people with mental illnesses received prayers in church from their religious leaders, as was done for people who had physical illnesses. It didn't necessarily require a complete overall of the social system. We learned how to work with community groups and create practice networks. We also learned the importance of becoming sustainable, and how to do so. Most importantly, we learned how to make sure that people with lived experience of a mental or substance use disorder were driving the bus, not sitting in the back seat.

As anti-stigma programs have increasingly targeted their activities to specific groups and recognized that interventions need to be culturally and socially situated to resonate within these groups (one size does *not* fit all), the field has blossomed. In *Paradigms Lost, Paradigms Found* we presented how our thinking, and the field, has expanded to include a growing emphasis on structural and internalized stigma. We also examined a broader range of anti-stigma tools and approaches.

Table 13.1 summarizes some of the key messages of this book by contrasting them with the situation described in the earlier *Paradigms Lost* volume. By providing a "then and now" perspective, it highlights the extent to which current approaches have grown in breadth and complexity.

Stigma was once synonymous with a negative or stereotypical attitude, and people talked (and still do talk) about stigma and discrimination as if they were different animals. More recently, advocates and researchers have adopted a much broader understanding of stigma and use the term as an umbrella to refer to the entire stigmatization process, including aspects of individual-level, interpersonal-level, and structural-level barriers to social inclusion. We recently heard of a hospital CEO who banned the word "stigma" from the hospital vocabulary, insisting instead that they talk about discrimination. As more people begin to understand that stigmatization is a broad and complex social process, these vocabulary divides will no longer be necessary. Perhaps one thing that we could do to get everyone on the same page is to educate colleagues about the nature of stigma and how the concept has evolved over time. We could also help individuals understand that removing discrimination, marginalization, and social inequities is the natural denouement of anti-stigma advocacy and programming.

Most articles and books about stigma make the broad claim that stigma is universal. By promoting universal thinking, it may also promote the idea the solutions are generic and can be universally applied. Universal thinking may also give the impression that stigma is unfixable. We have shown that there have been many times and places where stigmatization has *not* been the dominant reaction to people with a mental illness or substance use disorder. Countries fall on a broad spectrum of social intolerance, as reported by World Value Survey participants. We have also shown that stigma is culture-bound and intimately tied to lay understandings of the nature of mental illnesses. This means that anti-stigma programs will have to be increasingly culturally nuanced to maximize their effectiveness. This is true globally, but equally

Table 13.1 THEN AND NOW

Description	Paradigms lost	Paradigms lost, paradigms found
Stigma	Often used synonymously with a negative attitude, leaving critics to argue for a shift in focus to discrimination	A much broader conceptualization, including multiple levels and types of stigmas. Stigma has become an umbrella term for individual, interpersonal, and structural aspects.
The nature of stigma	Stigma is universal, suggesting that it is unbeatable.	There have been times and places where stigmatization has not been the dominant reaction to people with a mental illness. Stigma is historically and culturally situated, and anti-stigma work can be undertaken in any culture with culturally specific and adapted tools and methods.
Anti-stigma messaging	Top-down approaches; often generic and "one size fits all"	Programs are targeted, specific, and culturally situated to harness the resources of local community stakeholders.
Theories of change	Most anti-stigma programs do not build on viable theories of change.	Interventions must be evidence-based and logical and build on a strong theory about why the intervention could be expected to work.
Knowledge—action—behavior model	Improving knowledge will change attitudes, which in turn will change behaviors.	Knowledge and positive attitudes are not associated with improved social tolerance or structural inequities, so the latter should be primary targets for anti-stigma interventions.
Approach to stigma reduction	Structured and based on long-term plans	Enlightened opportunism allows grassroots groups to take advantage of windows of opportunities for targeted action.
Funding for anti-stigma programs	To be successful, anti-stigma programs need large budgets.	Anti-stigma programs may be mounted with limited funding and resources. Including key stakeholders in planning and implementation ensures access to a wide range of community resources.

Continued

Table 13.1 CONTINUED

Description	Paradigms lost	Paradigms lost, paradigms found
Active ingredients	Often literacy-based, medically oriented, presenting facts about mental illnesses and substance use disorders	Contact-based education relies on storytelling by someone with lived experience of a mental or substance use condition who is trained to offer an engaging learning opportunity. Provision of information may enhance stigma unless included in the framework of a comprehensive anti-stigma program. Also, selective perception may ensure that only the things that support prejudices are attended to and remembered.
Human rights frameworks	Anti-stigma activities emphasize stereotype replacement and focus on individual cognitions.	Increasingly, human rights frameworks are used to guide anti-stigma efforts. Stigma is viewed through a social justice lens.
Discrimination	Often considered too difficult to change so not a target of anti-stigma programming	The success of anti-stigma programs should be judged by changes in behavior, laws, and regulations and greater social inclusion of people with mental and substance use disorders as full members of society.
Media	Media create and maintain negative imagery in support of stigma.	Growing understanding of how to use the media, particularly social media, as a source of positive imagery and as a platform for change
Healthcare settings	Structure and culture of healthcare settings not a key target for anti-stigma activities	Greater effort to understand the implicit and explicit biases of healthcare workers and to create healthcare environments that are person-centered and recovery-oriented
Educational settings	Programs typically target older students in high school or postsecondary institutions.	In the future, we must develop a continuum of interventions that begin prior to preschool (with the parents) and move along the life course to postsecondary students. Programming will be developmentally appropriate.

Table 13.1 CONTINUED

Description	Paradigms lost	Paradigms lost, paradigms found
Workplaces	Workplaces are not often targeted, and employers have been hard to engage.	A number of evidence-based programs exist to assist people with mental or substance use disorders return to work. Employers are increasingly interested in promoting mentally healthy workplaces. Researchers have demonstrated a return on investment for workplace programs.
Technology	Use of videos, radio, theater, etc.	The explosion of digital and other new technologies offers many new avenues for program development and implementation to reach large populations.
Research	Mental health and anti-stigma research is inequitably funded.	As the evidence base for anti-stigma activities grows, research results will become an important advocacy tool in support of sustainable funding.
Substance use	Public health officials use stigma to deter "deviant" behavior and promote prosocial norms.	As harm-reduction strategies are increasingly used, and as more countries decriminalize personal substance use, substance users will experience less stigma. Proponents of decriminalization argue that by destigmatizing the substances themselves, they will also destigmatize the users.

applicable to multicultural societies. The "what matters most" within a particular culture may be the most useful way to gain a better understanding about how to redress stigma in local contexts. When approaches are not nuanced, they can create stigma where none existed. In Egypt, for example, Bedouins were caring for an individual who had a mental illness. They believed he was changed because of a curse that had been put upon him by an enemy tribe. Once they learned that he was mentally ill, they left him behind in the desert. Affixing a diagnostic label on someone or some behavior (using Western medical model thinking) is only likely to increase the possibility of stigma, making the consequences of stigma worse than the condition itself. We also know of examples where people with schizophrenia have pretended to be intoxicated ("simple drunkards") in order to remain a part of their community. If they were considered to be mentally ill, they would have been excluded.

Top-down approaches to anti-stigma programming have been the norm, typically associated with large social marketing or educational campaigns. Generic, one-sized messages and factoids do not resonate with cultural perspectives, nor do they give target audiences the skillsets necessary to address stigma within their specific settings. What we want a police officer to do when faced with a disturbed individual wielding a knife is not what we want a kindergarten teacher or a priest to do. In addition to creating understanding and empathy in these target groups, we must consider what behavioral changes should occur and how to empower people to make these changes. We must replace stigmatizing behaviors with ones that are affirming and empowering.

We have made mistakes in the past because we have done things on assumptions alone without testing out whether those assumptions hold. "Mental illness is an illness like any other" or "mental illnesses are brain diseases" are examples of well-meaning but ultimately toxic approaches to stigma reduction. In addition to ensuring that interventions are evidence-based, we need to have a clear understanding of the chain of reactions that the intervention will produce, and these have to be logical and, if possible, evidence-based. For example, why would understanding mental illnesses as brain diseases improve social inclusion when members of the public may deem this a hereditary taint or an unfixable flaw? Why would they welcome someone like "this," who is irredeemably broken, into their workplace or family?

Social science research has shown that the variance in behavioral outcomes explained by changes in knowledge or attitudes is small. We know that many of our most knowledgeable citizens (healthcare providers) are experienced as among the most stigmatizing of any group. We must have our sights clearly set on behavioral change at the individual or organizational level. It is probably time for the knowledge—action—behavior model of change to be retired. It is time to replace this paradigm with one that aims to change behaviors, laws, policies, and other social and structural barriers that discriminate against people with mental and substance use disorders and prevent them from being full and effective members of society.

Enlightened opportunism is our model to guide anti-stigma interventions. It recognizes that windows of opportunities will open, and anti-stigma programmers must be ready to jump in. Recently an important hockey player in Canada stepped away from the ice in order to enter a program to address his mental health. Anti-stigma activists could make hay with this, given that most news stations are covering the story. Interestingly enough, because hockey figures in Canada are superheroes, and he happens to be a good one, the press has been highly sympathetic, and colleagues have been overtly congratulatory about his decision. There's not much from the anti-stigma community as yet. Through the emphasis on the extreme stressors that elite athletes face, the press has knowingly or unknowingly normalized mental illness and made it seem like anyone would "crack under similar pressure." Programs that are based on highly structured and long-term plans would not be in a position to pounce on this situation or others like it.

In our own work with the World Psychiatric Association, we have seen many important and successful activities implemented with limited budgets or in-kind resources. Many times, organizations have stigma reduction as one of their goals, so it is possible for them to lend staff to coordinated community-based anti-stigma activities (but not solo efforts). Public health–oriented organizations typically have equity goals, so it is easy to appeal to their interests if a viable anti-stigma team can be formed. Public health–oriented organizations also highly appreciate the value of networks and coalitions. Including key stakeholders such as these in planning and implementation can ensure access to a wide range of community resources. Of course, large budgets are preferable, but the point to be made is that having a limited budget is not a reason to do nothing.

Many times, medical students or other health professional students who want to make a dent in stigma plan to offer local high school students medically oriented information about the signs, symptoms, and treatments for specific disorders such as depression or anxiety. While students may find this interesting, it will do little to change the way they behave toward people with mental or substance use disorders and it will not solidify an appreciation of neurodiversity. It may also prompt them to worry about their own mental health and wonder if they (or a friend) have any one of the disorders discussed. Educational encounters that rely on contact with someone who has experienced a mental illness or substance use disorder is the preferred and evidence-based approach. Medical information might better be offered in the context of psychoeducational groups for parents or caregivers who are often left bewildered by the healthcare system or don't know how to support their family members.

Thinking more broadly about stigma reduction, we now have powerful international declarations and tools, such as the Convention on the Rights of Persons with Disabilities, that adopt a human rights perspective on stigma. It should be an impetus to move beyond attempting to change individual stereotypes or cognitions to changing the social structures that create and maintain inequities. What we don't necessarily have are the mechanisms through which people with mental or substance use disorders can redress the stigmatizing behaviors of others. Some countries have human rights commissions or patient advocates to fulfill this role, but these are often insufficient or out of reach for people with serious mental health or substance use challenges. Nor do they exist in many low- and middle-income countries, where the bulk of the world's population lives. Perhaps a way forward is to begin to establish legal or other oversight bodies that could react to discrimination and respond to people who have been stigmatized. These could exist at any level in the system (local, organizational, regional, national). For example, in Hong Kong, there was an office in the government where people could lodge complaints if they felt wronged by the healthcare system or by others (e.g., employers) because of a mental illness or other impairment. A companion piece could be the development of guides and toolkits to help recognize and eliminate structural stigma in the legislative and policy realms. It also would be useful to develop a stigma thermometer or report card that could inform these bodies about the location and severity of stigma in support of targeted programming.

The media have long been identified as key culprits in presenting negative and gripping images of people with mental health or substance use disorders. In the case of the opioid epidemic, news media often show someone who has overdosed being revived on the street by paramedics with a gaggle of police standing around (just in case!), sometimes in full view of family members or neighbors (Figure 13.1). Increasingly, however, we can see how the media can be used as a source of positive energy and a platform for change. Social media may be the game changer in this regard, as people can post directly. We have seen how a single individual's protest has gone viral and resulted in important social changes.

Traditionally, healthcare settings have not been targets of anti-stigma interventions, largely because programs were not sufficiently targeted to key groups. As we have learned the importance of targeting our programs, the culture and processes of care in health and mental health settings, as well as the health professionals who work within them, have become important targets

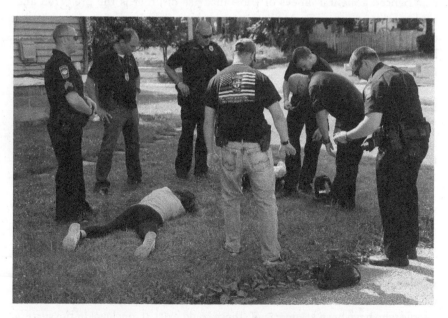

Figure 13.1 Response to opioid overdose. Photo by Spencer Platt/Getty Images
Source: BBC News, https://www.bbc.com/news/world-us-canada-43305340. Accessed October 19, 2021.

for change. There has been a growing effort to understand implicit biases and how these may affect healthcare. Healthcare providers who are well-intentioned and believe they don't stigmatize are surprised to learn that they do hold implicit biases. This type of awareness-raising may help them understand the need for, and increase the acceptance of, anti-stigma programming targeted toward them. It may also support efforts to create healthcare environments that are person-centered and recovery-oriented, and may even affect the choice of professional development activities. It is important for healthcare providers who are supporting anti-stigma programming to be clear about their own feelings about people with mental illnesses or substance use disorders, as the potential for conscious and unconscious biases can seep into and undermine anti-stigma activities. Thus, as a first step in contributing to a program, healthcare providers and other potential supporters should ask themselves the hard questions: Would they employ a person with a mental illness? Would they have that person in their home? Would they want them as a friend?

In our model, people with lived experience of a mental illness or substance use disorder would be the natural leaders for anti-stigma activities. However, to make this occur, it will be necessary to assist them with leadership training and other logistical supports, such as transportation to and from meetings, access to equipment such as computers or telephones, and administrative support to ensure that activity notes and minutes are collected and circulated. It is also worth noting that considerable support and training is required for people with lived experiences of mental illness or substance use to become speakers who deliver contact-based education, and burnout is always a risk.

We have identified a need to consider educational interventions much more broadly than is the current case. We take a life-course view and recommend that anti-stigma programming begin as soon as stereotypes and pre-prejudices begin—that is, among preschoolers. Age-appropriate information must then be developed for each subsequent educational level. In addition to helping students accept people with mental or substance use problems, it could also promote dignity and respect for all persons with impairments (eyesight, hearing, stutter, mobility problems, etc.) and greater appreciation for ethnic, religious, and racial diversity. Alongside these student-focused initiatives, there should be teacher-focused initiatives to promote the confidence and skills teachers will need to create and manage curricular change. We consider this to be a pressing need and one that should be prioritized for future consideration.

With respect to education, we have also talked about changing educational curricula for healthcare providers to help them better understand issues such as opioid prescribing and dependence, but also to highlight the potential for implicit biases seeping into day-to-day activities, and the importance of recovery-oriented and culturally respectful care. As many evidence-based programs exist, what must be done now is to convince the holders of health-care curricula that changes should be made. This will take considerable advocacy, as we are competing for prime real estate. Epidemiological data showing the prevalence and burden of mental illnesses may be helpful in arguing that the intensity of healthcare providers' training should match the burden of disease caused by mental and substance use disorders. Family doctors, nurses, and emergency room personnel are particularly well suited for these programs, as they will be the ones most frequently coming into contact with people who have mental or substance use disorders.

Workplaces offer excellent locations for anti-stigma activities, and employers are increasingly getting on board with workplace mental health programs, particularly as a result of post-pandemic return-to-work planning. Scientists have convincingly made the argument that mental health problems translate into lost productivity and that there is a return on investment for providing workplace programs and access to external employee assistance programs. A number of evidence-based workplace programs now exist both to address issues of prevention and promotion and to help create a smooth return to work. It is not known how these will work in small- and medium-sized businesses or in low- and middle-income countries that may still have a large part of their economy in family-run businesses or in small farming communities.

It is important to note that the knowledge and practices gained from the work conducted in the fields of mental and substance use to remove stigma are likely transferable or adaptable to other stigmatized conditions, such as racialized groups, cultural groups, the elderly, and other non-disease states. Thus, what is being done about stigma in our field may be a source of tools and methods (and inspiration) that could be used to make societies more humane and better places for all.

In conclusion, while it will take some time before stigma is reduced, in the meantime we may be able to help people with mental and substance uses disorders acquire skills that will assist them in managing stigma, particularly self-stigma. Traditional treatment regimens do not address this problem, and practitioners are often oblivious to the psychological effects of being diagnosed with a mental illness or substance use problem on individuals or their family members. Training modules that could be accessed as part of professional development may be an effective and efficient way to reach healthcare providers across a range of settings. It may also be useful to develop measurement tools that address sources of stigma associated with healthcare cultures and organizational processes that contribute to self-stigma and disempowerment so that these might be highlighted for targeted intervention.

Given that we now have numerous approaches and programs that have been demonstrated to reduce social intolerance and promote social inclusion for people with mental and substance use disorders, it will be important to ensure that these are more widely scaled up and funded. We must continue to develop new interventions and create a stronger evidence base so that this information can be used to advocate for better-quality services and more equitable social and health outcomes for people with mental and substance use disorders as well as members of other stigmatized groups. The visibility of the "Together Against Stigma" conference is helpful in this regard because it brings together multiple communities and often has high-profile policy-makers or politicians in attendance. As the conference moves from country to country, it draws attention to the matter of stigma in areas that are seeking a higher profile for their own anti-stigma activities, or places where anti-stigma activities are just beginning and the expert opinion and knowledge from conference delegates are helpful in kickstarting local activities.

As we have pointed out repeatedly in this book, we must never forget about the power of human testimony as a powerful stigma-reduction tool. With the advent of social media, we now have unlimited opportunities to share experiences and stories with a broad audience. People with lived experiences of mental or substance use conditions who post their personal stories have the means to reach out independently, far beyond what traditional live contact-based education has been able to do, and with no risk of burnout. How we can appropriately leverage these stories and systematically judge the impact they have on the lives of others is a topic for future research.

Finally, it is worth remembering that civilizations can be judged by the amount of support they give to their most feeble members—the disabled, elderly, children, and those who are ill. Wherever stigma is an obstacle to this happening, it also decivilizes society. Thus, removing stigma does not only help people with mental illness and their families, but it also contributes to make society a more civilized place for all its members.

APPENDIX
Stigma Section Bibliography

The Stigma Section of the World Psychiatric Association (WPA), through its network of international members, engages in scholarly, scientific, and public health activities designed to reduce stigma and discrimination because of mental disorders and improve social inclusion for people with mental illness and their families. More specifically, the Stigma Section:

- Disseminates information about stigma and discrimination because of mental disorders through academic and technical publications, and through symposia and courses offered at WPA regional meetings and congresses.
- Advances scientific knowledge about stigma through collaborative research and evaluation.
- Provides training opportunities to support the development of effective programs to fight stigma and discrimination because of mental disorders.

This bibliography represents the scholarly work of Stigma Section members for peer-reviewed articles, book chapters, and books published between 2019 and 2020. It is updated yearly and available from the WPA site under the Stigma Section materials.

BIBLIOGRAPHY

Bakolis, Ioannis, Graham Thornicroft, Silia Vitoratou, Nicolas Rüsch, Chiara Bonetto, Antonio Lasalvia, and Sara Evans-Lacko. "Development and Validation of the DISCUS Scale: A Reliable Short Measure for Assessing Experienced Discrimination in People with Mental Health Problems on a Global Level." *Schizophrenia Research* 212 (2019): 213–20. https://doi.org/10.1016/j.sch res.2019.07.018.

Barber, S., P. C. Gronholm, S. Ahuja, N. Rüsch, and G. Thornicroft. "Microaggressions towards People Affected by Mental Health Problems: A Scoping Review."

Epidemiology and Psychiatric Sciences 29, May (2019). https://doi.org/10.1017/S2045796019000763.

Bates, Sage, Andrew J. De Leonardis, Patrick W. Corrigan, and Gregory S. Chasson. "Buried in Stigma: Experimental Investigation of the Impact of Hoarding Depictions in Reality Television on Public Perception." *Journal of Obsessive-Compulsive and Related Disorders* 26, February (2020): 100538. https://doi.org/10.1016/j.jocrd.2020.100538.

Beattie, Tara S., Boryana Smilenova, Shari Krishnaratne, and April Mazzuca. "Mental Health Problems among Female Sex Workers in Low- and Middle-Income Countries: A Systematic Review and Meta-Analysis." *PLoS Medicine* 17 (2020). https://doi.org/10.1371/journal.pmed.1003297.

Bogaers, Rebecca, Elbert Geuze, Jaap van Weeghel, Fenna Leijten, Dike van de Mheen, Piia Varis, Andrea Rozema, and Evelien Brouwers. "Barriers and Facilitators for Treatment-Seeking for Mental Health Conditions and Substance Misuse: Multi-Perspective Focus Group Study within the Military." *BJPsych Open* 6, no. 6 (2020): 1–8. https://doi.org/10.1192/bjo.2020.136.

Bond, Kathy S., Nicola J. Reavley, Betty A. Kitchener, Claire M. Kelly, Jane Oakes, and Anthony F. Jorm. "Evaluation of the Effectiveness of Online Mental Health First Aid Guidelines for Helping Someone Experiencing Gambling Problems." *Advances in Mental Health* Advance online publication, (2020). https://doi.org/10.1080/18387357.2020.1763815.

Brouwers, E. P. M., M. C. W. Joosen, C. van Zelst, and J. Van Weeghel. "To Disclose or Not to Disclose: A Multi-Stakeholder Focus Group Study on Mental Health Issues in the Work Environment." *Journal of Occupational Rehabilitation* 30, no. 1 (2020): 84–92. https://doi.org/10.1007/s10926-019-09848-z.

Campo-Arias, Adalberto, Isabel Álvarez-Solorza, Andrés Felipe Tirado-Otálvaro, and Carlos Arturo Cassiani-Miranda. "Proposal of a Scale for COVID-19 Stigma-Discrimination toward Health Workers." *Journal of Investigative Medicine* 69, no. 1 (2021): 100–1. https://doi.org/10.1136/jim-2020-001647.

Campo-Arias, Adalberto, Guillermo A. Ceballos-Ospino, and Edwin Herazo. "Barriers to Access to Mental Health Services among Colombia Outpatients." *International Journal of Social Psychiatry* 66, no. 6 (2020): 600–6. https://doi.org/10.1177/0020764020925105.

Campo-Arias, Adalberto, Guillermo Ceballos-Ospino, and Edwin Herazo-Acevedo. "Denominaciones Para Trastornos Mentales Conocidas Por Estudiantes de Medicina: Un Estudio Cualitativo." *IPSA Scientia, Revista Científica Multidisciplinaria* 5, no. 1 (2020): 72–8. https://doi.org/10.25214/27114406.968.

Campo-Arias, Adalberto, Edwin Herazo, and Guillermo Augusto Ceballos-Ospino. "Stigma-Discrimination Complex Associated with Major Depressive Disorder." *Revista Facultad de Medicina* 67, no. 4 (2019): 531–2. https://doi.org/10.15446/revfacmed.v67n4.72529.

Cassiani-Miranda, Carlos Arturo, Adalberto Campo-Arias, Andrés Felipe Tirado-Otálvaro, Luz Adriana Botero-Tobón, Luz Dary Upegui-Arango, María Soledad Rodríguez-Verdugo, María Elena Botero-Tobón, et al. "Stigmatisation Associated with COVID-19 in the General Colombian Population." *International Journal of Social Psychiatry* 67, no. 6 (2020). https://doi.org/10.1177/0020764020972445.

Chang, Chih Cheng, Kun Chia Chang, Wen Li Hou, Cheng Fang Yen, Chung Ying Lin, and Marc N. Potenza. "Measurement Invariance and Psychometric Properties of Perceived Stigma toward People Who Use Substances (PSPS) among Three

Types of Substance Use Disorders: Heroin, Amphetamine, and Alcohol." *Drug and Alcohol Dependence* 216, no. June (2020): 108319. https://doi.org/10.1016/j.drugalcdep.2020.108319.

Chang, Chih Cheng, Yu Min Chen, Tai Ling Liu, Ray C. Hsiao, Wen Jiun Chou, and Cheng Fang Yen. "Affiliate Stigma and Related Factors in Family Caregivers of Children with Attention-Deficit/Hyperactivity Disorder." *International Journal of Environmental Research and Public Health* 17, no. 2 (2020). https://doi.org/10.3390/ijerph17020576.

Chang, Chih Cheng, Jian An Su, Kun Chia Chang, Chung Ying Lin, Mirja Koschorke, Nicolas Rüsch, and Graham Thornicroft. "Development of the Family Stigma Stress Scale (FSSS) for Detecting Stigma Stress in Caregivers of People with Mental Illness." *Evaluation and the Health Professions* 42, no. 2 (2019): 148–68. https://doi.org/10.1177/0163278717745658.

Chang, Kun Chia, Chung Ying Lin, Chih Cheng Chang, Shuo Yen Ting, Ching Ming Cheng, and Jung Der Wang. "Psychological Distress Mediated the Effects of Self-Stigma on Quality of Life in Opioid-Dependent Individuals: A Cross-Sectional Study." *PLoS ONE* 14, no. 2 (2019): 1–15. https://doi.org/10.1371/journal.pone.0211033.

Cheetham, Ali, Anthony F. Jorm, Coralie Wilson, Bonita J. Berridge, Fiona Blee, and Dan I. Lubman. "Stigmatising Attitudes towards Depression and Alcohol Misuse in Young People: Relationships with Help-Seeking Intentions and Behavior." *Adolescent Psychiatry* 9, no. 1 (2018): 24–32. https://doi.org/10.2174/2210676608666180913130616.

Chen, Yi Lung, Chih Cheng Chang, Yu Min Chen, Tai Ling Liu, Ray C. Hsiao, Wen Jiun Chou, and Cheng Fang Yen. "Association between Affiliate Stigma and Depression and Its Moderators in Caregivers of Children with Attention-Deficit/Hyperactivity Disorder." *Journal of Affective Disorders* 279 (2021): 59–65. https://doi.org/10.1016/j.jad.2020.09.121.

Cheng, Ching Ming, Chih Cheng Chang, Jung Der Wang, Kun Chia Chang, Shuo Yen Ting, and Chung Ying Lin. "Negative Impacts of Self-Stigma on the Quality of Life of Patients in Methadone Maintenance Treatment: The Mediated Roles of Psychological Distress and Social Functioning." *International Journal of Environmental Research and Public Health* 16, no. 7 (2019). https://doi.org/10.3390/ijerph16071299.

Chou, Wen Jiun, Tai Ling Liu, Ray C. Hsiao, Yu Min Chen, Chih Cheng Chang, and Cheng Fang Yen. "Application and Perceived Effectiveness of Complementary and Alternative Intervention Strategies for Attention-Deficit/Hyperactivity Disorder: Relationships with Affiliate Stigma." *International Journal of Environmental Research and Public Health* 17, no. 5 (2020). https://doi.org/10.3390/ijerph17051505.

Cogollo-Milanés, Zuleima, Edna Gómez-Bustamante, Edwin Herazo, Margarita Montoya-Hernández, and Adalberto Campo-Arias. "Relación Entre Autorreconocimiento Étnico-Racial, Experiencias de Discriminación y Consumo Problemático de Alcohol En Recicladores de Residuos Urbanos." *Duazary* 16, no. 2 (2019): 10–18. https://doi.org/10.21676/2389783X.3151.

Corrigan, Patrick W. "Beware the Progressive's Zeal." *Stigma and Health* 4, no. 2 (2019): 117.

Corrigan, Patrick W. "Beware the Word Police." *Psychiatric Services* 70, no. 3 (2019): 234–6. https://doi.org/10.1176/appi.ps.201800369.

Corrigan, Patrick W. "Challenges to Welcoming People with Mental Illnesses into Faith Communities." *British Journal of Psychiatry* 217, no. 5 (2020): 595–6. https://doi.org/10.1192/bjp.2020.83.

Corrigan, Patrick W., and Maya A. Al-Khouja. "Reactions to Solidarity versus Normalcy Messages for Antistigma Campaigns." *Journal of Nervous and Mental Disease* 207, no. 12 (2019): 1001–4. https://doi.org/10.1097/NMD.0000000000001062.

Corrigan, Patrick W., and Katherine Nieweglowski. "Difference as an Indicator of the Self-Stigma of Mental Illness." *Journal of Mental Health* 30, no. 4 (2019): 417–23. https://doi.org/10.1080/09638237.2019.1581351.

Corrigan, Patrick W., and Katherine Nieweglowski. "How Does Familiarity Impact the Stigma of Mental Illness?" *Clinical Psychology Review* 70, February (2019): 40–50. https://doi.org/10.1016/j.cpr.2019.02.001.

Corrigan, Patrick W., Katherine Nieweglowski, and Janis Sayer. "Self-Stigma and the Mediating Impact of the 'Why Try' Effect on Depression." *Journal of Community Psychology* 47, no. 3 (2019): 698–705. https://doi.org/10.1002/jcop.22144.

Corrigan, Patrick W., Sang Qin, Larry Davidson, Georg Schomerus, Valery Shuman, and David Smelson. "How Does the Public Understand Recovery from Severe Mental Illness versus Substance Use Disorder?" *Psychiatric Rehabilitation Journal* 42, no. 4 (2019): 341–9. https://doi.org/10.1037/prj0000380.

Corrigan, Patrick W., Sang Qin, Larry Davidson, Georg Schomerus, Valery Shuman, and David Smelson. "Public Perceptions of Recovery Prospects and Peer Style (Support and Confrontation) in Services for Serious Mental Illness versus Substance Use Disorder." *Journal of Dual Diagnosis* 15, no. 4 (2019): 226–32. https://doi.org/10.1080/15504263.2019.1635292.

Corrigan, Patrick W., Binoy Biren Shah, Juana Lorena Lara, Kathleen T. Mitchell, Peggy Combs-Way, Diana Simmes, and Kenneth L. Jones. "Stakeholder Perspectives on the Stigma of Fetal Alcohol Spectrum Disorder." *Addiction Research and Theory* 27, no. 2 (2019): 170–7. https://doi.org/10.1080/16066359.2018.1478413.

Cottrill, Fairlie A., Kathy S. Bond, Fiona L. Blee, Claire M. Kelly, Betty A. Kitchener, Anthony F. Jorm, and Nicola J. Reavley. "Offering Mental Health First Aid to a Person Experiencing Psychosis: A Delphi Study to Redevelop the Guidelines Published in 2008." *BMC Psychology* 9, no. 1 (2021): 1–10. https://doi.org/10.1186/s40359-021-00532-7.

DeLuca, Joseph S., Junseon Hwang, Lauren Stepinski, and Philip T. Yanos. "Understanding Explanatory Mechanisms for Racial and Ethnic Differences in Mental Health Stigma: The Role of Vertical Individualism and Right-Wing Authoritarianism." *Journal of Mental Health* (2020). https://doi.org/10.1080/09638237.2020.1836556.

DeLuca, Joseph S., Janet Tang, Sarah Zoubaa, Brandon Dial, and Philip T. Yanos. "Reducing Stigma in High School Students: A Cluster Randomized Controlled Trial of the National Alliance on Mental Illness' Ending the Silence Intervention." *Stigma and Health* 6, no. 2 (2020): 228–42. https://doi.org/10.1037/sah0000235.

Dewa, Carolyn S., Jaap Van Weeghel, Margot C. W. Joosen, and Evelien P. M. Brouwers. "What Could Influence Workers' Decisions to Disclose a Mental Illness at Work?" *International Journal of Occupational and Environmental Medicine* 11, no. 3 (2020): 119–27. https://doi.org/10.34172/ijoem.2020.1870.

Dey, M., L. Marti, and A. F. Jorm. "The Swiss Youth Mental Health Literacy and Stigma Survey: Study Methodology, Survey Questions/Vignettes, and Lessons Learned." *European Journal of Psychiatry* 33, no. 2 (2019): 72–82. https://doi.org/10.1016/j.ejpsy.2018.12.001.

Dey, Michelle, Raquel Paz Castro, Anthony Francis Jorm, Laurent Marti, Michael Patrick Schaub, and Andrew Mackinnon. "Stigmatizing Attitudes of Swiss Youth towards Peers with Mental Disorders." *PLoS ONE* 15, no. 7 (2020): 1–18. https://doi.org/10.1371/journal.pone.0235034.

Djamali, Julia, Luise Nehf, Anna Sama-, Nicolas Rüsch, Michael Kempter, Michele Noterdaeme, and Isabel Böge Ravensburg-Weissenau. "In Würde Zu Sich Stehen." *Soziale Psychiatrie* 2 (2019): 37–8.

Eaton, Kim, Jeneva L. Ohan, Werner G.K. Stritzke, and Patrick W. Corrigan. "The Parents' Self-Stigma Scale: Development, Factor Analysis, Reliability, and Validity." *Child Psychiatry and Human Development* 50, no. 1 (2019): 83–94. https://doi.org/10.1007/s10578-018-0822-8.

Erp, Nicole Van, Philippe Delespaul, Jaap Van Weeghel, and Joyce J. P. A. Bierbooms. "Positieve Effecten van Voorlichting over Psychiatrische Aandoeningen in de Algemene Bevolking." *Tijdschrift Voor Psychiatrie* 52, no. 6 (2020): 481–7.

Fegert, Jörg M., Harald Baumeister, Peter Brieger, Jürgen Gallinat, Hans J. Grabe, Harald Gündel, Martin Härter, et al. "Greifswalder Erklarung Zur Gesellschaftlichen Bedeutung Des Bereichs Psychische Gesundheit in Der Gesundheitsforschung—'Lost in Translation?' [Mental Health Research—'Lost in Translation?']" *Psychiatrische Praxis* 46 (2019): 70–72.

Fiorillo, Andrea, Mario Luciano, Maurizio Pompili, and Norman Sartorius. "Editorial: Reducing the Mortality Gap in People with Severe Mental Disorders: The Role of Lifestyle Psychosocial Interventions." *Frontiers in Psychiatry* 10 (2019): 1–3. https://doi.org/10.3389/fpsyt.2019.00434.

Fischer, Melanie W., Annalee V. Johnson-Kwochka, Ruth L. Firmin, Lindsay Sheehan, Patrick W. Corrigan, and Michelle P. Salyers. "Patient, Client, Consumer, or Service User? An Empirical Investigation into the Impact of Labels on Stigmatizing Attitudes." *Psychiatric Rehabilitation Journal* 43, no. 3 (2020): 1–8. https://doi.org/10.1037/prj0000406.

Fokuo, J. K., M. M. MaronLeey, and P. Corrigan. "Pilot of a Consumer Based Anti-Stigma Mentorship Program for Nursing Students." *Journal of Public Mental Health* 19, no. 1 (2019): 51–61.

Forthal, Sarah, Abebaw Fekadu, Girmay Medhin, Medhin Selamu, Graham Thornicroft, and Charlotte Hanlon. "Rural vs Urban Residence and Experience of Discrimination among People with Severe Mental Illnesses in Ethiopia." *BMC Psychiatry* 19, no. 1 (2019): 4–13. https://doi.org/10.1186/s12888-019-2345-7.

Hart, Laura M., Penny Cropper, Amy J. Morgan, Claire M. Kelly, and Anthony F. Jorm. "Teen Mental Health First Aid as a School-Based Intervention for Improving Peer Support of Adolescents at Risk of Suicide: Outcomes from a Cluster Randomised Crossover Trial." *Australian and New Zealand Journal of Psychiatry* 54, no. 4 (2020): 382–92. https://doi.org/10.1177/0004867419885450.

Hartog, Kim, Carly D. Hubbard, Angelica F. Krouwer, Graham Thornicroft, Brandon A. Kohrt, and Mark J. D. Jordans. "Stigma Reduction Interventions for Children and Adolescents in Low- and Middle-Income Countries: Systematic Review of Intervention Strategies." *Social Science and Medicine* 246 (2020): 112749. https://doi.org/10.1016/j.socscimed.2019.112749.

Heim, E., C. Henderson, B. A. Kohrt, M. Koschorke, M. Milenova, and G. Thornicroft. "Reducing Mental Health-Related Stigma among Medical and Nursing Students in Low- and Middle-Income Countries: A Systematic Review." *Epidemiology and Psychiatric Sciences* 1, no. 29 (2019): e28. https://doi.org/10.1017/S2045796019000167.

Huang, Debbie, Lawrence H. Yang, and Bernice A. Pescosolido. "Understanding the Public's Profile of Mental Health Literacy in China: A Nationwide Study." *BMC Psychiatry* 19, no. 20 (2019): 1–12.

Janssens, K. M. E., J. Van Weeghel, C. Henderson, M. C. W. Joosen, and E. P. M. Brouwers. "Evaluation of an Intervention to Support Decisions on Disclosure in the Employment Setting (DECIDES): Study Protocol of a Longitudinal Cluster-Randomized Controlled Trial." *Trials* 21, no. 1 (2020): 1–10. https://doi.org/10.1186/s13063-020-04376-1.

Johnson, C. L., L. M. Hart, A. Rossetto, A. J. Morgan, and A. F. Jorm. "Lessons Learnt from the Field: A Qualitative Evaluation of Adolescent Experiences of a Universal Mental Health Education Program." *Health Education Research* 36, no. 1 (2021): 126–39. https://doi.org/10.1093/her/cyaa050.

Jorm, A. F., A. J. Mackinnon, L. M. Hart, N. J. Reavley, and A. J. Morgan. "Effect of Community Members' Willingness to Disclose a Mental Disorder on Their Psychiatric Symptom Scores: Analysis of Data from Two Randomised Controlled Trials of Mental Health First Aid Training." *Epidemiology and Psychiatric Sciences* 9, no. 29 (2019): e46. https://doi.org/10.1017/S2045796019000404.

Jorm, Anthony F. "Effect of Contact-Based Interventions on Stigma and Discrimination: A Critical Examination of the Evidence." *Psychiatric Services* 71, no. 7 (2020): 735–7. https://doi.org/10.1176/appi.ps.201900587.

Jorm, Anthony F., Betty A. Kitchener, and Nicola J. Reavley. "Mental Health First Aid Training: Lessons Learned from the Global Spread of a Community Education Program." *World Psychiatry* 18, no. 2 (2019): 142–3. https://doi.org/10.1002/wps.20621.

Kaur, Amanpreet, Sudha Kallakuri, Brandon A. Kohrt, Eva Heim, Petra C. Gronholm, Graham Thornicroft, and Pallab K. Maulik. "Systematic Review of Interventions to Reduce Mental Health Stigma in India." *Asian Journal of Psychiatry* 55 (2021): 102466. https://doi.org/10.1016/j.ajp.2020.102466.

Kikuzawa, Saeko, Bernice Pescosolido, Mami Kasahara-kiritani, Tomoko Matoba, Chikako Yamaki, and Katsumi Sugiyama. "Mental Health Care and the Cultural Toolboxes of the Present-Day Japanese Population: Examining Suggested Patterns of Care and Their Correlates." *Social Science & Medicine* 228 (2019): 252–61. https://doi.org/10.1016/j.socscimed.2019.03.004.

Knaak, Stephanie, Romie Christie, Sue Mercer, and Heather Stuart. "Harm Reduction, Stigma and the Problem of Low Compassion Satisfaction." *Journal of Mental Health and Addiction Nursing* 3, no. 1 (2019): e8–e21. https://doi.org/10.22374/jmhan.v3i1.37.

Kosyluk, Kristin A., Kyaien O. Conner, Maya Al-Khouja, Andrea Bink, Blythe Buchholz, Sarah Ellefson, Konadu Fokuo, et al. "Factors Predicting Help Seeking for Mental Illness among College Students." *Journal of Mental Health* (2020), e1–8. https://doi.org/10.1080/09638237.2020.1739245.

Krendl, Anne C., and Bernice A Pescosolido. "Countries and Cultural Differences in the Stigma of Mental Illness: The East–West Divide." *Journal of Cross-Cultural Psychology* 51, no. 2 (2020): 149–67. https://doi.org/10.1177/0022022119901297.

Kudva, Kundadak Ganesh, Samer El Hayek, Anoop Krishna Gupta, Shunya Kurokawa, Liu Bangshan, Maria Victoria C. Armas-Villavicencio, Kengo Oishi, Saumya Mishra, Saratcha Tiensuntisook, and Norman Sartorius. "Stigma in Mental Illness: Perspective from Eight Asian Nations." *Asia-Pacific Psychiatry* 12, no. 2 (2020). https://doi.org/10.1111/appy.12380.

Lang, Anne, Nicolas Rüsch, Peter Brieger, and Johannes Hamann. "Disclosure Management when Returning to Work after a Leave of Absence due to Mental Illness." *Psychiatric Services* 71, no. 8 (2020): 855–7. https://doi.org/10.1176/appi.ps.201900617.

Li, J., Yu Fan, Hua Qing Zhong, Xiao Ling Duan, Wen Chen, Sara Evans-Lacko, and Graham Thornicroft. "Effectiveness of an Anti-Stigma Training on Improving Attitudes and Decreasing Discrimination towards People with Mental Disorders among Care Assistant Workers in Guangzhou, China." *International Journal of Mental Health Systems* 13, no. 1 (2019): 1–10. https://doi.org/10.1186/s13033-018-0259-2.

Li, Wenjing, Anthony F. Jorm, Yan Wang, Shurong Lu, Yanling He, and Nicola Reavley. "Development of Chinese Mental Health First Aid Guidelines for Psychosis: A Delphi Expert Consensus Study." *BMC Psychiatry* 20, no. 1 (2020): 1–10. https://doi.org/10.1186/s12888-020-02840-5.

Lu, Shurong, Wenjing Li, Brian Oldenburg, Yan Wang, Anthony F. Jorm, Yanling He, and Nicola J. Reavley. "Cultural Adaptation of the Mental Health First Aid Guidelines for Assisting a Person at Risk of Suicide to China: A Delphi Expert Consensus Study." *BMC Psychiatry* 20, no. 1 (2020. https://doi.org/10.1186/s12888-020-02858-9.

Lu, Shurong, Wenjing Li, Brian Oldenburg, Yan Wang, Anthony F. Jorm, Yanling He, and Nicola J. Reavley. "Cultural Adaptation of the Mental Health First Aid Guidelines for Depression Used in English-Speaking Countries for China: A Delphi Expert Consensus Study." *BMC Psychiatry* 20, no. 1 (2020): 336. https://doi.org/10.1186/s12888-020-02736-4.

Manago, Bianca, Bernice A. Pescosolido, and Sigrun Olafsdottir. "Icelandic Inclusion, German Hesitation and American Fear: A Cross-Cultural Comparison of Mental-Health Stigma and the Media." *Scandinavian Journal of Public Health* 47, no. 2 (2019): 90–98. https://doi.org/10.1177/1403494817750337.

Martinelli, Thomas F., Gert Jan Meerkerk, Gera E. Nagelhout, Evelien P. M. Brouwers, Jaap van Weeghel, Gerdien Rabbers, and Dike van de Mheen. "Language and Stigmatization of Individuals with Mental Health Problems or Substance Addiction in the Netherlands: An Experimental Vignette Study." *Health and Social Care in the Community* 28, no. 5 (2020): 1504–13. https://doi.org/10.1111/hsc.12973.

Mascayano, Franco, Josefina Toso-Salman, Yu Chak Sunny Ho, Saloni Dev, Thamara Tapia, Graham Thornicroft, Leopoldo J. Cabassa, et al. "Including Culture in Programs to Reduce Stigma toward People with Mental Disorders in Low- and Middle-Income Countries." *Transcultural Psychiatry* 57, no. 1 (2020): 140–60. https://doi.org/10.1177/1363461519890964.

Maulik, Pallab K., Siddhardha Devarapalli, Sudha Kallakuri, Anadya Prakash Tripathi, Mirja Koschorke, and Graham Thornicroft. "Longitudinal Assessment of an Anti-Stigma Campaign Related to Common Mental Disorders in Rural India." *British Journal of Psychiatry* 214, no. 2 (2019): 90–5. https://doi.org/10.1192/bjp.2018.190.

Mayer, Lea, Nicolas Rüsch, Laura M. Frey, Michael R. Nadorff, Chris W. Drapeau, Lindsay Sheehan, and Nathalie Oexle. "Anticipated Suicide Stigma, Secrecy, and Suicidality among Suicide Attempt Survivors." *Suicide and Life-Threatening Behavior* 50, no. 3 (2020): 706–13. https://doi.org/10.1111/sltb.12617.

Mills, Harriet, Nadine Mulfinger, Sophie Raeder, Nicolas Rüsch, Henry Clements, and Katrina Scior. "Self-Help Interventions to Reduce Self-Stigma in People with

Mental Health Problems: A Systematic Literature Review." *Psychiatry Research* 284 (2020): 112702. https://doi.org/10.1016/j.psychres.2019.112702.

Mittal, Dinesh, Richard R. Owen, Songthip Ounpraseuth, Lakshminarayana Chekuri, Karen L. Drummond, Matthew B. Jennings, Jeffrey L. Smith, J. Greer Sullivan, and Patrick W. Corrigan. "Targeting Stigma of Mental Illness among Primary Care Providers: Findings from a Pilot Feasibility Study." *Psychiatry Research* 284 (2020). https://doi.org/10.1016/j.psychres.2019.112641.

Moll, S., S. B. Patten, H. Stuart, B. Kirsh, and J. C. MacDermid. "Beyond Silence: Protocol for a Randomized Parallel-Group Trial Comparing Two Approaches to Workplace Mental Health Education for Healthcare Employees." *BMC Medical Education* 15, no. 1 (2015). https://doi.org/10.1186/s12909-015-0363-9.

Moll, S. E., S. Patten, H. Stuart, J. C. MacDermid, and B. Kirsh. "Beyond Silence: A Randomized, Parallel-Group Trial Exploring the Impact of Workplace Mental Health Literacy Training with Healthcare Employees." *Canadian Journal of Psychiatry* 63, no. 12 (2018). https://doi.org/10.1177/0706743718766051.

Morgan, Amy J., Julie Anne A. Fischer, Laura M. Hart, Claire M. Kelly, Betty A. Kitchener, Nicola J. Reavley, Marie B. H. Yap, and Anthony F. Jorm. "Long-Term Effects of Youth Mental Health First Aid Training: Randomized Controlled Trial with 3-Year Follow-Up." *BMC Psychiatry* 20, no. 1 (2020). https://doi.org/10.1186/s12888-020-02860-1.

Mulfinger, Nadine, Nicolas Rüsch, Philipp Bayha, Sabine Müller, Isabel Böge, Vehbi Sakar, and Silvia Krumm. "Secrecy versus Disclosure of Mental Illness among Adolescents: I. The Perspective of Adolescents with Mental Illness." *Journal of Mental Health* 28, no. 3 (2019): 296–303. https://doi.org/10.1080/09638237.2018.1487535.

Mulfinger, Nadine, Nicolas Rüsch, Philipp Bayha, Sabine Müller, Isabel Böge, Vehbi Sakar, and Silvia Krumm. "Secrecy versus Disclosure of Mental Illness among Adolescents: II. The Perspective of Relevant Stakeholders." *Journal of Mental Health* 28, no. 3 (2019): 304–11. https://doi.org/10.1080/09638237.2018.1487537.

Mutiso, V. N., K. M. Pike, C. N. Musyimi, T. J. Rebello, A. Tele, I. Gitonga, G. Thornicroft, and D. M. Ndetei. "Changing Patterns of Mental Health Knowledge in Rural Kenya after Intervention Using the WHO MhGAP-Intervention Guide." *Psychological Medicine* 49, no. 13 (2019): 2227–36. https://doi.org/10.1017/S0033291718003112.

Mutiso, Victoria, Christine Musyimi, Albert Tele, Isaiah Gitonga, and David Ndetei. "Feasibility Study on the MhGAP-IG as a Tool to Enhance Parental Awareness of Symptoms of Mental Disorders in Lower Primary (6-10 Year Old) School-Going Children: Towards Inclusive Child Mental Health Services in a Kenyan Setting." *Early Intervention in Psychiatry* 27, August (2020): 486–96. https://doi.org/10.1111/eip.12963.

Nakamura, Yuko, Naohiro Okada, Shuntaro Ando, Kazusa Ohta, Yasutaka Ojio, Osamu Abe, Akira Kunimatsu, Sosei Yamaguchi, Kiyoto Kasai, and Shinsuke Koike. "The Association Between Amygdala Subfield-Related Functional Connectivity and Stigma Reduction 12 Months After Social Contacts: A Functional Neuroimaging Study in a Subgroup of a Randomized Controlled Trial." *Frontiers in Human Neuroscience* 14 (2020): 1–9. https://doi.org/10.3389/fnhum.2020.00356.

Nieweglowski, Katherine, Rachel Dubke, Nadine Mulfinger, Lindsay Sheehan, and Patrick W. Corrigan. "Understanding the Factor Structure of the Public Stigma of Substance Use Disorder." *Addiction Research and Theory* 27, no. 2 (2019): 156–61. https://doi.org/10.1080/16066359.2018.1474205.

O'Connor, L. K., and P. T. Yanos. "Stigma." In *The Cambridge Handbook of Psychology, Health and Medicine*, edited by C. D. Llewellyn, S. Ayers, C. McManus, S. Newman, K. J. H. Petrie, T. A. Revenson, and J. Weinman (Cambridge: Cambridge University Press, 2019), 145–9.

Oexle, N., L. Mayer, and N. Rüsch. "Suicide Stigma and Suicide Prevention [German]." *Nervenarzt* 91 (2020): 779–84. https://doi.org/10.1007/s00115-020-00961-6.

Oexle, Nathalie, Katharina Herrmann, Tobias Staiger, Lindsay Sheehan, Nicolas Rüsch, and Silvia Krumm. "Stigma and Suicidality among Suicide Attempt Survivors: A Qualitative Study." *Death Studies* 43, no. 6 (2019): 381–8. https://doi.org/10.1080/07481187.2018.1474286.

Oexle, Nathalie, Wagner Ribeiro, Helen L. Fisher, Petra C. Gronholm, Kristin R. Laurens, Pedro Pan, Shanise Owens, Renee Romeo, Nicolas Rüsch, and Sara Evans-Lacko. "Childhood Bullying Victimization, Self-Labelling, and Help-Seeking for Mental Health Problems." *Social Psychiatry and Psychiatric Epidemiology* 55, no. 1 (2020): 81–8. https://doi.org/10.1007/s00127-019-01743-5.

Ojio, Yasutaka, Sosei Yamaguchi, Shuntaro Ando, and Shinsuke Koike. "Impact of Parents' Mental-Health-Related Stigma on Their Adolescent Children' Response to Anti-Stigma Interventions over 24 Months: Secondary Exploratory Analysis of a Randomized Controlled Trial." *Psychiatry and Clinical Neurosciences* 74, no. 9 (2020): 508–10. https://doi.org/10.1111/pcn.13085.

Pelleboer-Gunnink, Hannah A., Wietske M. W. J. van Oorsouw, Jaap van Weeghel, and Petri J. C. M. Embregts. "Stigma Research in the Field of Intellectual Disabilities: A Scoping Review on the Perspective of Care Providers." *International Journal of Developmental Disabilities* 67, no. 3 (2019): 168–87. https://doi.org/10.1080/20473869.2019.1616990.

Pelleboer-Gunnink, Hannah A., Wietske van Oorsouw, Jaap van Weeghel, and Petri Embregts. "Familiarity with People with Intellectual Disabilities, Stigma, and the Mediating Role of Emotions among the Dutch General Public." *Stigma and Health* 6, no. 2 (2020): 173–83. https://doi.org/10.1037/sah0000228.

Perry, Brea L., Bernice A. Pescosolido, and Anne C. Krendl. "The Unique Nature of Public Stigma toward Non-Medical Prescription Opioid Use and Dependence: A National Study." *Addiction*, 115, no. 12 (2020): 2317–26. https://doi.org/10.1111/add.15069.

Pescosolido, Bernice A. "Stigma as a Mental Health Policy Controversy: Positions, Options, and Strategies for Change." In *The Palgrave Handbook of American Mental Health Policy*, edited by H. Goldman, R. Frank, and J. Morrissey (London, UK: Palgrave Macmillan, Cham, 2019), 543–72.

Pescosolido, Bernice A., Bianca Manago, and John Monahan. "Evolving Public Views on the Likelihood of Violence from People with Mental Illness: Stigma and Its Consequences." *Health Affairs* 38, no. 10 (2019): 1735–43. https://doi.org/10.1377/hlthaff.2019.00702.

Pescosolido, Bernice A., Brea L. Perry, and Anne C. Krendl. "The College Toolbox Project." *Journal of the American Academy of Child & Adolescent Psychiatry* 59, no. 4 (2020): 519–30. https://doi.org/10.1016/j.jaac.2019.06.016.Ralston, A., J. van Weeghel, N. van Erp, G. Kienhorst, S. Oudejans, and L. Koppen. "Destigmatiserend Werken in de GGZ." *OstEpert Maart* 1 (2020): 40–49.

Reavley, Nicola J., Amy J. Morgan, Dennis Petrie, and Anthony F. Jorm. "Does Mental Health-Related Discrimination Predict Health Service Use 2 Years

Later? Findings from an Australian National Survey." *Social Psychiatry and Psychiatric Epidemiology* 55, no. 2 (2020): 197–204. https://doi.org/10.1007/s00127-019-01762-2.

Reneses, B., S. Ochoa, R. Vila-Badia, F. Lopez-Mico, R. Garcia-Andrade, R. Rodriguez, I. Argudo, C. Carrascosa, and G. Thornicroft. "Validation of the Spanish Version of the Discrimination and Stigma Scale (DISC 12)." *Actas Espanolas de Psiquiatria* 47, no. 4 (2019): 137–48.

Reneses, B., J. Sevilla-Llewellyn-Jones, R. Vila-Badia, T. Palomo, C. Lopez-Mico, M. Pereira, M. J. Regatero, and S. Ochoa. "The Relationship between Sociodemographic, Psychosocial and Clinical Variables with Personal-Stigma in Patients Diagnosed with Schizophrenia." *Actas Espanolas de Psiquiatria* 48, no. 3 (2020): 116–25.

Roe, James, Susan Brown, Caroline Yeo, Stefan Rennick-Egglestone, Julie Repper, Fiona Ng, Joy Llewelyn-Beardsley, et al. "Opportunities, Enablers, and Barriers to the Use of Recorded Recovery Narratives in Clinical Settings." *Frontiers in Psychiatry* 11 (2020): 1–11. https://doi.org/10.3389/fpsyt.2020.589731.

Ross, A. M., Amy Morgan, Anthony F. Jorm, and Nicola J. Reavley. "A Systematic Review of the Impact of Media Reports of Severe Mental Illness on Stigma and Discrimination, and Interventions that Aim to Mitigate Any Adverse Impact." *Social Psychiatry and Psychiatric Epidemiology* 54, no. 1 (2019): 11–31.

Rüsch, Nicolas, and Markus Kösters. "Honest, Open, Proud to Support Disclosure Decisions and to Decrease Stigma's Impact among People with Mental Illness: Conceptual Review and Meta-analysis of Program Efficacy." *Social Psychiatry and Psychiatric Epidemiology* 56 (2021) 1513–26. https://doi.org/10.1007/s00127-021-02076-y.

Rüsch, Nicolas, Alexandra Malzer, Nathalie Oexle, Tamara Waldmann, Tobias Staiger, Andreas Bahemann, Moritz E. Wigand, Thomas Becker, and Patrick W. Corrigan. "Disclosure and Quality of Life among Unemployed Individuals with Mental Health Problems: A Longitudinal Study." *Journal of Nervous and Mental Disease* 207, no. 3 (2019): 137–9. https://doi.org/10.1097/NMD.0000000000000914.

Rüsch, Nicolas, Luise Nehf, Julia Djamali, Nadine Mulfinger, and Sabine Müller. "Honest, Open, Proud: A Peer-Led Group Program for Adolescents with Mental Illness." *Nervenheilkunde* 38 (2019): 30–34. https://doi.org/10.1055/a-0813-9493.

Rüsch, Nicolas, Nathalie Oexle, Lea Reichhardt, and Stephanie Ventling. "In Würde Zu Sich Stehen—Konzept Und Wirksamkeit Eines Peergeleiteten Programms Zu Offenlegung Und Stigmabewältigung [Honest, Open, Proud: Concept and Efficacy of a Peer-Led Program to Provide Support with Disclosure Decisions and Coping with Stigma]." *Psychiatrische Praxis* 46, no. 2 (2019): 97–102. http://search.ebscohost.com/login.aspx?direct=true&AuthType=&db=psyh&AN=2019-14784-004&site=ehost-live.

Rüsch, Nicolas, Nathalie Oexle, Graham Thornicroft, Johannes Keller, Christiane Waller, Ines Germann, Christina A. Regelmann, Michael Noll-Hussong, and Roland Zahn. "Self-Contempt as a Predictor of Suicidality: A Longitudinal Study." *Journal of Nervous and Mental Disease* 207, no. 12 (2019): 1056–7. https://doi.org/10.1097/NMD.0000000000001079.

Rüsch, Nicolas, Tobias Staiger, Tamara Waldmann, Marie Christine Dekoj, Thorsten Brosch, Lisa Gabriel, Andreas Bahemann, et al. "Efficacy of a Peer-Led Group Program for Unemployed People with Mental Health Problems: Pilot

Randomized Controlled Trial." *International Journal of Social Psychiatry* 65, no. 4 (2019): 333–7. https://doi.org/10.1177/0020764019846171.

Saavedra, Javier, Samuel Arias-Sánchez, Patrick Corrigan, and Marcelino López. "Assessing the Factorial Structure of the Mental Illness Public Stigma in Spain." *Disability and Rehabilitation* 43, no. 18 (2020): 2656–62. https://doi.org/10.1080/09638288.2019.1710769.

Sapag, Jaime C., Rachel Klabunde, Luis Villarroel, Paola R. Velasco, Cinthia Álvarez, Claudia Parra, Sireesha J. Bobbili, et al. "Validation of the Opening Minds Scale and Patterns of Stigma in Chilean Primary Health Care." *PLoS ONE* 14, no. 9 (2019): 1–14. https://doi.org/10.1371/journal.pone.0221825.

Sartorius, N. "Early Interventions to Prevent Stigmatization and Its Consequences." In *Early Intervention in Psychiatric Disorders Across Cultures*, edited by E. Y. H. Chan, A. Ventriglio, and D. Bhugra (Oxford: Oxford University Press, 2019), 9–15.

Sartorius, Norman. "Fighting Stigma 2020: Synopsis of the Presentation of the Yves Pelicier Prize Lecture at the World Congress of Social Psychiatry, Bucharest, October 2019." *World Social Psychiatry* 2, no. 3 (2020): 181–3. https://doi.org/10.4103/wsp.wsp.

Sartorius, Norman. "Norman Sartorius: A Personal History of Psychiatry." *Global Psychiatry* 3, no. 1 (2020): 1–8. https://doi.org/10.2478/gp-2020-0007.

Sartorius, Vera, and Norman Sartorius. "The WPA Celebrates Its 70th Birthday." *World Psychiatry* 19, no. 3 (2020): 403–4. https://doi.org/10.1002/wps.20787.

Schulz, Michael. "Es Hilft Bei Stigma-Bewältigung." *Psychiatrische Pflege* 5, no. 1 (2020): 32–3.

Scior, Katrina, Nicolas Rüsch, Chris White, and Patrick W. Corrigan. "Supporting Mental Health Disclosure Decisions: The Honest, Open, Proud Programme." *British Journal of Psychiatry* 216, no. 5 (2020): 243–45. https://doi.org/10.1192/bjp.2019.256.

Scocco, P., A. Preti, S. Totaro, P. W. Corrigan, and C. Castriotta. "Stigma, Grief and Depressive Symptoms in Help-Seeking People Bereaved through Suicide." *Journal of Affective Disorders* 244 (2019): 223–30. https://doi.org/10.1016/j.jad.2018.10.098.

Shah, Binoy B., Katherine Nieweglowski, and Patrick W. Corrigan. "Perceptions of Difference and Disdain on the Self-Stigma of Mental Illness." *Journal of Mental Health* 31, no. 1 (2020): 22–28. https://doi.org/10.1080/09638237.2020.1803231.

Shefer, Guy, Claire Henderson, Louise M. Howard, Joanna Murray, and Graham Thornicroft. "Diagnostic Overshadowing and Other Challenges Involved in the Diagnostic Process of Patients with Mental Illness Who Present in Emergency Departments with Physical Symptoms: A Qualitative Study." *PLoS ONE* 9, no. 11 (2014): 1–8. https://doi.org/10.1371/journal.pone.0111682.

Sinha, Moitreyee, Manasi Kumar, Lian Zeitz, Pamela Y Collins, Steve Fisher, Nathaniel Foote, Norman Sartorius, et al. "Towards Mental Health Friendly Cities during and after COVID-19." *Cities & Health* (2020). https://doi.org/10.1080/23748834.2020.1790251.

Soomro, S., and P. T. Yanos. "Predictors of Mental Health Stigma among Police Officers: The Role of Trauma and PTSD." *Journal of Police and Criminal Psychology* 34 (2019): 175–83.

Sørensen, Kristine. "Defining Health Literacy: Exploring Differences and Commonalities." In *International Handbook of Research, Practice and Policy Across the Lifespan*, edited by O. Okan, U. Bauer, P. Pinheiro, Kristine Sørensen, and D. Levin (Bristol, UK: Policy Press, 2019).

Stuart, H. "Managing the Stigma of Opioid Use." *Healthcare Management Forum* 32, no. 2 (2019). https://doi.org/10.1177/0840470418798658.

Stuart, Heather, Brooke Linden, and Norman Sartorius. "Stigma: An Old Unmet Need in Psychiatric Practice." In *New Directions in Psychiatry*, edited by M. Pompili, R. McIntyre, A. Fiorilo, and N. Sartorius (Cham, Switzerland: Springer, 2020), 205–30.

Stuart, Heather, Norman Sartorius, and Graham Thornicroft. "Fighting Mental Illness-Related Stigma: What We Have Learned." In *Advances in Psychiatry*, edited by A. Javed and K. Fountoulakis (Cham, Switzerland: Springer, 2019), 621–36.

Su, Jian An, and Chih Cheng Chang. "Association between Family Caregiver Burden and Affiliate Stigma in the Families of People with Dementia." *International Journal of Environmental Research and Public Health* 17, no. 8 (2020), 2772. https://doi.org/10.3390/ijerph17082772.

Šumskienė, Eglė, and Monika Nemanyte. "Discursive Exploitation or Actual Impact: Mental Health Anti-Stigma Campaigns in the Post-Communist Area." *Archives of Psychiatry and Psychotherapy* 22, no. 1 (2020): 22–33. https://doi.org/10.12740/APP/116654.

Tan, Denise P.W., Amy J. Morgan, Anthony F. Jorm, and Nicola J. Reavley. "Emotional Impacts of Participation in an Australian National Survey on Mental Health-Related Discrimination." *Ethics and Behavior* 29, no. 6 (2019): 438–58. https://doi.org/10.1080/10508422.2019.1593844.

Thornicroft, Graham, Ioannis Bakolis, Sara Evans-Lacko, Petra C Gronholm, Claire Henderson, Brandon A. Kohrt, Mirja Koschorke, et al. "Key Lessons Learned from the INDIGO Global Network on Mental Health Related Stigma and Discrimination." *World Psychiatry* 18, no. 2 (2019): 229–30. https://doi.org/10.1002/wps.20628.

Turan, Janet M., Melissa A. Elafros, Carmen H. Logie, Swagata Banik, Bulent Turan, Kaylee B. Crockett, Bernice Pescosolido, and Sarah M. Murray. "Challenges and Opportunities in Examining and Addressing Intersectional Stigma and Health." *BMC Medicine* 17, no. 1 (2019): 1–15. https://doi.org/10.1186/s12916-018-1246-9.

Van Weeghel, J. "Stigma Als Comorbide Probleem Is Normalisering de Oplossing?" *Tijdschrift Participatie En Herstel* 29, no. 1 (2020): 19–22.

Waldmann, Tamara, Tobias Staiger, Nathalie Oexle, and Nicolas Rüsch. "Mental Health Literacy and Help-Seeking among Unemployed People with Mental Health Problems." *Journal of Mental Health* 29, no. 3 (2020): 270–6. https://doi.org/10.1080/09638237.2019.1581342.

Wasserman, D., G. Apter, C. Baeken, S. Bailey, J. Balazs, C. Bec, P. Bienkowski, et al. "Compulsory Admissions of Patients with Mental Disorders: State of the Art on Ethical and Legislative Aspects in 40 European Countries." *European Psychiatry* 63, no. 1 (2020). https://doi.org/10.1192/j.eurpsy.2020.79.

Wigand, Moritz E., Nathalie Oexle, Tobias Staiger, Tamara Waldmann, and Nicolas Rüsch. "Causal Attributions and Secrecy in Unemployed People with Mental Health Problems." *Psychiatry Research* 272 (2019): 447–9. https://doi.org/10.1016/j.psychres.2018.12.160.

Wigand, Moritz E., Nathalie Oexle, Tamara Waldmann, Tobias Staiger, Thomas Becker, and Nicolas Rüsch. "Predictors of Help-Seeking in Unemployed People with

Mental Health Problems." *International Journal of Social Psychiatry* 65, no. 7–8 (2019): 543–7. https://doi.org/10.1177/0020764019868262.

Xu, Z., B. Lay, N. Oexle, T. Drack, M. Bleiker, S. Lengler, C. Blank, et al. "Involuntary Psychiatric Hospitalisation, Stigma Stress and Recovery: A 2-Year Study." *Epidemiology and Psychiatric Sciences* 28, no. 4 (2019): 458–65. https://doi.org/10.1017/S2045796018000021.

Yamaguchi, S., Y. Ojio, S. Ando, P. Bernick, K. Ohta, K. I. Watanabe, G. Thornicroft, T. Shiozawa, and S. Koike. "Long-Term Effects of Filmed Social Contact or Internet-Based Self-Study on Mental Health-Related Stigma: A 2 Year Follow-up of a Randomised Controlled Trial." *Social Psychiatry and Psychiatric Epidemiology* 54, no. 1 (2019): 33–42.

Yamaguchi, Satoshi, Yasutaka Ojio, Jerome Clifford Foo, Emiko Michigami, Satoshi Usami, Taruto Fuyama, Kumiko Onuma, et al. "A Quasi-Cluster Randomized Controlled Trial of a Classroom-Based Mental Health Literacy Educational Intervention to Promote Knowledge and Help-Seeking/Helping Behavior in Adolescents." *Journal of Adolescence* 82 (2020): 58–66. https://doi.org/10.1016/j.adolescence.2020.05.002.

Yanos, Philip T., Joseph S. DeLuca, David Roe, and Paul H. Lysaker. "The Impact of Illness Identity on Recovery from Severe Mental Illness: A Review of the Evidence." *Psychiatry Research* 288 (2020): 112950. https://doi.org/10.1016/j.psychres.2020.112950.

Yanos, Philip T., Joseph S. DeLuca, Michelle P. Salyers, Melanie W. Fischer, Jennifer Song, and Juliana Caro. "Cross-Sectional and Prospective Correlates of Associative Stigma among Mental Health Service Providers." *Psychiatric Rehabilitation Journal* 43, no. 2 (2020): 85–90. https://doi.org/10.1037/prj0000378.

Yanos, Philip T., Paul H. Lysaker, Steven M. Silverstein, Beth Vayshenker, Lauren Gonzales, Michelle L. West, and David Roe. "A Randomized-Controlled Trial of Treatment for Self-Stigma among Persons Diagnosed with Schizophrenia-Spectrum Disorders." *Social Psychiatry and Psychiatric Epidemiology* 54, no. 11 (2019): 1363–78. https://doi.org/10.1007/s00127-019-01702-0.

Yanos, Philip T., David Roe, and Paul H. Lysaker. "The Impact of Illness Identity on Recovery from Severe Mental Illness." *American Journal of Psychiatric Rehabilitation* 13, no. 2 (2010): 73–93. https://doi.org/10.1080/15487761003756860.

Young, Daniel K. W., Petrus Y. N. Ng, Patrick Corrigan, Renee Chiu, and Shuyan Yang. "Self-Stigma Reduction Group for People with Depression: A Randomized Controlled Trial." *Research on Social Work Practice* 30, no. 8 (2020): 846–57. https://doi.org/10.1177/1049731520941594.

Zehnder, Mara, Jochen Mutschler, Wulf Rössler, Michael Rufer, and Nicolas Rüsch. "Stigma as a Barrier to Mental Health Service Use among Female Sex Workers in Switzerland." *Frontiers in Psychiatry* 10 (2019): 7–9. https://doi.org/10.3389/fpsyt.2019.00032.

Zoubaa, Sarah, Sarah Dure, and Philip T. Yanos. "Is There Evidence for Defensive Projection? The Impact of Subclinical Mental Disorder and Self-Identification on Endorsement of Stigma." *Stigma and Health* 5, no. 4 (2020): 434–41. https://doi.org/10.1037/sah0000217.

REFERENCES

1. Stuart H, Arboleda-Flórez J, Sartorius N. *Paradigms Lost: Fighting Stigma and the Lessons Learned.* Oxford: Oxford University Press, 2012.
2. Arboleda-Flórez J, Stuart H. From sin to science: Fighting the stigmatization of mental illnesses. *Can J Psychiatry* 2012;**57**:457–63.
3. Sayce L. *From Psychiatric Patient to Citizen.* London: Macmillan Press Ltd., 2000.
4. Link BG, Phelan JC. Conceptualizing stigma. *Annu Rev Sociol* 2001;**27**:363–85.
5. Stangor C. Book overview. In: Stangor C (ed.). *Stereotypes and Prejudice.* Philadelphia: Taylor & Francis, 2000, 1–19.
6. Allport G. The nature of prejudice. In: Stangor C (ed.). *Stereotypes and Prejudice.* Philadelphia: Taylor & Francis, 2000, 20–48.
7. Bourget Management Consulting. Mental health literacy: A review of the literature. Canadian Alliance on Mental Illness and Mental Health, 2007. www.camimh.ca/key-reports/mental-health-literacy
8. Pescosolido BA, Monahan J, Link BG et al. The public's view of the competence, dangerousness, and need for legal coercion of persons with mental health problems. *Am J Public Health* 1999;**89**(9):1339–45.
9. Link BG, Bresnahan M, Stueve A et al. Public conceptions of mental illness: Labels, causes, dangerousness, and social distance. *Am J Public Health* 1999;**89**:1328–33.
10. Jorm AF. Mental health literacy: Public knowledge and beliefs about mental disorders. *Br J Psychiatry* 2000;**177**:396–401.
11. Haslam N. Folk psychiatry: Lay thinking about mental disorder. *Soc Res (New York)* 2003;**70**:621–44.
12. Giosan E, Glovsky V, Haslam N. The lay concept of "mental disorder": A cross-cultural study. *Transcultural Psychiatry* 2001;**38**:317–32.
13. Patel P. Forced sterilization of women as discrimination. *Public Health Rev* 2017;**38**:1–12.
14. Goffman E. *Stigma: Notes on the Management of Spoiled Identity.* Englewood Cliffs, NJ: Prentice-Hall, 1963.
15. Goffman E. *Asylums: Essays on the Social Situation of Mental Patients and Other Inmates.* Garden City, NY: Anchor Books, 1961.
16. Crossley NRD. Laing and the British anti-psychiatry movement: A socio-historical analysis. *Soc Sci Med* 1998;**47**:877–89.
17. Weinstein RM. Goffman's asylums and the social situation of mental patients. *J Orthomol Psychiatry* 1982;**11**:267–74.
18. Scull AT. Madness and segregative control: The rise of the insane asylum. *Soc Probl* 1977;**24**:337–51.

19. Cooper J, Sartorius N. Cultural and temporal variations in schizophrenia: A speculation on the importance of industrialization. *Br J Psychiatry* 1977;**130**:50–5.

20. Turner T. The history of deinstitutionalization and reinstitutionalization. *Psychiatry* 2004;**3**(9):1–4.

21. Dear M, Taylor S. *Not on Our Street*. London, UK: Pion Limited, 1982.

22. Dear M. Understanding and overcoming the NIMBY syndrome. *J Am Plan Assoc* 1992;**58**:288–300.

23. Sayce L. Stigma, discrimination and social exclusion: What's in a word? *J Mental Health* 1998;**7**:331–43.

24. Zippay AL. Psychiatric residences: Notification, NIMBY, and neighborhood relations. *Psychiatr Serv* 2007;**58**:109–13.

25. Arens DA. What do the neighbors think now? Community residences on Long Island, New York. *Community Mental Health J* 1993;**29**:235–45.

26. Wolff G, Pathare S, Craig T et al. Public education for community care: A new approach. *Br J Psychiatry* 1996;**168**:441–47.

27. Fazel S, Danesh J. Serious mental disorder in 23000 prisoners: A systematic review of 62 surveys. *Lancet* 2002;**359**:545–50.

28. Fazel S, Lubbe S. Prevalence and characteristics of mental disorders in jails and prisons. *Curr Opin Psychiatry* 2005;**18**:550–54.

29. Toynbee M. The Penrose hypothesis in the 21st century: Revisiting the asylum. *Evid Based Mental Health* 2015;**18**:76.

30. Hartvig P, Kjelsberg E. Penrose's Law revisited: The relationship between mental institution beds, prison population and crime rate. *Nord J Psychiatry* 2009;**63**:51–56.

31. Large MM, Nielssen O. The Penrose hypothesis in 2004: Patient and prisoner numbers are positively correlated in low-and-middle income countries but are unrelated in high-income countries. *Psychol Psychother Theory, Res Pract* 2009;**82**:113–19.

32. Kaliski S. Reinstitutionalization by stealth: The forensic mental health service is the new chronic system. *African J Psychiatry (South Africa)* 2013;**16**:13–17.

33. Amering M, Schmolke M. *Recovery in Mental Health*. Oxford: Wiley-Blackwell, 2009.

34. Davidson L, O'Connel M, Tondora J et al. The top ten concerns about recovery encountered in mental health system transformation. *Psychiatr Serv* 2006;**57**:640–45.

35. Stuart H. What we need is person-centred care. *Perspect Med Educ* 2017;**6**:146–47.

36. Chen SP, Krupa T, Lysaght R et al. The development of recovery competencies for in-patient mental health providers working with people with serious mental illness. *Administration & Policy in Mental Health & Mental Health Services Research* 2013;**40**:96–116.

37. Roberts M, Bell A. Recovery in mental health and substance misuse services: A commentary on recent policy development in the United Kingdom. *Adv Dual Diagn* 2013;**6**:76–83.

38. Timpson H, Eckley L, Sumnall H et al. "Once you've been there, you're always recovering": Exploring experiences, outcomes, and benefits of substance misuse recovery. *Drugs & Alcohol Today* 2016;**16**:29–38.

39. Repper J, Carter T. A review of the literature on peer support in mental health services. *J Mental Health* 2011;**20**:392–411.

40. Stein CH, Aguirre R, Hunt MG. Social networks and personal loss among young adults with mental illness and their parents: A family perspective. *Psychiatr Rehabil J* 2013;**36**:15–21.

41. Gillard S, Foster R, Gibson S et al. Describing a principles-based approach to developing and evaluating peer worker roles as peer support moves into mainstream mental health services. *Mental Health Soc Incl* 2017;**21**:133–43.

42. Shefer G, Henderson C, Howard LM et al. Diagnostic overshadowing and other challenges involved in the diagnostic process of patients with mental illness who present in emergency departments with physical symptoms: A qualitative study. *PLoS One* 2014;**9**:1–8.

43. Jones S, Howard L, Thornicroft G. "Diagnostic overshadowing": Worse physical health care for people with mental illness. *Acta Psychiatr Scand* 2008;**118**(3):169–71.

44. Van Nieuwenhuizen A, Henderson C, Kassam A et al. Emergency department staff views and experiences on diagnostic overshadowing related to people with mental illness. *Epidemiol Psychiatr Sci* 2013;**22**:255–62.

45. Nash M. Diagnostic overshadowing: A potential barrier to physical health care for mental health service users. *Mental Health Pract* 2013;**17**:22–26.

46. Zun LS, Rozel J. Looking past labels: Effective care of the psychiatric patient. In: Martin ML, Heron SL, Moreno-Walton L et al. (eds.). *Diversity and Inclusion in Quality Patient Care*. Switzerland: Springer, 2016, 121–29.

47. Clarke DE, Dusome D, Hughes L. Emergency department from the mental health client's perspective: Feature article. *Int J Mental Health Nurs* 2007;**16**:1126–31.

48. Roy T, Lloyd CE, Pouwer F et al. Screening tools used for measuring depression among people with type 1 and type 2 diabetes: A systematic review. *Diabet Med* 2012;**29**:164–75.

49. Corrigan PW, Markowitz FE, Watson AC. Structural levels of mental illness stigma and discrimination. *Schizophr Bull* 2004;**30**:481–91.

50. Bhugra D, Pathare S, Joshi R et al. Right to property, inheritance, and contract and persons with mental illness. *Int Rev Psychiatry* 2016;**28**:402–408.

51. Link BG, Phelan J. Stigma power. *Soc Sci Med* 2014;**103**:24–32.

52. Stuart H. Reducing the stigma of mental illness. *Global Mental Health* 2016;**3**:1–14.

53. Canadian Institute for Health Information. *Summary Report: Physicians in Canada 2018*. Ottawa, ON: Canadian Institute for Health Information, 2019.

54. Chang CK, Hayes RD, Perera G et al. Life expectancy at birth for people with serious mental illness and other major disorders from a secondary mental health care case register in London. *PLoS One* 2011;**6**(5):e19590.

55. John A, McGregor J, Jones I et al. Premature mortality among people with severe mental illness: New evidence from linked primary care data. *Schizophr Res* 2018;**199**:154–62.

56. Lesage A, Rochette L, Émond V et al. A surveillance system to monitor excess mortality of people with mental illness in Canada. *Can J Psychiatry* 2015;**60**:571–79.

57. Kilbourne AM, Beck K, Spaeth-Rublee B et al. Measuring and improving the quality of mental health care: A global perspective. *World Psychiatry* 2018;**17**:30–38.

58. Stuart H. Media portrayal of mental illness and its treatments: What effect does it have on people with mental illness? *CNS Drugs* 2006;**20**:99–106.

59. Leduc A. *Disfigured: On Fairy Tales, Disability, and Making Space*. Toronto: Coach House Books, 2020.

60. Corrigan PW, Kuwabara SA, O'Shaughnessy J. The public stigma of mental illness and drug addiction: Findings from a stratified random sample. *J Soc Work* 2009;**9**:139–47.

61. Martin JK, Pescosolido BA, Tuch SA. Of fear and loathing: The role of "disturbing behavior," labels, and causal attributions in shaping public attitudes toward people with mental illness. *J Health Soc Behav* 2000;**41**:208–23.

62. Stuart H, Patten SB, Koller M et al. Stigma in Canada: Results from a rapid response survey. *Can J Psychiatry* 2014;**59**:S27–33.

63. Lasalvia A, Zoppei S, Van Bortel T et al. Global pattern of experienced and anticipated discrimination reported by people with major depressive disorder: A cross-sectional survey. *Lancet* 2013;

64. Angermeyer MC, Dietrich S. Public beliefs about and attitudes towards people with mental illness: A review of population studies. *Acta Psychiatr Scand* 2006;**113**:163–79.

65. Simmie S, Nunes J. *The Last Taboo: A Survival Guide to Mental Health Care in Canada*. Toronto: McClelland and Stewart, Ltd., 2001.

66. Corrigan PW, Larson JE, Rüsch N. Self-stigma and the "why try" effect: Impact on life goals and evidence-based practices. *World Psychiatry* 2009;**8**:75–81.

67. Stringer SA, Williams SL, Ault KE et al. A fulcrum of change: From self-stigma to resilience. *Stigma Health* 2018;**3**:315–24.

68. Brohan E, Elgie R, Sartorius N et al. Self-stigma, empowerment and perceived discrimination among people with schizophrenia in 14 European countries: The GAMIAN-Europe study. *Schizophr Res* 2010;**122**:232–38.

69. Sartorius N, Schulze H. *Reducing the Stigma of Mental Illness*. Cambridge: Cambridge University Press, 2005.

70. Yoles S. *From Witchcraft and Sorcery To Head Shrinking: Society's Concern About Mental Health*. Washington, DC: US Department of Health, Education, and Welfare, 1969.

71. Ahonen M. Ancient philosophers on mental illness. *Hist Psychiatry* 2019;**30**:3–18.

72. Jones C. Stigma: Tattooing and branding in Graeco-Roman antiquity. *J Rom Stud* 1987;**77**:139–55.

73. Simon B. Shame, stigma, and mental illness in ancient Greece. In: Fink PJ, Tasman A (eds.). *Stigma and Mental Illness*. Washington DC: American Psychiatric Press, Inc., 1992, 29–40.

74. Tzeferakos G, Douzenis A. Sacred psychiatry in ancient Greece. *Ann Gen Psychiatry* 2014;**13**:1–9.

75. Cheng TO. Hippocrates, cardiology, Confucius and the Yellow Emperor. *Int J Cardiol* 2001;**81**:219–33.

76. Mora G. Stigma during the medival and renaissance periods. In: Fink PJ, Tasman A (eds.). *Stigma and Mental Illness*. Washington DC: American Psychiatric Press, Inc., 1992, 41–58.

77. Turi Z. "Border liners": The ship of fools tradition in sixteenth-century England. *Trans* 2010;**10**. doi:10.4000/trans.421

78. Maher WB, Maher B. The ship of fools: Stultifera navis or ignis fatuus? *Am Psychol* 1982;**37**:756–61.

79. Pérez J, Girón-Irueste F, Gurpegui M et al. The lions of Granada Maristan. *Am J Psychiatry* 2013;**170**:152–53.

80. Moussaoui D, Glick ID. The maristan "Sidi Fredj" in Fez, Morocco. *Am J Psychiatry* 2015;**172**:838–39.

81. Perez J, Baldessarini RJ, Undurraga J et al. Origins of psychiatric hospitalization in medieval Spain. *Psychiatr Q* 2012;**83**:419–30.

82. Hare EH. *On the History of Lunacy: The 19th Century and After*. Dulwich, London: Gabbay, 1998.

83. Covey HC. Western Christianity's two historical treatments of people with disabilities or mental illness. *Soc Sci J* 2005;**42**:107–14.

84. Li Parry-Jones W. Asylum for the mentally ill in historical perspective. *Bull R Coll Psychiatr* 1988;**12**:407–10.
85. Wing JK. The functions of asylum. *Br J Psychiatry* 1990;**157**:822–27.
86. Woods E, Carlson E. The psychiatry of Philippe Pinel. *Bull Hist Med* 1961;**35**:14–25.
87. Rothman D. *The Discovery of the Asylum Social Order and Disorder in the New Republic*. Boston: Little Brown & Company, 1971.
88. Ozarin L. Moral treatment and the mental hospital. *Am J Psychiatry* 1954;**111**:371–78.
89. Tuntiya N. Free-air treatment for mental patients: The deinstitutionalization debate of the nineteenth century. *Sociol Perspect* 2007;**50**:469–88.
90. Earle P. Gheel. *Am J Insanity* 1851;**8**:67–78.
91. Sibbald J. Gheel and Lierneux, the asylum-colonies for the insane in Belgium. *J Mental Sci* 1897;**182**:435–61.
92. Kilgour AJ. Colony Gheel. *Am J Psychiatry* 1936;**92**:959–65.
93. Lloyd M. Book review: Mental Health Policy and Practice Across Europe, edited by M. Knapp, D. McDaid, E. Mossialos and G. Thornicroft. *Crit Public Health* 2010;**20**:267–69.
94. Laosebikan S. Mental health in Nigeria: The promise of a behavioral approach in treatment and rehabilitation. *J Black Stud* 1973;**4**:221–28.
95. Okasha A, Arboleda-Flórez J, Sartorius N eds. *Ethics, Culture and Psychiatry*. Washington DC: APPI, 2000.
96. Okasha A. Mental health in the Middle East: An Egyptian perspective. *Clin Psychol Rev* 1999;**19**:917–33.
97. Coker EM. Selfhood and social distance: Toward a cultural understanding of psychiatric stigma in Egypt. *Soc Sci Med* 2005;**61**:920–30.
98. Fabrega H. Psychiatric stigma in the classical and medieval period: A review of the literature. *Compr Psychiatry* 1990;**31**:289–306.
99. Youssef HA, Youssef FA. Evidence for the existence of schizophrenia in medieval Islamic society. *Hist Psychiatry* 1996;**7**:55–62.
100. Sewilam AM, Watson AMM, Kassem AM et al. Suggested avenues to reduce the stigma of mental illness in the Middle East. *Int J Soc Psychiatry* 2015;**61**:111–20.
101. Zolezzi M, Alamri M, Shaar S et al. Stigma associated with mental illness and its treatment in the Arab culture: A systematic review. *Int J Soc Psychiatry* 2018;**64**:597–609.
102. Kadri N, Manoudi F, Berrada S et al. Stigma impact on Moroccan families of patients with schizophrenia. *Can J Psychiatry* 2004;**49**:625–29.
103. Ng CH. The stigma of mental illness in Asian cultures. *Aust N Z J Psychiatry* 1997;**31**(3):382–90.
104. Tsang HWH, Angell B, Corrigan PW et al. A cross-cultural study of employers' concerns about hiring people with psychotic disorder: Implications for recovery. *Soc Psychiatry Psychiatr Epidemiol* 2007;**42**:723–33.
105. Pearson V. The Chinese equation in mental health policy and practice: Order plus control equal stability. *Int J Law Psychiatry* 1996;**19**:437–58.
106. Verwaal R. *Hippocrates Meets the Yellow Emperor: On the Reception of Chinese and Japanese Medicine in Early Modern Europe*. Utrecht University Faculty of Humanities, Master's thesis, 2010.
107. Fàbrega H. Mental health and illness in traditional India and China. *Psychiatr Clin North Am* 2001;**24**:555–67.
108. Weiss MG, Desai A, Jadhav S et al. Humoral concepts of mental illness in India. *Soc Sci Med* 1988;**27**:471–77.

109. Kapur RL. The role of traditional healers in mental health care in rural India. *Soc Sci Med Part B Med Anthropol* 1979;**13**:27–31.

110. Bhattacharyya DP. Psychiatric pluralism in Bengal, India. *Soc Sci Med* 1983;**17**:947–56.

111. Raguram R, Weiss MG, Channabasavanna SM et al. Stigma, depression, and somatization in South India. *Am J Psychiatry* 1996;**153**:1043–49.

112. Krishnamurthy K, Venugopal D, Alimchandani AK. Mental hospitals in India. *Indian J Psychiatry* 2000;**42**:125–32.

113. Yang LH, Thornicroft G, Alvarado R et al. Recent advances in cross-cultural measurement in psychiatric epidemiology: Utilizing "what matters most" to identify culture-specific aspects of stigma. *Int J Epidemiol* 2014;**43**:494–510.

114. Pescosolido BA, Olafsdottir S, Martin JK et al. Cross-cultural aspects of the stigma of mental illness. In: Arboleda-Flórez J, Sartorius N (eds.). *Understanding the Stigma of Mental Illness: Theory and Interventions*. Wiley Online, 2008,19–35.

115. Seeman N, Tang S, Brown AD et al. World survey of mental illness stigma. *J Affect Disord* 2016;**190**:115–21.

116. Inglehart R, Haerpfer A, Moreno C et al. World Values Survey: Round Four—Country-Pooled Datafile. 2018. doi.org/10.14281/18241.5

117. Thornicroft G, Brohan E, Rose D et al. Global pattern of experienced and anticipated discrimination against people with schizophrenia: A cross-sectional survey. *Lancet* 2009;**373**:408–15.

118. Lasalvia A, Van Bortel T, Bonetto C et al. Cross-national variations in reported discrimination among people treated for major depression worldwide: The ASPEN/INDIGO international study. *Br J Psychiatry* 2015;**207**:507–14.

119. Stuart H, Chen S-P, Christie R et al. Opening minds in Canada: Background and rationale. *Can J Psychiatry* 2014;**59**:S8–S12.

120. Stuart H, Chen S-P, Christie R et al. Opening minds in Canada: Targeting change. *Can J Psychiatry* 2014;**59**:S13–18.

121. Callard F, Sartorius N, Arboleda-Flórez J et al. *Mental Illness, Discrimination and the Law: Fighting for Social Justice*. Oxford: Wiley-Blackwell, 2012.

122. Gostin LO, Gable L. The human rights of persons with mental disabilities: A global perspective on the application of human rights principles to mental health. *Maryl Law Rev* 2004;**63**:20–118.

123. Jellinek G. *Declaration of the rights of man and of citizens*. New York: Henry Holt and Company, 1901.

124. Ludwikowski R. The French declaration of the rights of man and citizen and the American constitutional development. *Am J Comp Law* 1990;**38**:445–62.

125. Shamoo AE. Human rights in reference to persons with mental illness. *Account Res* 1996;**4**:207–16.

126. Karados G. Universality, progressive realization, economic crises: The ICERS fifty years on. In: Langford M (ed.). *Social Rights Jurisprudence: Emerging Trends in International and Comparative Law*. Cambridge: Cambridge University Press, 2008, 3–13.

127. Alston P, Quinn G. The nature and scope of states parties' obligations under the International Covenant on Economic, Social and Cultural Rights. *Hum Rights Q* 1987;**9**:156.

128. Harris D. Commentary by the rapporteur on the consideration of states parties' reports and international co-operation. *Hum Rights Q* 1987;**9**:147.

129. Szmukler G, Daw R, Callard F. Mental health law and the UN Convention on the rights of persons with disabilities. *Int J Law Psychiatry* 2014;**37**:245–52.

130. Stuart H. United Nations Convention on the rights of persons with disabilities: A roadmap for change. *Curr Opin Psychiatry* 2012;**25**:365–69.
131. Brody EB. The World Federation for Mental Health: Its origins and contemporary relevance to WHO and WPA policies. *World Psychiatry* 2004;**3**:54–55.
132. Sartorius V, Sartorius N. The WPA celebrates its 70th birthday . *World Psychiatry* 2020;**19**:403–404.
133. Newell K (ed.). *Health by the People.* Geneva, 1975.
134. Mental health care in developing countries: A critical appraisal of research findings. *World Health Organization Technical Report Series* 1984;**698**:1–34.
135. Bertolote JM. The roots of the concept of mental health. *World Psychiatry* 2008;**7**:113–16.
136. World Health Organization. *Stop Exclusion: Dare to Care.* Geneva, Switzerland, 2001.
137. Merieau L. *World Health Day. 7 April 2001.* Geneva, Switzerland, 2001.
138. Curran WJ, Harding TW. *The Law and Mental Health: Harmonizing Objectives.* Geneva, Switzerland, 1978.
139. World Health Organization. *WHO QualityRights Tool Kit.* Geneva, Switzerland, 2012.
140. World Health Organization. *Mental Health Action Plan 2013–2020.* Geneva, Switzerland, 2013.
141. World Health Organization. *Mental Health Atlas.* Geneva, Switzerland, 2018.
142. Stuart H, Sartorius N. Opening doors: The global programme to fight stigma and discrimination because of schizophrenia. In: Gaebel W, Rössler W, Sartorius N (eds.). *The Stigma of Mental Illness: End of the Story?* Springer Link, 2016, 227–35.
143. Stuart H, Linden B, Sartorius N. Stigma: An old unmet need in psychiatric practice. In: Pompili M, McIntyre R, Fiorillo A, Sartorius N. *New Directions in Psychiatry.* Springer Link, 2020, 205–30.
144. Beldie A, den Boer JA, Brain C et al. Fighting stigma of mental illness in midsize European countries. *Soc Psychiatry Psychiatr Epidemiol* 2012;**47**:1–38.
145. Allport G. *The Nature of Prejudice.* Reading, MA: Addison-Wesley, 1954.
146. McKay C. The value of contact: Unpacking Allport's contact theory to support inclusive education. *Palaestra* 2018;**32**:21–25.
147. Moskos CC Jr. Racial integration in the armed forces. *Am J Sociol* 1966;**72**:132–48.
148. Corrigan PW, Morris SB, Michaels PJ et al. Challenging the public stigma of mental illness: A meta-analysis of outcome studies. *Psychiatr Serv* 2012;**63**:963–73.
149. Chen S-P, Koller M, Krupa T et al. Contact in the classroom: Developing a program model for youth mental health contact-based anti-stigma education. *Community Mental Health J* 2016;**52**:281–93.
150. Gronholm PC, Henderson C, Deb T et al. Interventions to reduce discrimination and stigma: The state of the art. *Soc Psychiatry Psychiatr Epidemiol* 2017;**52**:249–58.
151. Jorm AF. Effect of contact-based interventions on stigma and discrimination: A critical examination of the evidence. *Psychiatr Serv* 2020;**71**:735–37.
152. Ashton LJ, Gordon SE, Reeves RA. Key ingredients—target groups, methods and messages, and evaluation—of local-level, public interventions to counter stigma and discrimination: A lived experience informed selective narrative literature review. *Community Mental Health J* 2018;**54**:312–33.
153. Fisher WR. Clarifying the narrative paradigm. *Communication Monogr* 1989;**56**:55–58.

154. Djikic M, Oatley K. The art in fiction: From indirect communication to changes of the self. *Psychology of Aesthetics and the Creative Arts* 2014;**8**:498–505.
155. Corrigan PW. *The Stigma Effect: Unintended Consequences of Mental Health Campaigns*. New York: Columbia University Press, 2018.
156. Keen S. Introduction: Narrative and the emotions. *Poetics Today* 2011;**32**(1):1–53.
157. Mar RA, Oatley K. The function of fiction is the abstraction and simulation of social experience. *Perspect Psychol Sci* 2008;**3**:173–92.
158. McKee R, Fryer B. Storytelling that moves people. *Harv Bus Rev* 2003;**81**:1–7.
159. Corrigan PW, Rao D. On the self-stigma of mental illness: Stages, disclosure, and strategies for change. *Can J Psychiatry* 2012;**57**:464–69.
160. Corrigan PW, Kosyluk KA, Rüsch N. Reducing self-stigma by coming out proud. *Am J Public Health* 2013;**103**:794–800.
161. Rüsch N, Kösters M. Honest, Open, Proud to support disclosure decisions and to decrease stigma's impact among people with mental illness: Conceptual review and meta-analysis of program efficacy. *Soc Psychiatry Psychiatr Epidemiol* 2021;**56**(9):1513–26.
162. Russinova Z, Rogers ES, Gagne C et al. A randomized controlled trial of a peer-run antistigma photovoice intervention. *Psychiatr Serv* 2014;**65**:242–46.
163. Tsang HWH, Ching SC, Tang KH et al. Therapeutic intervention for internalized stigma of severe mental illness: A systematic review and meta-analysis. *Schizophr Res* 2016;**173**:45–53.
164. Yanos PT, Lucksted A, Drapalski AL et al. Interventions targeting mental health self-stigma: A review and comparison. *Psychiatr Rehabil J* 2015;**38**:171–78.
165. Aragonès E, López-Muntaner J, Ceruelo S et al. Reinforcing stigmatization: Coverage of mental illness in Spanish newspapers. *J Health Communication* 2014;**19**:1248–58.
166. Bilić B, Georgaca E. Representations of "mental illness" in Serbian newspapers: A critical discourse analysis. *Qual Res Psychol* 2007;**4**:167–86.
167. Gwarjanski AR, Parrott S. Schizophrenia in the news: The role of news frames in shaping online reader dialogue about mental illness. *Health Communication* 2018;**33**:954–61.
168. Schmidtke A, Hafner H. The Werther effect after television films: New evidence for an old hypothesis. *Psychol Med* 1988;**18**:665–76.
169. Pirkis J, Machlin A. Differing perspectives on what is important in media reporting of suicide. *Br J Psychiatry* 2013;**203**:168–69.
170. Everymind. *Guidelines on Media Reporting of Severe Mental Illness in the Context of Violence and Crime*. Newcastle, Australia, 2020.
171. Canadian Journalism Forum on Violence and Trauma. *MINDSET: Reporting on Mental Health*, 3rd ed., 2020. https://www.mindset-mediaguide.ca/
172. Mental Health Foundation of New Zealand. *Media Guidelines*, 2018. https://mentalhealth.org.nz/media/media-guidelines
173. Time to Change. *Media Guidelines*, 2012. https://www.time-to-change.org.uk/sites/default/files/Time%20to%20Change%20Media%20Guidelines.pdf
174. Whitley R, Berry S. Trends in newspaper coverage of mental illness in Canada: 2005–2010. *Can J Psychiatry* 2013;**58**:107–12.
175. Whitley R, Wang JW. Good news? A longitudinal analysis of newspaper portrayals of mental illness in Canada, 2005 to 2015. *Can J Psychiatry* 2017;**62**:278–85.
176. Rhydderch D, Krooupa AM, Shefer G et al. Changes in newspaper coverage of mental illness from 2008 to 2014 in England. *Acta Psychiatr Scand* [Special

issue: Effectiveness of national anti-stigma programmes: Canada, England and Sweden] 2016;**134**(S446):45–52.

177. Goulden R, Corker E, Evans-Lacko S et al. Newspaper coverage of mental illness in the UK, 1992–2008. *BMC Public Health* 2011;**11**: Article number 796.

178. Clement S, Foster N. Newspaper reporting on schizophrenia: A content analysis of five national newspapers at two time points. *Schizophr Res* 2008;**98**:178–83.

179. Bowen ML. Stigma: Content analysis of the representation of people with personality disorder in the UK popular press, 2001–2012. *Int J Mental Health Nurs* 2016;**25**:598–605.

180. Chen M, Lawrie S. Newspaper depictions of mental and physical health. *Br J Psych Bull* 2017;**41**:308–13.

181. Burridge K. Euphemism and language change: The sixth and seventh ages. *Lexis* 2012. doi:10.4000/lexis.355

182. Cheung I. Minding our language. *Philos Forum* 2018;**49**:5–7.

183. Aoki A, Aoki Y, Goulden R et al. Change in newspaper coverage of schizophrenia in Japan over 20-year period. *Schizophr Res* 2016;**175**:193–97.

184. Sartorius N, Chiu H, Heok KE et al. Name change for schizophrenia. *Schizophr Bull* 2014;**40**:255–58.

185. Lasalvia A, Penta E, Sartorius N et al. Should the label "schizophrenia" be abandoned? *Schizophr Res* 2015;**162**:276–84.

186. Cape GS. Addiction, stigma and movies. *Acta Psychiatr Scand* 2003;**107**:163–69.

187. Hersey C. Script(ing) treatment: Representations of recovery from addiction in Hollywood film. *Contemp Drug Probl* 2005;**32**:467–93.

188. Bhugra D. Mad tales from Bollywood: The impact of social, political, and economic climate on the portrayal of mental illness in Hindi films. *Acta Psychiatr Scand* 2005;**112**:250–56.

189. Owen PR. Portrayals of schizophrenia by entertainment media: A content analysis of contemporary movies. *Psychiatr Serv* 2012;**63**:655–59.

190. Lawson A, Fouts G. Mental illness in Disney animated films. *Can J Psychiatry* 2004;**49**:310–14.

191. Gharaibeh NM. The psychiatrist's image in commercially available American movies. *Acta Psychiatr Scand* 2005;**111**:316–19.

192. Pirkis J, Blood RW, Francis C et al. On-screen portrayals of mental illness: Extent, nature, and impacts. *J Health Communication* 2006;**11**:523–41.

193. Maiorano A, Lasalvia A, Sampogna G et al. Reducing stigma in media professionals: Is there room for improvement? Results from a systematic review. *Can J Psychiatry* 2017;**62**:702–15.

194. Stuart H. Stigma and the daily news: Evaluation of a newspaper intervention. *Can J Psychiatry* 2003;**48**(10):651–56.

195. Stark C, Paterson B, Devlin B. Newspaper coverage of a violent assault by a mentally ill person. *J Psychiatr Mental Health Nurs* 2004;**11**:635–43.

196. Campbell NN, Heath J, Bouknight J et al. Speaking out for mental health: Collaboration of future journalists and psychiatrists. *Acad Psychiatry* 2009;**33**:166–68.

197. Li A, Jiao D, Zhu T. Detecting depression stigma on social media: A linguistic analysis. *J Affect Disord* 2018;**232**:358–62.

198. Robinson P, Turk D, Jilka S et al. Measuring attitudes towards mental health using social media: Investigating stigma and trivialisation. *Soc Psychiatry Psychiatr Epidemiol* 2019;**54**:51–58.

199. Betton V, Borschmann R, Docherty M et al. The role of social media in reducing stigma and discrimination. *Br J Psychiatry* 2015;**206**:443–44.
200. The Entertainment Industries Council TEAM Up. Social Media Guidelines for Mental Health Promotion and Suicide Prevention. teamup-mental-health-social-media-guidelines.pdf
201. Thornicroft G. *Shunned: Discrimination Against People with Mental Illness*. Oxford: Oxford University Press, 2006.
202. Stuart H, Knaak S. *Mental Illness and Structural Stigma in Canadian Healthcare Settings: Results of a Focus Group Study*. Ottawa, 2020.
203. Bil JS. Stigma and architecture of mental health facilities. *Br J Psychiatry* 2016;**208**:499–500.
204. Sine DM. The architecture of madness and the good of paternalism. *Psychiatr Serv* 2008;**59**:1060–62.
205. Kohn R, Saxena S, Levav I et al. The treatment gap in mental health care. *Bull World Health Organ* 2004;**82**:858–66.
206. Knapp M, Funk M, Curran C et al. Economic barriers to better mental health practice and policy. *Health Policy Plan* 2006;**21**:157–70.
207. Kathol RG, Butler M, McAlpine DD et al. Barriers to physical and mental condition integrated service delivery. *Psychosom Med* 2010;**72**:511–18.
208. Cunningham PJ. Beyond parity: Primary care physicians' perspectives on access to mental health care. *Health Aff* 2009;**28**:490–501.
209. Globerman S (ed.). *Reducing Wait Times for Health Care: What Canada Can Learn from Theory and International Experience*. Fraser Institute, 2013. https://www.fraserinstitute.org/sites/default/files/reducing-wait-times-for-health-care.pdf
210. Schneider EC, Shah A, Doty MM et al. *Mirror, Mirror 2021: Reflecting Poorly: Health Care in the U.S. Compared to Other High-Income Countries*, 2021. The Commonwealth Fund. https://www.commonwealthfund.org/sites/default/files/2021-08/Schneider_Mirror_Mirror_2021.pdf
211. Kelly TM, Daley DC. Integrated treatment of substance use and psychiatric disorders. *Soc Work Public Health* 2013;**28**:388–406.
212. Canaway R, Merkes M. Barriers to comorbidity service delivery: The complexities of dual diagnosis and the need to agree on terminology and conceptual frameworks. *Aust Health Rev* 2010;**34**:262–68.
213. Mannion R, Davies H. Culture in health care organizations. In: Ferlie E, Montgomery K, Pedeersen AR (eds.). *The Oxford Handbook of Health Care Management*. Oxford Handbooks Online, 2016. doi:10.1093/oxfordhb/9780198705109.001.0001
214. Gillin N, Taylor R, Walker S. Exploring the concept of "caring cultures": A critical examination of the conceptual, methodological and validity issues with the "caring cultures" construct. *J Clin Nurs* 2017;**26**:5216–23.
215. Bhugra D, Malik A. Introduction. In: Bhugra D, Malik A (eds.). *Professionalism in Mental Healthcare: Experts, Expertise and Expectations*. Cambridge: Cambridge University Press, 2011;1–5.
216. Rafferty AM, Philippou J, Fitzpatrick JM et al. Development and testing of the "Culture of Care Barometer" (CoCB) in healthcare organisations: A mixed methods study. *BMJ Open* 2017;**7**:1–8.
217. Scott T, Mannion R, Davies HTO et al. Implementing culture change in health care: Theory and practice. *Int J Qual Health Care* 2003;**15**:111–18.
218. Thomas P, Bracken P, Timimi S. The limits of evidence-based medicine in psychiatry. *Philos Psychiatry Psychol* 2012;**19**:295–308.

219. Livingston JD. *Structural Stigma in Health-Care Contexts for People with Mental Health and Substance Use Issues: A Literature Review*. Mental Health Commission of Canada, 2020. https://mentalhealthcommission.ca/wp-content/uploads/2021/09/structural_stigma_in_healthcare_eng.pdf

220. Høyer G. Involuntary hospitalization in contemporary mental health care: Some (still) unanswered questions. *J Mental Health* 2008;**17**:281–92.

221. Danzer G, Wilkus-Stone A. The give and take of freedom: The role of involuntary hospitalization and treatment in recovery from mental illness. *Bull Menninger Clin* 2015;**79**:255–80.

222. World Health Organisation. *Guidance on Community Mental Health Services*, 2021. https://www.who.int/publications/i/item/9789240025707

223. O'Donoghue B, Roche E, Shannon S et al. Perceived coercion in voluntary hospital admission. *Psychiatry Res* 2014;**215**:120–26.

224. Eytan A, Chatton A, Safran E et al. Impact of psychiatrists' qualifications on the rate of compulsory admissions. *Psychiatr Q* 2013;**84**:73–80.

225. Khazaal Y, Manghi R, Delahaye M et al. Psychiatric advance directives, a possible way to overcome coercion and promote empowerment. *Front Public Health* 2014;**2**:1–5.

226. Lay B, Kawohl W, Rössler W. Outcomes of a psycho-education and monitoring programme to prevent compulsory admission to psychiatric inpatient care: A randomised controlled trial. *Psychol Med* 2018;**48**:849–60.

227. Goldman A. Continued overreliance on involuntary commitment: The need for a less restrictive alternative. *J Leg Med* 2015;**36**:233–51.

228. Cornwall JK, Deeney R. Exposing the myths surrounding preventive outpatient commitment for individuals with chronic mental illness. *Psychol Public Policy Law* 2003;**9**:209–32.

229. Link B, Castille DM, Stuber J. Stigma and coercion in the context of outpatient treatment for people with mental illnesses. *Soc Sci Med* 2008;**67**:409–19.

230. Swanson JW, Swartz MS, Borum R et al. Involuntary out-patient commitment and reduction of violent behaviour in persons with severe mental illness. *Br J Psychiatry* 2000;**176**:324–31.

231. Swanson JW, Swartz MS, Elbogen EB et al. Effects of involuntary outpatient commitment on subjective quality of life in persons with severe mental illness. *Behav Sci Law* 2003;**21**:473–91.

232. Swartz MS, Swanson JW, Monahan J. Endorsement of personal benefit of outpatient commitment among persons with severe mental illness. *Psychol Public Policy Law* 2003;**9**:70–93.

233. Latimer E, Farmer O, Crocker A et al. Perceived coercion, client-centredness, and positive and negative pressures in an assertive community treatment program: An exploratory study. *Can J Community Mental Health* 2010;**29**:35–50.

234. Bond GR, Drake RE, Mueser KT et al. Assertive community treatment for people with severe mental illness: Critical ingredients and impact on patients. *Dis Manag Health Outcomes* 2001;**9**:141–59.

235. Steinert T, Lepping P, Bernhardsgrütter R et al. Incidence of seclusion and restraint in psychiatric hospitals: A literature review and survey of international trends. *Soc Psychiatry Psychiatr Epidemiol* 2010;**45**:889–97.

236. Mayers P, Keet N, Winkler G et al. Mental health service users? Perceptions and experiences of sedation, seclusion and restraint. *Int J Soc Psychiatry* 2010;**56**:60–73.

237. Kontio R, Joffe G, Putkonen H et al. Seclusion and restraint in psychiatry: Patients' experiences and practical suggestions on how to improve practices and use alternatives. *Perspect Psychiatr Care* 2012;**48**:16–24.

238. Georgieva I, Mulder CL, Wierdsma A. Patients' preference and experiences of forced medication and seclusion. *Psychiatr Q* 2012;**83**:1–13.

239. Chieze M, Hurst S, Kaiser S et al. Effects of seclusion and restraint in adult psychiatry: A systematic review. *Front Psychiatry* 2019;**10**:1–19.

240. Bernstein R. Commentary on the "choice" between seclusion and forced medication. *Psychiatr Serv* 2008;**59**:212.

241. Kalisova L, Raboch J, Nawka A et al. Do patient and ward-related characteristics influence the use of coercive measures? Results from the EUNOMIA international study. *Soc Psychiatry Psychiatr Epidemiol* 2014;**49**:1619–29.

242. Scanlan JN. Interventions to reduce the use of seclusion and restraint in inpatient psychiatric settings: What we know so far a review of the literature. *Int J Soc Psychiatry* 2010;**56**:412–23.

243. Jacobson N, Greenley D. What is Recovery? A conceptual model. *Psychiatr Serv* 2001;**52**:482–85.

244. Robb J, Stone J. Implicit bias toward people with mental illness: A systematic literature review. *J Rehabil* 2016;**82**:3–13.

245. Fitzgerald C, Hurst S. Implicit bias in healthcare professionals: A systematic review. *BMC Med Ethics* 2017;**18**(1):19.

246. Ungar T, Knaak S, Mantler E. Making the implicit explicit: A visual model for lowering the risk of implicit bias of mental/behavioural disorders on safety and quality of care. *Healthc Manag Forum* 2021;**34**:72–6.

247. Merino Y, Adams L, Hall WJ. Implicit bias and mental health professionals: Priorities and directions for research. *Psychiatr Serv* 2018;**69**:723–25.

248. Byrne A, Tanesini A. Instilling new habits: Addressing implicit bias in healthcare professionals. *Adv Health Sci Educ* 2015;**20**:1255–62.

249. Boscardin CK. Reducing implicit bias through curricular interventions. *J Gen Intern Med* 2015;**30**:1726–28.

250. Sukhera J, Watling CJ, Gonzalez CM. Implicit bias in health professions: From recognition to transformation. *Acad Med* 2020;**95**:717–23.

251. Vuletich HA, Payne BK. Stability and change in implicit bias. *Psychol Sci* 2019;**30**:854–62.

252. Pritlove C, Juando-Prats C, Ala-leppilampi K et al. The good, the bad, and the ugly of implicit bias. *Lancet* 2019;**393**:502–504.

253. Livingston JD. *Structural Stigma in Healthcare Contexts for People with Mental Health and Substance Use Issues: A Literature Review*. Ottawa, Ontario, 2019.

254. Knaak S, Patten S. A grounded theory model for reducing stigma in health professionals in Canada. *Acta Psychiatr Scand* 2016;**134**:53–62.

255. Knaak S, Modgill G, Patten SB. Key ingredients of anti-stigma programs for health care providers: A data synthesis of evaluative studies. *Can J Psychiatry* 2014;**59**:S19–S26.

256. Kohrt BA, Jordans MJD, Turner EL et al. Reducing stigma among healthcare providers to improve mental health services (RESHAPE): Protocol for a pilot cluster randomized controlled trial of a stigma reduction intervention for training primary healthcare workers in Nepal. *Pilot Feasibility Stud* 2018;**4**:1–18.

257. Linden B, Stuart H. Preliminary analysis of validation evidence for two new scales assessing teachers' confidence and worries related to delivering mental health content in the classroom. *BMC Psychol* 2019;**7**:32.

258. Economou M, Louki E, Peppou LE et al. Fighting psychiatric stigma in the classroom: The impact of an educational intervention on secondary school students' attitudes to schizophrenia. *Int J Soc Psychiatry* 2012;**58**:544–51.

259. Pitre N, Stewart S, Adams S et al. The use of puppets with elementary school children in reducing stigmatizing attitudes towards mental illness. *J Mental Health* 2007;**16**:415–29.

260. Hennessy E, Swords L, Heary C. Children's understanding of psychological problems displayed by their peers: A review of the literature. *Child Care Health Dev* 2008;**34**:4–9.

261. Sartorius N. Early interventions to prevent stigmatization and its consequences. In: Chan E, Ventriglio A, Bhugra D (eds.). *Early Intervention in Psychiatric Disorders Across Cultures*. Oxford: Oxford University Press, 2019, 9–15.

262. Degner J, Wentura D. Automatic prejudice in childhood and early adolescence. *J Pers Soc Psychol* 2010;**98**:356–74.

263. Wahl OE. Children's views of mental illness: A review of the literature. *Psychiatr Rehabil Skills* 2002;**6**:134–58.

264. Araujo L, Strasser J. Confronting prejudice in the early childhood classroom. *Kappa Delta Pi Record* 2003;**39**:178–82.

265. Weiss MF. Children's attitudes toward the mentally ill: A developmental analysis. *Psychol Rep* 1986;**58**:11–20.

266. Weiss MF. Children's attitudes toward the mentally ill: An eight-year longitudinal follow-up. *Psychol Rep* 1994;**74**:51–56.

267. Ventieri D, Clarke DM, Hay M. The effects of a school-based educational intervention on preadolescents' knowledge of and attitudes towards mental illness. *Adv Sch Mental Health Promot* 2011;**4**:5–17.

268. Wahl O, Susin J, Lax A et al. Knowledge and attitudes about mental illness: A survey of middle school students. *Psychiatr Serv* 2012;**63**:649–54.

269. Favazza PC, Phillipsen L, Kumar P. Measuring and promoting acceptance of young children with disabilities. *Except Child* 2000;**66**:491–508.

270. Painter K, Phelan JC, DuPont-Reyes MJ et al. Evaluation of antistigma interventions with sixth-grade students: A school-based field experiment. *Psychiatr Serv* 2017;**68**:345–52.

271. Link BG, DuPont-Reyes MJ, Barkin K et al. A school-based intervention for mental illness stigma: A cluster randomized trial. *Pediatrics* 2020;**145**(6):e20190780.

272. Wahl OF, Susin J, Kaplan L et al. Changing knowledge and attitudes with a middle school mental health education curriculum. *Stigma Res Action* 2011;**1**:44–53.

273. Watson AC, Otey E, Westbrook AL et al. Changing middle schoolers' attitudes about mental illness through education. *Schizophr Bull* 2004;**30**:563–72.

274. Larkings JS, Brown PM. Do biogenetic causal beliefs reduce mental illness stigma in people with mental illness and in mental health professionals? A systematic review. *Int J Mental Health Nurs* 2018;**27**:928–41.

275. Harrist AW, Bradley KD. "You can't say you can't play": Intervening in the process of social exclusion in the kindergarten classroom. *Early Child Res Q* 2003;**18**:185–205.

276. Sakellari E, Leino-Kilpi H, Kalokerinou-Anagnostopoulou A. Educational interventions in secondary education aiming to affect pupils' attitudes towards mental illness: A review of the literature. *J Psychiatr Mental Health Nurs* 2011;**18**:166–76.

277. Koller M, Stuart H. Reducing stigma in high school youth. *Acta Psychiatr Scand* 2016;**134**(Suppl 446):63–70.

278. Murman NM, Buckingham KCE, Fontilea P et al. Let's Erase the Stigma (LETS): A quasi-experimental evaluation of adolescent-led school groups intended to reduce mental illness stigma. *Child Youth Care Forum* 2014;**43**:621–37.

279. Wada M, Suto MJ, Lee M et al. University students' perspectives on mental illness stigma. *Mental Health Prev* 2019;**14**:200159.

280. Boucher LA, Campbell DG. An examination of the impact of a biological anti-stigma message for depression on college students. *J College Stud Psychother* 2014;**28**:74–81.

281. Mezuk B, Needham B, Joiner K et al. What elephant? Pedagogical approaches to addressing stigma toward mental disorders in undergraduate public health education. *Pedagogy in Health Promotion* 2020;**7**(3):183–90.

282. Finkelstein J, Lapshin O, Wasserman E. Randomized study of different anti-stigma media. *Patient Educ Couns* 2008;**71**:204–14.

283. Yamaguchi S, Wu SI, Biswas M et al. Effects of short-term interventions to reduce mental health-related stigma in university or college students: A systematic review. *J Nerv Mental Dis* 2013;**201**:490–503.

284. Linden B, Stuart H. Post-secondary stress and mental well-being: A scoping review of the academic literature. *Can J Community Mental Health* 2020;**39**:1–32.

285. Monaghan C, Linden B, Stuart H. Postsecondary mental health policy in Canada: A scoping review of the grey literature. *Can J Psychiatry* 2020;**66**(7):603–15.

286. Pescosolido BA, Perry BL, Krendl AC. Empowering the next generation to end stigma by starting the conversation: Bring change to mind and the college toolbox project. *J Am Acad Child Adolesc Psychiatry* 2020;**59**:519–30.

287. Masedo A, Grandón P, Saldivia S et al. A multicentric study on stigma towards people with mental illness in health sciences students. *BMC Med Educ* 2021;**21**:324.

288. Mino Y, Yasuda N, Kanazawa S et al. Effects of medical education on attitudes towards mental illness among medical students: A five-year follow-up study. *Acta Med Okayama* 2000;**54**:127–32.

289. Gouthro TJ, Gouthro TJ, East C et al. Issues in mental health nursing: Recognizing and addressing the stigma associated with mental health nursing: A critical perspective. *Issues Mental Health Nurs* 2009;**30**:669–76.

290. Higashi RT, Tillack A, Steinman MA et al. The worthy patient: Rethinking the hidden curriculum in medical education. *Anthropol Med* 2013;**20**:13–23.

291. Stuart H, Sartorius N, Liinamaa T et al. Images of psychiatry and psychiatrists. *Acta Psychiatr Scand* 2015;**131**:21–28.

292. Peck C, McCall M, McLaren B et al. Professional development: International comparisons. *BMJ* 2000;**320**:432–35.

293. Pinto-Foltz MD, Logsdon MC. Reducing stigma related to mental disorders: Initiatives, interventions, and recommendations for nursing. *Arch Psychiatr Nurs* 2009;**23**:32–40.

294. Davis DA, Thomson MA, Oxman AD et al. Changing physician performance: A systematic review of the effect of continuing medical education strategies. *J Am Med Assoc* 1995;**274**:700–705.

295. MacCarthy D. Mental health practice and attitudes can be changed. *Permanente Journal* 2013;**17**:14–17.

296. Ungar T, Knaak S, Szeto ACH. Theoretical and practical considerations for combating mental illness stigma in health care. *Community Mental Health J* 2016;**52**:262–71.

297. Khenti A, Bobbili SJ, Sapag JC. Evaluation of a pilot intervention to reduce mental health and addiction stigma in primary care settings. *J Community Health* 2019;**44**:1204–13.

298. Mittal D, Owen RR, Ounpraseuth S et al. Targeting stigma of mental illness among primary care providers: Findings from a pilot feasibility study. *Psychiatry Res* 2020;**284**:112641.

299. Hansson L, Markström U. The effectiveness of an anti-stigma intervention in a basic police officer training programme: A controlled study. *BMC Psychiatry* 2014;**14**:1–8.

300. Silverstone PH, Krameddine YI, DeMarco D et al. A novel approach to training police officers to interact with individuals who may have a psychiatric disorder. *J Am Acad Psychiatry Law* 2013;**41**:344–55.

301. Krameddine YI, DeMarco D, Hassel R et al. A novel training program for police officers that improves interactions with mentally ill individuals and is cost-effective. *Front Psychiatry* 2013;**4**:1–10.

302. Mansfield R, Patalay P, Humphrey N. A systematic literature review of existing conceptualisation and measurement of mental health literacy in adolescent research: Current challenges and inconsistencies. *BMC Public Health* 2020;**20**:1–14.

303. Stuart H. Stigma and work. *Healthcare Papers* 2004;**5**(2):100–11.

304. Stuart H. Mental illness and employment discrimination. *Curr Opin Psychiatry* 2006;**19**(5):522–26.

305. Goss D, Goss F, Adam-Smith D. Disability and employment: A comparative critique of UK legislation. *Int J Hum Resour Manag* 2000;**11**:807–21.

306. Aizawa K, Hisanaga F. Employment support services in Japan. *Int J Mental Health* 2012;**41**:48–60.

307. Colker R. The Americans with Disabilities Act: A windfall for defendants. *Harvard Civil Rights-Civil Liberties Law Review* 1999;**34**(1):

308. Vilchinsky N, Findler L. Attitudes toward Israel's equal rights for people with disabilities law: A multiperspective approach. *Rehabil Psychol* 2004;**49**:309–16.

309. Henderson C, Williams P, Little K et al. Mental health problems in the workplace: Changes in employers' knowledge, attitudes and practices in England 2006–2010. *Br J Psychiatry* 2013;**202**:70–76.

310. Heijbel B, Josephson M, Jensen I et al. Employer, insurance, and health system response to long-term sick leave in the public sector: Policy implications. *J Occup Rehabil* 2005;**15**:167–76.

311. Long A. Introducing the new and improved Americans with Disabilities Act: Assessing the ADA Amendments Act of 2008. *Northwest Univ Law Rev* 2008;**103**:217.

312. Agocs C. Canada's employment equity legislation and policy, 1987–2000: The gap between policy and practice. *Int J Manpower* 2002;**23**(3):256–76.

313. Krupa T, Kirsh B, Cockburn L et al. Understanding the stigma of mental illness in employment. *Work* 2009;**33**:413–25.

314. Rao D, Horton RA, Tsang HWH et al. Does individualism help explain differences in employers' stigmatizing attitudes toward disability across Chinese and American cities? *Rehabil Psychol* 2010;**55**:351–59.

315. Hipes C, Lucas J, Phelan JC et al. The stigma of mental illness in the labor market. *Soc Sci Res* 2016;**56**:16–25.

316. Gayed A, Milligan-Saville JS, Nicholas J et al. Effectiveness of training workplace managers to understand and support the mental health needs of employees: A systematic review and meta-analysis. *Occup Environ Med* 2018;**75**:462–70.

317. Szeto ACH, Dobson KS. Reducing the stigma of mental disorders at work: A review of current workplace anti-stigma intervention programs. *Appl Prev Psychol* 2010;**14**:41–56.

318. Malachowski C, Kirsh B. Workplace antistigma initiatives: A scoping study. *Psychiatr Serv* 2013;**64**:694–702.

319. LaMontagne AD, Martin A, Page KM et al. Workplace mental health: Developing an integrated intervention approach. *BMC Psychiatry* 2014;**14**:1–11.

320. Szeto A, Dobson KS, Knaak S. The road to mental readiness for first responders: A meta-analysis of program outcomes. *Can J Psychiatry* 2019;**64**:18S–29S.

321. Dobson KS, Szeto A, Knaak S. The working mind: A meta-analysis of a workplace mental health and stigma reduction program. *Can J Psychiatry* 2019;**64**:39S–47S.

322. Moll SE, Patten S, Stuart H et al. Beyond Silence: A randomized, parallel-group trial exploring the impact of workplace mental health literacy training with healthcare employees. *Can J Psychiatry* 2018;**63**(12):826–33.

323. Moll SE, VandenBussche J, Brooks K et al. Workplace mental health training in health care: Key ingredients of implementation. *Can J Psychiatry* 2018;**63**(12):834–41.

324. Sayers E, Rich J, Rahman MM et al. Does help-seeking behavior change over time following a workplace mental health intervention in the coal mining industry? *J Occup Environ Med* 2019;**61**:E282–90.

325. Tynan RJ, James C, Considine R et al. Feasibility and acceptability of strategies to address mental health and mental ill-health in the Australian coal mining industry. *Int J Mental Health Syst* 2018;**12**:1–10.

326. Moffitt J, Bostock J, Cave A. Promoting well-being and reducing stigma about mental health in the fire service. *J Public Mental Health* 2014;**13**:103–13.

327. Dewa CS, Hoch JS. When could a stigma program to address mental illness in the workplace break even? *Can J Psychiatry* 2014;**59**:S34–39.

328. McDowell C, Fossey E. Workplace accommodations for people with mental illness: A scoping review. *J Occup Rehabil* 2015;**25**:197–206.

329. Dewa CS. Worker attitudes towards mental health problems and disclosure. *Int J Occup Environ Med* 2014;**5**:175–86.

330. Corbiere M, Lecomte T. Vocational services offered to people with severe mental illness. *J Mental Health* 2009;**18**:38–50.

331. Vick A. "A place to work like any other?" Sheltered workshops in Canada, 1970–1985. *Can J Disabil Stud* 2015;**5**:100–11.

332. Luo K, Yu D. Enterprise-based sheltered workshops in Nanjing: A new model for the community rehabilitation of mentally ill workers. *Br J Psychiatry* 1994;**164**:89–95.

333. McKay C, Nugent KL, Johnsen M et al. A systematic review of evidence for the clubhouse model of psychosocial rehabilitation. *Administration & Policy in Mental Health & Mental Health Services Research* 2018;**45**:28–47.

334. Phillips JR, Biller EF. Transitional employment program for persons with long-term mental illness: A review. *Psychosoc Rehabil J* 1993;**17**:101–106.

335. Warner R, Mandiberg J. An update on affirmative businesses or social firms for people with mental illness. *Psychiatr Serv* 2006;**57**:1488–92.

336. Krupa T, Lagarde M, Carmichael K. Transforming sheltered workshops into affirmative businesses: An outcome evaluation. *Psychiatr Rehabil J* 2003;**26**:359–67.

337. Lysaght R, Jakobsen K, Granhaug B. Social firms: A means for building employment skills and community integration. *Work* 2012;**41**:455–63.

338. Krupa T, Sabetti J, Lysaght R. How work integration social enterprises impact the stigma of mental illness: Negotiating perceptions of legitimacy, value and competence. *Soc Enterp J* 2019;**15**:475–94.

339. Drake RE, Bond GR, Rapp C. Explaining the variance within supported employment programs: Comment on "What predicts supported employment outcomes?" *Community Mental Health J* 2006;**42**:315–18.

340. Mueser KT. Supported employment for persons with serious mental illness: Current status and future directions. *Encephale* 2014;**40**:S45–S56.

341. Wedding D, Boyd MA, Niemiec RM. *Movies and Mental Illness*, 2nd ed. Cambridge, MA: Hogrefe & Huber Publishers, 2005.

342. Corrigan PW, Larson J, Sells M et al. Will filmed presentations of education and contact diminish mental illness stigma? *Community Mental Health J* 2007;**43**:171–81.

343. Tergesen CL, Gurung D, Dhungana S et al. Impact of service user video presentations on explicit and implicit stigma toward mental illness among medical students in Nepal: A randomized controlled trial.*Int J Environ Res Public Health* 2021;**18**:1–23.

344. Winkler P, Janoušková M, Kožený J et al. Short video interventions to reduce mental health stigma: A multi-centre randomised controlled trial in nursing high schools. *Soc Psychiatry Psychiatr Epidemiol* 2017;**52**:1549–57.

345. Whitley R, Sitter KC, Adamson G et al. Can participatory video reduce mental illness stigma? Results from a Canadian action-research study of feasibility and impact. *BMC Psychiatry* 2020;**20**(1):16.

346. Tippin GK, Maranzan KA. Efficacy of a Photovoice-based video as an online mental illness anti-stigma intervention and the role of empathy in audience response: A randomized controlled trial. *J Appl Soc Psychol* 2019;**49**:381–94.

347. Janoušková M, Tušková E, Weissová A et al. Can video interventions be used to effectively destigmatize mental illness among young people? A systematic review. *Eur Psychiatry* 2017;**41**:1–9.

348. Hamblen JL, Grubaugh AL, Davidson TM et al. An online peer educational campaign to reduce stigma and improve help seeking in veterans with posttraumatic stress disorder. *Telemed e-Health* 2019;**25**:41–47.

349. Yamaguchi S, Ojio Y, Ando S et al. Long-term effects of filmed social contact or internet-based self-study on mental health-related stigma: A 2-year follow-up of a randomised controlled trial. *Soc Psychiatry Psychiatr Epidemiol* 2019;**54**:33–42.

350. Moyer-Gusé E. Toward a theory of entertainment persuasion: Explaining the persuasive effects of entertainment-education messages. *Communications Theory* 2008;**18**:407–25.

351. Ritterfeld U, Jin S-A. Addressing media stigma for people experiencing mental illness using an entertainment-education strategy. *J Health Psychol* 2006;**11**:247–67.

352. Ferrari M, McIlwaine SV, Jordan G et al. Gaming with stigma: Analysis of messages about mental illnesses in video games. *J Med Internet Res* 2019;**21**:1–22.

353. Cangas AJ, Navarro N, Parra JMA et al. Stigma-Stop: A serious game against the stigma toward mental health in educational settings. *Front Psychol* 2017;**8**:1385.

354. Ferchaud A, Seibert J, Sellers N et al. Reducing mental health stigma through identification with video game avatars with mental illness. *Front Psychol* 2020. doi:10.3389/fpsyg.2020.02240

355. Mullor D, Sayans-Jimé Nez P, Cangas AJ et al. Effect of a serious game (Stigma-Stop) on reducing stigma among psychology students: A controlled study. *Cyberpsychol Behav Soc Netw* 2019;**22**:205–11.

356. Hanisch SE, Birner UW, Oberhauser C et al. Development and evaluation of digital game-based training for managers to promote employee mental health and reduce mental illness stigma at work: Quasi-experimental study of program effectiveness. *JMIR Mental Health* 2017;**4**:e31.

357. Griffiths KM, Christensen H, Jorm AF et al. Effect of web-based depression literacy and cognitive-behavioural therapy interventions on stigmatising attitudes to depression: Randomised controlled trial. *Br J Psychiatry* 2004;**185**:342–49.

358. Shann C, Martin A, Chester A et al. Effectiveness and application of an online leadership intervention to promote mental health and reduce depression-related stigma in organizations. *J Occup Health Psychol* 2019;**24**:20–35.

359. Poushter J, Bishop C, Chwe H. *Social Media Use Continues to Rise in Developing Countries But Plateaus Across Developed Ones: Smartphone Ownership on the Rise in Emerging Economies.* Pew Research Center, 2018. http://www.pewglobal.org/2018/06/19/2-smartphone-ownership-on-the-rise-in-emerging-economies/

360. Maher CA, Lewis LK, Ferrar K et al. Are health behavior change interventions that use online social networks effective? A systematic review. *J Med Internet Res* 2014;**16**:1–13.

361. Livingston JD, Tugwell A, Korf-Uzan K et al. Evaluation of a campaign to improve awareness and attitudes of young people towards mental health issues. *Soc Psychiatry Psychiatr Epidemiol* 2013;**48**:965–73.

362. Livingston JD, Cianfrone M, Korf-Uzan K et al. Another time point, a different story: One year effects of a social media intervention on the attitudes of young people towards mental health issues. *Soc Psychiatry Psychiatr Epidemiol* 2014;**49**:985–90.

363. Maunder RD, White FA, Verrelli S. Modern avenues for intergroup contact: Using E-contact and intergroup emotions to reduce stereotyping and social distancing against people with schizophrenia. *Group Processes & Intergroup Relations* 2019;**22**:947–63.

364. Rodríguez-Rivas ME, Cangas AJ, Fuentes-Olavarría D. Controlled study of the impact of a virtual program to reduce stigma among university students toward people with mental disorders. *Front Psychiatry* 2021;**12**:1–9.

365. White FA, Maunder R, Verrelli S. Text-based E-contact: Harnessing cooperative Internet interactions to bridge the social and psychological divide. *Eur Rev Soc Psychol* 2020;**31**:76–119.

366. Ando S, Clement S, Barley EA et al. The simulation of hallucinations to reduce the stigma of schizophrenia: A systematic review. *Schizophr Res* 2011;**133**:8–16.

367. Brown SA. Implementing a brief hallucination simulation as a mental illness stigma reduction strategy. *Community Mental Health J* 2010;**46**:500–504.

368. Craig TK, Rus-Calafell M, Ward T et al. AVATAR therapy for auditory verbal hallucinations in people with psychosis: A single-blind, randomised controlled trial. *Lancet Psychiatry* 2018;**5**:31–40.

369. Sebastian J, Richards D. Changing stigmatizing attitudes to mental health via education and contact with embodied conversational agents. *Comput Human Behav* 2017;**73**:479–88.

370. Kirschner B, Goetzl M, Curtin L. Mental health stigma among college students: Test of an interactive online intervention. *J Am Coll Health* 2020 [online ahead of print]. doi:10.1080/07448481.2020.1826492

371. Wind TR, Rijkeboer M, Andersson G et al. The COVID-19 pandemic: The "black swan" for mental health care and a turning point for e-health. *Internet Interv* 2020;**20**:100317.

372. Dowling M, Rickwood D. Online counseling and therapy for mental health problems: A systematic review of individual synchronous interventions using chat. *J Technol Hum Serv* 2013;**31**:1–21.

373. Twomey C, O'Reilly G. Effectiveness of a freely available computerised cognitive behavioural therapy programme (MoodGYM) for depression: Meta-analysis. *Aust N Z J Psychiatry* 2017;**51**:260–69.

374. Murray CJL, Lopez AD, World Health Organization, World Bank & Harvard School of Public Health. *The Global Burden of Disease: A Comprehensive Assessment of Mortality and Disability from Diseases, Injuries, and Risk Factors in 1990 and Projected to 2020*. Geneva: World Health Organization, 1996. https://apps.who.int/iris/handle/10665/41864

375. Mathers CD, Loncar D. Projections of global mortality and burden of disease from 2002 to 2030. *PLoS Med* 2006;**3**:2011–30.

376. Srithanaviboonchai K, Stockton M, Pudpong N et al. Building the evidence base for stigma and discrimination-reduction programming in Thailand: Development of tools to measure healthcare stigma and discrimination. *BMC Public Health* 2017;**17**:1–11.

377. Lundell-Smith K, Grant J, Kemmer D. *The Inequities of Mental Health Research Funding*. 2020. https://digitalscience.figshare.com/articles/report/The_Inequities_of_Mental_Health_Research_IAMHRF_/13055897

378. Woelbert E, Kirtley A, Balmer N et al. How much is spent on mental health research: Developing a system for categorising grant funding in the UK. *Lancet Psychiatry* 2019;**6**:445–52.

379. Hoagwood KE, Atkins M, Kelleher K et al. Trends in children's mental health services research funding by the National Institute of Mental Health from 2005 to 2015: A 42% reduction. *J Am Acad Child Adolesc Psychiatry* 2018;**57**:10–13.

380. Christensen H, Batterham PJ, Hickie IB et al. Funding for mental health research: The gap remains. *Med J Aust* 2011;**195**:681–84.

381. Woelbert E, White R, Lundell-Smith K et al. *The Inequities of Mental Health Research Funding*. Montreal, Canada, 2020.

382. Larivière V, Diepeveen S, Ni Chonaill S et al. International comparative performance of mental health research, 1980–2011. *Eur Neuropsychopharmacol* 2013;**23**:1340–47.

383. Wellcome Trust. *Annual Report and Financial Statements 2020 Table of Contents*. 2020. https://wellcome.org/reports/wellcome-annual-report-2020

384. Stuart H. Building an evidence base for anti-stigma programming. In: Arboleda-Flórez J, Sartorius N (eds.). *Understanding the Stigma of Mental Illness: Theory and Interventions*. Chichester, West Sussex: John Wiley & Sons, Ltd., 2008, 135–45.

385. Stuart H. What has proven effective in anti-stigma programming. In: Gaebel W, Rossler W, Sartorius N (eds.). *The Stigma of Mental Illness—End of the Story?* Zurich, Switzerland: Springer, 2016, 497–514.

386. Thornicroft G, Bakolis I, Evans-Lacko S et al. Key lessons learned from the INDIGO global network on mental health related stigma and discrimination. *World Psychiatry* 2019;**18**:229–30.

387. Morselli PL, Elgie R. GAMIAN-Europe*/BEAM survey I—Global analysis of a patient questionnaire circulated to 3450 members of 12 European advocacy groups operating in the field of mood disorders. *Bipolar Disord* 2003;**5**:265–78.

388. Cumming E, Cumming J. *Closed Ranks: An Experiment in Mental Health Education.* Cambridge, MA: Harvard University Press, 1957.
389. Link BG, Yang LH, Phelan JC et al. Measuring mental illness stigma. *Schizophr Bull* 2004;**30**:511–41.
390. Willits F, Theodori G, Luloff A. Another look at Likert scales. *J Rural Soc Sci* 2016;**31**:6.
391. Kassam A, Papish A, Modgill G et al. The development and psychometric properties of a new scale to measure mental illness related stigma by health care providers: The Opening Minds Scale for Health Care Providers (OMS-HC). *BMC Psychiatry* 2012;**12**:62.
392. Loo R, Thorpe K. Confirmatory factor analyses of the full and short versions of the Marlowe-Crowne social desirability scale. *J Soc Psychol* 2000;**140**:628–35.
393. Pescosolido BA, Monahan J, Link BG et al. The public's view of the competence, dangerousness, and need for legal coercion of persons with mental health problems. *Am J Public Health* 1999;**89**:1339–45.
394. Streiner DL, Kottner J. Recommendations for reporting the results of studies of instrument and scale development and testing. *J Adv Nurs* 2014;**70**:1970–79.
395. Polit DF. Getting serious about test-retest reliability: A critique of retest research and some recommendations. *Qual Life Res* 2014;**23**:1713–20.
396. Hallgren K. Computing inter-rater reliability for observational data: An overview and tutorial. *Quant Methods Psychol* 2012;**8**:23–34.
397. Bajpai S, Bajpai RC, Chaturvedi HK. Evaluation of inter-rater agreement and inter-rater reliability for observational data: An overview of concepts and methods. *J Indian Acad Appl Psychol* 2015;**41**:20–27.
398. Tsang S, Royse CF, Terkawi AS. Guidelines for developing, translating, and validating a questionnaire in perioperative and pain medicine. *Saudi J Anaesth* 2017;**11**:S80–89.
399. Beatty PC, Willis GB. Research synthesis: The practice of cognitive interviewing. *Public Opin Q* 2007;**71**:287–311.
400. Alexander LA, Link BG. The impact of contact on stigmatizing attitudes toward people with mental illness. *J Mental Health* 2003;**12**:271–89.
401. Evans-Lacko S, Rose D, Little K et al. Development and psychometric properties of the Reported and Intended Behaviour Scale (RIBS): A stigma-related behaviour measure. *Epidemiol Psychiatr Sci* 2011;**20**:263–71.
402. Pingani L, Evans-Lacko S, Luciano M et al. Psychometric validation of the Italian version of the Reported and Intended Behaviour Scale (RIBS). *Epidemiol Psychiatr Sci* 2016;**25**:485–92.
403. Ribeiro WS, Gronholm PC, Silvestre de Paula C et al. Development and validation of the Brazilian Portuguese Version of the Reported and Intended Behaviour Scale (RIBS-BP). *Stigma Health* 2021;**6**:163–72.
404. Yamaguchi S, Koike S, Watanabe KI et al. Development of a Japanese version of the Reported and Intended Behaviour Scale: Reliability and validity. *Psychiatry Clin Neurosci* 2014;**68**:448–55.
405. Koller M, Stuart H. Stereotype and social distance scales for youth. In: Dobson K, Stuart H (eds.). *The Stigma of Mental Illness.* New York: Oxford University Press, 2021, 81–89.
406. Link BG. Understanding labeling effects in the area of mental disorders: An assessment of the effects of expectations of rejection. *Am Sociol Rev* 1987;**52**:96–112.
407. Stuart H. *Stigma and Discrimination Module Background Document Table of Contents.* 2008.

408. Patten SB, Williams JVA, Lavorato DH et al. Perceived stigma among recipients of mental health care in the general Canadian population. *Can J Psychiatry* 2016;**61**(8):480–88.

409. Brohan E, Clement S, Rose D et al. Development and psychometric evaluation of the Discrimination and Stigma Scale (DISC). *Psychiatry Res* 2013;**208**:33–40.

410. Bakolis I, Thornicroft G, Vitoratou S et al. Development and validation of the DISCUS scale: A reliable short measure for assessing experienced discrimination in people with mental health problems on a global level. *Schizophr Res* 2019;**212**:213–20.

411. Ritsher JB, Otilingam PG, Grajales M. Internalized stigma of mental illness: Psychometric properties of a new measure. *Psychiatry Res* 2003;**121**:31–49.

412. Chang CC, Chang KC, Hou WL et al. Measurement invariance and psychometric properties of Perceived Stigma toward People who use Substances (PSPS) among three types of substance use disorders: Heroin, amphetamine, and alcohol. *Drug Alcohol Depend* 2020;**216**:108319.

413. Boyd JE, Adler EP, Otilingam PG et al. Internalized Stigma of Mental Illness (ISMI) scale: A multinational review. *Compr Psychiatry* 2014;**55**:221–31.

414. Corrigan PW, Michaels PJ, Vega E et al. Self-Stigma of Mental Illness Scale-Short Form: Reliability and validity. *Psychiatry Res* 2012;**199**:65–69.

415. Brohan E, Slade M, Clement S, Thornicroft G. Experiences of mental illness stigma, prejudice and discrimination: A review of measures. *BMC Health Serv Res* 2010;**10**:80.

416. Stuart H. *Measuring Structural Stigma in Healthcare Settings from the Perspective of Service Users*. Mental Health Commission of Canada, 2020. https://mental-healthcommission.ca

417. Harding E, Wait S, Scrutton J. *The State of Play in Person-Centred Care: Report Summary*. London: Health Policy Partnership, 2015. https://www.healthpolicy-partnership.com/app/uploads/The-state-of-play-in-person-centred-care-summary.pdf

418. Bayer R. Stigma and the ethics of public health: Not can we but should we. *Soc Sci Med* 2008;**67**:463–72.

419. Crisp AH, Gelder MG, Rix S et al. Stigmatisation of people with mental illnesses. *Br J Psychiatry* 2000;**177**:4–7.

420. Crisp A, Gelder M, Goddard E et al. Stigmatization of people with mental illnesses: A follow-up study within the Changing Minds campaign of the Royal College of Psychiatrists. *World Psychiatry* 2005;**4**:106–13.

421. Lloyd C. The stigmatization of problem drug users: A narrative literature review. *Drugs Educ Prev Policy* 2013;**20**:85–95.

422. Stuart H. Managing the stigma of opioid use. *Healthc Manag Forum* 2019;**32**(2):78–83.

423. Janulis P, Ferrari JR, Fowler P. Understanding public stigma toward substance dependence. *J Appl Soc Psychol* 2013;**43**:1065–72.

424. Room R. Stigma, social inequality and alcohol and drug use. *Drug Alcohol Rev* 2005;**24**:143–55.

425. Dikötter F, Laamann L, Xun Z. Narcotic culture: A social history of drug consumption in China. *Br J Criminol* 2002;**42**:317–36.

426. Kandall SR. Women and drug addiction: A historical perspective. *J Addict Dis* 2010;**29**:117–26.

427. Wakeman SE. Using science to battle stigma in addressing the opioid epidemic: Opioid agonist therapy saves lives. *Am J Med* 2016;**129**:455–56.

428. Pearlman J. Combatting Massachusetts's opioid epidemic: Reducing the social stigma of addiction through increased access to voluntary treatment services and expansion of mandatory clinician education programs. *Am J Law Med* 2016;**42**:835–57.

429. Fischer B. Some notes on the use, concept and socio-political framing of "stigma" focusing on an opioid-related public health crisis. *Subst Abuse Treat Prev Policy* 2020;**15**:1–7.

430. Holbrook AM. Methadone versus buprenorphine for the treatment of opioid abuse in pregnancy: Science and stigma. *Am J Drug Alcohol Abuse* 2015;**41**:371–73.

431. Kennedy-Hendricks H, Barry C, Gollust S, Ensminger, Margaret E. Chisolm, Margaret S. McGinty, Emma E. Social stigma toward persons with prescription opioid use disorder: Associations with public support for punitive and public health-oriented policies. *Psychiatr Serv* 2017;**68**(5):462–69.

432. Cooper S, Nielsen S. Stigma and social support in pharmaceutical opioid treatment populations: A scoping review. *Int J Mental Health Addict* 2017;**15**:452–69.

433. McGinty EE, Stone EM, Kennedy-Hendricks A, Barry CL. Stigmatizing languate in news media coverage of the opioid epidemic: Implications for public health. *Prev Med* 2019;**124**:110–14.

434. Schomerus G, Lucht M, Holzinger A et al. The stigma of alcohol dependence compared with other mental disorders: A review of population studies. *Alcohol Alcoholism* 2011;**46**:105–12.

435. Reio T, Ghosh R. Antecedents and outcomes of workplace incivility. *Hum Resour Dev Q* 2012;**23**(1):129–132.

436. Griffiths S, Murray SB, Mond JM. The stigma of anabolic steroid use. *J Drug Issues* 2016;**46**:446–56.

437. Rapoport M, Lantot K, Streiner D et al. Benzodiazepine use and driving: A meta-analysis. *J Clin Psychol* 2009;**21**:663–73.

438. Freeman S. The benzodiazepine stigma persists. *J Clin Psychol* 2009;**70**:12–13.

439. Halpern B, Halpern A. Why are anti-obesity drugs stigmatized? *Expert Opin Drug Saf* 2015;**14**:185–89.

440. Puhl R, Brownell KD. Ways of coping with obesity stigma: Review and conceptual analysis. *Eat Behav* 2003;**4**:53–78.

441. Mattoo SK, Sarkar S, Gupta S et al. Stigma towards substance use: Comparing treatment-seeking alcohol- and opioid-dependent men. *Int J Mental Health Addict* 2015;**13**:73–81.

442. Gunn A, Guarino H. "Not human, dead already": Perceptions and experiences of drug-related stigma among opioid-using young adults from the former Soviet Union living in the U.S. *Int J Drug Policy* 2016;**38**:63–72.

443. Ronzani TM, Higgins-Biddle J, Furtado EF. Stigmatization of alcohol and other drug users by primary care providers in Southeast Brazil. *Soc Sci Med* 2009;**69**:1080–84.

444. Guarnotta E. Drug Use in Religions. 2019. https://recovery.org/addiction/religions/

445. Deckenbach J. A brief history of physics and religion. *Physics World* 1999;**12**(12):69. https://www.winecellarinnovations.com/wine-racks/brief-history-wine-religion

446. Armstrong M. Foundations for a gender based treatment model for women in recovery from chemical dependency. *J Addict Nurs* 2008;**19**:77–82.

447. Grower SM, Floyd MR. Nurses' attitudes toward impaired practice and knowledge of peer assistance programs. *J Addict Nurs* 1998;**10**:70–76.

448. Darbro N. Alternative diversion programs for nurses with impaired practice: Completers and non-completers. *J Addict Nurs* 2005;**16**:169–85.

449. Smith L, Hughes T. Re-entry: When a chemically dependent colleague returns to work. *Am J Nurs* 1996;**96**:32–37.

450. Brewer MK, Nelms TP. Some recovering nurses' experiences of being labeled "impaired": A phenomenological inquiry. *J Addict Nurs* 1998;**10**:172–79.

451. Ahern J, Stuber J, Galea S. Stigma, discrimination and the health of illicit drug users. *Drug Alcohol Depend* 2007;**88**:188–96.

452. Marlatt G. Harm reduction: Come as you are. *Adict Behav* 1996;**21**:779–88.

453. Ashton M, Lenton S, Mitcheson L et al. A Review of the Evidence-Base for Harm Reduction Approaches to Drug Use. 2003. https://www.hri.global/files/2010/05/31/HIVTop50Documents11.pdf

454. Hedrich D, Pirona A, Wiessing L. From margin to mainstream: The evolution of harm reduction responses to problem drug use in Europe. *Drugs Educ Prev Policy* 2008;**15**:503–17.

455. Pauly B. Harm reduction through a social justice lens. *Int J Drug Policy* 2008;**19**:4–10.

456. Phelan JC, Link BG, Dovidio JF. Stigma and prejudice: One animal or two? *Soc Sci Med* 2008;**67**:358–67.

457. Williamson L, Thom B, Stimson GV et al. Stigma as a public health tool: Implications for health promotion and citizen involvement. *Int J Drug Policy* 2014;**25**:333–35.

458. Ritchie D, Amos A, Martin C. "But it just has that sort of feel about it, a leper": Stigma, smoke-free legislation and public health. *Nicotine Tobacco Res* 2010;**12**:622–29.

459. Guttman N, Salmon CT. Guilt, fear, stigma and knowledge gaps: Ethical issues in public health communication interventions. *Bioethics* 2004;**18**:531–52.

460. Livingston JD, Milne T, Fang ML et al. The effectiveness of interventions for reducing stigma related to substance use disorders: A systematic review. *Addiction* 2012;**107**:39–50.

461. Eastwood N, Fox E, Rosmarin A. A Quiet Revolution: Drug Decriminalisation Across the Globe. Release: Drugs, the Law, and Human Rights. 2016. https://www.release.org.uk/publications/drug-decriminalisation-2016

INDEX

For the benefit of digital users, indexed terms that span two pages (e.g., 52–53) may, on occasion, appear on only one of those pages.

Tables, figures, and boxes are indicated by *t*, *f*, and *b* following the page number

children (*cont.*)
    Science of Mental Illness teacher
        supplement, 136
    puppet plays, 132–33
    secondary school education, 137–38
    social distancing, 132–34
Chile, 140, 177, 188, 189*f*
China, 28–29, 104, 141–42, 160,
    185, 210
Chinese culture, 21, 28–29
Chisholm, Brock, 72–73
Christian cultures, 3, 34, 216–17. *See*
    also Western culture
churches, 227–28
civil rights, 67–68, 69–70
clubhouse model of psychosocial
    rehabilitation, 159–64
CNN effect, 101
coal mining industry, 156–57
cocaine dependence, 215–16
coerced sterilization laws, 3
coercive care practices, 117–21, 118*f*
    CRPD on, 113, 114–15, 118
    PTSD and, 119
    punitive cultures of care, 111–13,
        117–21, 118*f*
collective empowerment, 2–3
colloquialisms, 90–92, 93*t*
Coming Out Proud program, 84–85
communication
    anti-stigma programs, 65
    ethical considerations, 64
    generating enthusiasm for
        programs, 59
    program committees, 51–52
community-based service, 5
    anti-stigma interventions target, 55
    bias
        explicit, 126–29
        implicit, 123–25
        overview, 122–23
    Gheel colony, 25–26
    mental hospitals, 24–25
    NIMBY Syndrome, 5–7, 55
    outpatient commitment, 115–17
    staff sharing, 233
community mental health care
    movement, 24–25, 26,
    117, 222–23
concept formation, 130–31

Confucian ethics, 21, 28–29
Congress on Mental Hygiene, 71–72
consumer-survivor groups, 44–45
contact-based education, 81–83, 235
    effective storytelling, 83–84, 84*f*
    keys in implementing, 229*t*
    MHFA program, 154–57
    MIM program, 156–57
    for police recruits, 145–46
    R2MR/Working Mind
        intervention, 154–55
    videos, 166–70, 180–81
contract-based educational
    systems, 137–38
Convention on the Rights of Persons
    with Disabilities (CRPD), 233–34
    on coercive care practices, 113, 114–
        15, 118
    human rights legislation, 70–71
    QualityRights toolkit, 74
    workplace disability legislation, 149
Cooper, David, 4
correctional facilities, 23. *See also* prisons
Costs of Discrimination Assessment, 198
cough syrup, 214–15
courtesy stigma, 3–4
criminal justice system
    criminalization of mentally ill, 7–8
    fragmentation of care, 111
    police training, 145–46
crisis planning, 114–15
Croatia, 141–42
Cronbach's alpha statistic, 193–96,
    201, 203
cross-cultural studies, 30–34, 32*f*
CRPD. *See* Convention on the Rights of
    Persons with Disabilities
cultural rights, 67–69
cultural stereotypes, 2, 228–31
    entertainment media, 88, 98–
        100, 103–4
    movies, 88, 98–100
    news media, 88–90, 101–3, 105–6
    workplace, 151–53
culture, 19–20, 34, 228–31
    anti-stigma programs and, 227–
        28, 229*t*
    cross-cultural studies, 30–34, 32*f*
    non-Western
        Chinese culture, 21, 28–29

coerced/forced sterilization laws, 3
diagnostic term for
    schizophrenia, 97–98
postgraduate education, 140
social enterprises/affirmative
    businesses, 162
Jehovah's Witnesses, 216–17
jinn, 28
Jofré, Gilbert, 108–9, 109f
journalists, 88–90
    interventions targeting, 54
    media guidelines, 90–97, 93t
    Open the Doors schizophrenia anti-
        stigma program, 76t
    positive change by engaging
        with, 101–3
    program objectives, 57
    stigma from, 88
    survey results, 63
judges, 51–52, 76t

kava, 216–17
knowledge theory of change model, 43–
    46, 57b, 229t, 232–33
Koran, 28–29
Korea, 162

labeling theory, 192. See also social
    labeling
Laing, R. D., 4
Lambo, T. A., 26
language, 90–91, 97–98, 123–24
    guidelines, 91–92, 93t, 105
    person-first, 92, 93t, 97, 112, 234–35
    stigma measurement tools, 196–97
Latino culture, 30–31
law enforcement. See police officers
Law for Employment Promotion, 149
legislation, 55, 57, 88, 149–51. See also
    human rights legislation
Let's Erase the Stigma (LETS) focused
    intervention, 138
Let's Talk program, 77, 78t
liberty, right to, 67–68
life expectancy, 1, 8, 12–13
    diagnostic overshadowing and, 9–10
    drug-related infant, 217–18
    mental illness and, 12–13
    structural stigma and, 107–8
    therapeutic nihilism and, 8

Like Minds, Like Mine anti-stigma
    program, 78t, 91, 93t, 104–5, 175
Likert scale, 192
Lion King, The, 99–100
local community television channels, 59
locally implemented programs, 39,
    40b, 48
local programs, 53–55
longevity, 1, 8, 12–13
    diagnostic overshadowing and, 9–10
    drug-related infant, 217–18
    mental illness and, 12–13
    structural stigma and, 107–8
    therapeutic nihilism and, 8
Looking After Wellbeing at Work
    (LWW), 157
low-birthweight babies, 217–18
low-income nations
    cross-cultural studies, 30–34, 32f
    DISCUS scale, 201, 205t
    explicit bias, 128–29
    fragmentation of care, 110–11
    International Alliance of Mental
        Health Research Funders, 186,
        188f, 188, 189f
    property rights, 12
    social media use, 174–76
    successful anti-stigma programs, 126–
        29, 127f
LWW (Looking After Wellbeing at
    Work), 157

madhouses, 23. See also asylums
Madrid Declaration, 75–76
majnoon, 28
major depressive disorder, 7, 10, 12–15,
    32f, 33–34
Malleus Maleficarum, 22
marginalization, 3–4, 123–24, 228
marijuana, 213–14, 216–17
marijuana dependence, 215–16
maristans, 21–22, 23–24, 108–9, 109f
Marrakech maristan, 22
Massachusetts, 223
Mates in Mining (MIM), 156–57
media, 13, 88, 100–1, 105–6,
    229t, 232–33
    guidelines, 90–97, 93t
    language change, 90–91, 97–98
    language guidelines, 91–92, 93t